Medicinal and Aromatic Plants

Medicinal and Aromatic Plants

Editor: Holly Philips

MURPHY & MOORE
www.murphy-moorepublishing.com

Murphy & Moore Publishing,
1 Rockefeller Plaza,
New York City, NY 10020, USA

Visit us on the World Wide Web at:
www.murphy-moorepublishing.com

ISBN: 978-1-63987-361-6 (Hardback)

Cataloging-in-Publication Data

Medicinal and aromatic plants / edited by Holly Philips.
p. cm.
Includes bibliographical references and index.
ISBN 978-1-63987-361-6
1. Medicinal plants. 2. Aromatic plants--Therapeutic use. 3. Materia medica, Vegetable.
4. Botany, Medical. 5. Alternative medicine. I. Philips, Holly.

RS164 .M43 2022
615.321--dc23

Table of Contents

Preface

The plants which are used for therapeutic and medicinal purposes are known as medicinal and aromatic plants. Due to their aroma and flavor, they also find application in the field of culinary arts, cosmetics and health products. Phytochemicals which are pharmacologically active can be broadly classified into glycosides, polyphenols, terpenes and alkaloids. Production of medicinal plants requires intensive management. Some of them might be inert in their physical state and may require some chemical modification before being used as a medicine. Some common examples of medicinal and aromatic plants are Saint John's wort, saw palmetto, ginseng, echinacea and feverfew. This book explores all the important aspects of medicinal and aromatic plants in the present day scenario. Also included herein is a detailed explanation of the various concepts and applications of medicinal and aromatic plants. This book is a resource guide for experts as well as students.

The information shared in this book is based on empirical researches made by veterans in this field of study. The elaborative information provided in this book will help the readers further their scope of knowledge leading to advancements in this field.

Finally, I would like to thank my fellow researchers who gave constructive feedback and my family members who supported me at every step of my research.

Editor

1

Aromatic Compounds: From Plant to Nutraceuticals—An Example of Capsaicin

Adebayo Taiwo Ezekiel Jolayemi

Abstract

The current study is on extraction of capsaicin from capsicum using chromatography. Nuclear magnetic resonance was used to ascertain carbon structures of the extract, with the yield confirmed by nuclear magnetic resonance to be 98% pure capsaicin. The chemistry, pharmacological action, and side effects of capsaicin are thereafter discussed.

Keywords: aromatics, capsaicin, capsaicinoids, chromatography, nutraceuticals, solanaceae

1. Introduction

Capsicum frutescens Linn. (Family: Solanaceae) fruits were purchased from Warwick market in Durban, South Africa. The fruits were identified and authenticated by a botanist. A voucher specimen of the plant (with its ripe fruits) has been deposited in the University's Herbarium (JAT/01). The total weight of the dried red chili pepper fruits purchased from the local market was 3 kg. Following cleaning and subsequent pulverization, 2.5 kg of the chili powder was poured into a large conical flask. Thereafter, it was exhaustively extracted sequentially in hexane, dichloromethane, and ethyl acetate. Ethyl acetate extract was shown to contain active compounds (capsaicinoids) in preliminary pilot experiments. Using a rotary evaporator under reduced pressure, the ethyl acetate extract was concentrated to yield 298 g (10% yields) of the crude extract. Following further purification, nuclear magnetic resonance (NMR) analysis of the yield shows it to be 98% pure capsaicin.

2. Research methodology

Experimental procedures and protocols used in this study were approved by the Animal Ethics Committee of the University of Durban-Westville, Durban 4000, South Africa (now the University of KwaZulu-Natal, Westville Campus), and conform to the "*Guide to the care and use of animals in research and teaching*" (published by the University of Durban-Westville, Durban 4000, South Africa) [1–7]. Experimental protocols were written so as to lay down the organization of the study. The sequence of this study includes the purchase of *C. frutescens* from a local market, identification of *C. frutescens* by a Botanist, extraction and purification of *C. frutescens* fruit using liquid and paper chromatography.

A portion of the crude ethyl acetate extract was subjected to column chromatography over silica gel with gradient elution using 10% ethyl acetate in hexane to 40% ethyl acetate. On the basis of their thin-layer chromatography (TLC) similarities, a total of 51 eluates (25 ml each) were collected and combined into 15 fractions. These consisted of the non-polar fractions (one to three eluates), which were chlorophylls and its like, which were discarded. Next were the semi-polar/polar fractions (4–15 eluates). The latter were subjected to further column chromatography over silica gel with gradient elution (consisting of 30% ethyl acetate in hexane to 50% ethyl acetate). TLC was carried out on pre-coated aluminum plates by the use of Merck Si gel F254. Following further enhancement, the developed TLC plates were visualized under ultraviolet (UV) light (using wavelength of 254 and 366 nm), by spraying with anisaldehyde/sulfuric acid/alcohol solution, and heating at 110°C for 5 min. The presence of triterpenoids, as previously reported [8–10], was indicated by the appearance of blue to violet-blue coloration. NMR spectra (1D and 2D) were obtained on a Varian 300 (300-MHz) spectrometer, using the residual solvent peaks as internal standards.

In order to ensure that the chromatographic systems were up to standard, phase A of this study was conducted in the Chemistry Department under the supervision of a Professor of Analytical Chemistry. Finally, the identification of capsaicin from *C. frutescens* fruit extract was done by nuclear magnetic resonance in collaboration with the Chemistry Department of the University of KwaZulu-Natal to identify the final extract, that is, capsaicin.

3. Discussion

Phytochemical revolution took a positive turn in the 1970s onward, with the development of many laboratories that were involved in the production of bioactive nutraceuticals such as beta-carotene, omega-6, and other vitamins, with positive health-deriving values. Capsaicin is a chili pepper-derived spice. Apart from its spicy and flavorant properties, it has been found to be a digestive aid, a topical painkiller, and a potential cancer-fighting compound [11]. Capsicum is native to America, and the early Spanish explorers brought it to the "New World." It is cultivated in tropical regions of India, Nigeria, Japan, Southern Europe, Mexico, other African countries, and Sri Lanka.

Capsicum is 5–12 cm long, 2–4 cm wide, and could be globular, cylindrical, oval, or oblong in shape. It has a shriveled shape and could be orange, green, yellow, or red in color, with a prominent and bent pedicle. Internally, the fruits are divided into two halves by a membranous dissepiment to which the seeds are attached. Capsicum has a characteristic odor and an intense pungent taste. Although *Capsicum* can withstand tropical heat, it requires 3 months rainfall and thrives best in wet climate. The fruit yield is directly proportional to the manure of the cultivated farm.

The fruits are picked as they become fully ripe. The unripe fruits fade upon drying. The fruits are dried in sun and graded by color. The quality of the fruit is in part determined by its color, and they are occasionally oiled to give glossiness to their pericarps.

The pungent compounds of *C. frutescens* are capsaicin (69%), dihydrocapsaicin (22%), nordihydrocapsaicin (7%), homocapsaicin (1%), and homodihydrocapsaicin (1%). Capsaicin consists of an aromatic portion, which is derived from phenylalanine through frulic acid and vanillin—an aldehyde is a substrate for transamination to give vanillylamine. The acid portion of the amide structure in capsaicin is of polyketide origin, with a branched-chain fatty acyl-CoA, which is produced by a chain extension of 2-methylacetyl-CoA, with a starter unit, which is valine-derived.

In this study, vanilloid alkaloids otherwise known as capsaicinoids were extracted by sequentially in hexane, dichloromethane, and ethyl acetate. The extracts were later subjected to liquid, paper, gas chromatography, and high-performance liquid chromatography (HPLC).

The yield of 298 g (10% yields) of the 2.5-kg fruit is consistent with standard industrial yield. Following further purification, NMR analysis of the yield shows 98% capsaicin.

In 1912, Wilbur Scottville developed a dilution taste method, called "Scottville Organoleptic Test (SOT)," to measure the heat level of a chili pepper. This test consists of blended pure ground chilies with sugar water solution. In addition, there is a panel of testers who will sip the concoctions. Scottville increasingly diluted the concentrations until they reached the point at which the liquid no longer burned the mouth. Based on how much the chili needed to be diluted before one could taste no heat or burn the mouth, a number was then assigned to each chili to show its strength.

Measurement of the pungency of chili is done in multiples of 100 units. While the bell pepper measures zero Scottville units, the incendiary Habanero measures 300,000 Scottville units. For comparison, one part of chili "heat" per 1,000,000 drops of water rates as only 1.5 Scottville units. In another respect, while the substance that makes chili so hot and therefore so enjoyable is capsaicin, a pure capsaicin rates over 150,000,000 Scottville units. Red Savina Habanero is much hotter than the normal Habanero with "Guinness Book of Records" of 577,000 Scottville units while the Trinidad scorpion Moruga tests over two million Scottville units. The validity and accuracy of the Scoville Organoleptic Test (SOT) have been widely criticized. The Gillet method adopted by the American Spice Trade Association and the International Organization for Standardization is a modified version of the SOT. Although very costly, the high performance liquid chromatography is the most objective analysis method for obtaining the purest form of capsaicin. Capsaicin (N-vanillyl-8-methyl-6- (E)-nonenamide) is the most pungent of all the groups of compounds called "capsaicinoids" that can be isolated from chili peppers. It is sparingly soluble in water but very soluble in fats, oils, and alcohol.

Chromatographic separation can be achieved using three contrasting modes. They are column chromatography, thin-layer chromatography, and paper chromatography. In column chromatography, the stationary phase is attached to a suitable matrix (an inert, insoluble support) packed into a glass or a metal column. The mobile phase is passed through the column either by gravity feed (as in this study) or by the use of a pumping system, or applied gas pressure [9, 10]. This is the most common form of chromatographic modes. In thin-layer chromatography, the stationary matrix is coated thinly on to a glass, plastic, or metal foil plate. The mobile liquid phase across the thin-layer plate held either horizontally or vertically is by capillary action. Its advantage is that a large number of samples can be studied simultaneously. In paper chromatography, the stationary liquid phase is supported by the use of cellulose fibers of a paper sheet. Thin-layer and paper chromatography have several similarities. In both modes, the mobile phase passes along the paper sheet either by gravity feed or by capillary action and are the older forms of chromatography, with few current serious biochemical applications.

4. Conclusion

The result shows an extraction yield of 12%, which compares favorably with standard extraction process. An alternative source of the nutraceutical is shown in this study. NMR remains a gold standard in ascertaining the carbon-atom structure and high purity yield despite the use of high performance liquid chromatography (HPLC).

Author details

Adebayo Taiwo Ezekiel Jolayemi

Address all correspondence to: adebayoj@hotmail.com

Department of Anaesthesia and ICU, Goulburn Base Hospital, Australia National University, Golburn City, Australia

References

[1] Baler, A. Knowing our place in the animal world. In: Miller, H. and Williams, W. (eds). Ethics and animals. Clifton, NJ: Humana. 1983: 61–77.

[2] Baird, R.M. and Rosenbaum, S.E. (eds). Animal experimentation: The moral issues. Buffalo, NY: Prometheus Press. 1991.

[3] Brink H, (ed. By Van Der Walt C, Rensburg V) Fundamentals of Research Methodology for Health Care Professionals. 2nd ed. Lansdowne Juta and Co Ltd 2006.

[4] Hume. A Treatise on Human Nature (1739), ed. by L. A. Selby-Bigge, Oxford: Clarendon Press, 1967, I, III, 15,:175.

[5] Jasper, J.M. and Nelkin, D. The animal rights crusade: The growth of a moral protest. New York, NY: The Free Press. 1992.

[6] Midgeley, M. Animals and why they matter. Athens, GA: University of Georgia Press. 1983.

[7] Tannenbaum, J. Veterinary ethics. 2nd ed. St. Louis, MO: Mosby Press. 1995.

[8] Hostetman, K., Marston A. and Wolfender J. In: Hostetman, K., Marston, A., Maillard, M. and Hamburger M. (eds). Phytochemistry of plants used in traditional medicine. Oxford: Clarendon Press. 1995: 17–45.

[9] Musabayane, C.T, Mahlaleia, N., Shode, F.O., Ojewole, J.A. Effects of Syzgium (Hochst.) [Myrtaceae) leaf extract on plasma glucose and hepatic glycogen in streptozotocin-induced diabetic rats. Journal of Ethnopharmacology, 2005;97(3):485–490.

[10] Wilson, K., Walker, J. Chromatographic techniques. In: Principles and techniques of practical biochemistry. 4th ed. Cambridge: Cambridge University Press. 1999: 462–529.

[11] Winter, J., Bevan, S. and Campbell, E.A. Capsaicin and pain mechanisms. British Journal of Anaesthesia 1995;75:157–168.

2

Some Mexican Plants used in Traditional Medicine

Mayela Govea-Salas, Jésus Morlett-Chávez,
Raúl Rodriguez-Herrera and Juan Ascacio-Valdés

Abstract

In Mexico, there is an area known as semiarid region that is located in northern Mexico, and this region is rich in biodiversity (endemic flora and fauna). In the semiarid region of Mexico are more than 3500 species of plants that have been identified and used as natural alternatives to treat different ailments (digestive ailments, kidney problems, skin conditions, etc.). The use of plants for medicinal purposes was a common practice in Mexico before the arrival of the Spanish in the sixteenth century; although this knowledge was underestimated for a long time, now interest has reemerged in the use of plants as alternative remedies or traditional medicine. It is now known that the medicinal plant capacity is due to its biological properties, which are due to chemical compounds that are synthesized by the plant metabolisms, called phytochemicals. Phytochemicals are bioactive compounds that have important biological properties such as anticancer property, antimicrobial, antiparasitic, antioxidant, and interest in the recovery of these compounds has grown in recent years, in order to find natural alternatives to synthetic drugs, which they are used for different chronic conditions such as cancer.

Keywords: phytochemical, bioactive compounds, medicinal plant, antioxidant

1. Introduction

Mexico has diverse natural ecosystems that allow the development of a wide variety of flora and fauna; one of them is the semiarid ecosystem. Also, in Mexico, herbal medicine goes back beyond pre-Columbian times, representing a natural and inexpensive alternative for health care, having an important role in the system of traditional medicine. In this context, the plants that grow in Mexican semidesert have been used through the years as traditional medicinal agents and that practice and knowledge have been passed down from generation to generation. In according to data from the World Health Organization (WHO), about 75% of people use herbal medicinal plant extracts for primary health care worldwide.

Therefore, the interest in natural products has increased as a source of new medicines at the industrial and research level, where about 40% of modern drugs in use have been developed from natural products. Since these natural products have a wide structural diversity, mainly small molecules (<2000 Da), which are able to be absorbed and metabolized quickly in the body, called secondary metabolites, its interaction gives biological effects resulting in benefit to health [1]. About 39% of drugs approved between 1983 and 1994 were natural products or their derivatives, including a 60–80% antibacterial and anticancer agents from a natural source. For that reason scientific studies about chemical composition of plants from the Mexican semidesert have been developed, in order to understand and explain the medicinal effects of these plants. Now it is well known that the medicinal effects are due to the presence of phytochemicals with bioactive potential. This chapter provides an overview of the Mexican semidesert endemic plants that have been used in traditional medicine in order to project the opportunities for study and use of natural resources in Mexico.

2. *Jatropha dioica* Sessé (dragon's blood)

One of the plants used in Mexican traditional medicine is a plant called *Jatropha dioica* Sessé [1]. It is a plant native to the Mexican semidesert [2], is a small shrub (50–150 cm), and is commonly known by different names, such as batácora, coatli, dexthi, drago, felondilla, sangregado, and sangregada. In the Mexican semidesert, its most common name is dragon's blood [3] due to the fact that the plant contains a colorless liquid that turns red on contact with air (red-like blood) [2].

This plant grows in dry climates and rocky soils over the mountains; therefore, it is a unique specie of the Mexican semidesert [4, 5].

Dragon's blood has been used in Mexican traditional medicine to treat different diseases or to prevent hair loss. Actually, the stems of the plant are cooked in hot water, and the liquid is applied to the hair after washing [1, 6]. The liquid recovered from the cooking of dragon's blood stems is also used for the treatment of strokes, small wounds, acne, and also for other skin conditions [6, 7].

Also, it has been reported that this plant is useful for strengthening the gums, to keep the teeth in their sockets, acting on the fibers that sustains them [8]. Extracts from this plant have been used as antimicrobial agents. The plant is mainly used as medicinal infusions for the treatment of vaginitis, urethritis, gonorrhea, nephritis, gastroenteritis, conjunctivitis, renal congestion, and local antiseptic. The plant has also been used to treat ulcers and asthma [1].

In addition, there are few reports about the phytochemistry of *J. dioica*. It has been reported that from the root of the plant are extracted and identified terpenes, such as citlalitrione, jatrophone, riolosatrione, and sterols like R-sitosterol [2]. In addition, essential oils, resins, saponins, and alkaloids have been recovered [9].

The phytochemicals of *J. dioica* have been associated with important biological properties for traditional medicine. It has been reported that *J. dioica* contains secondary metabolites such as polyphenols or tannins, flavonoids, and terpenes, which help the defense mechanisms of the plant [10, 11]. Aguilera-Carbo *et al.* [12] reported the presence of important compounds such as ellagitannins and ellagic acid in the plant. These compounds are relevant because they posses biological activities such as antimicrobial and antioxidant.

Besides, this plant has antitumoral, antimicrobial, and antioxidant properties [13]. However, it has also been reported that the plant seeds produce toxic effects if they are consumed as infusions. The main toxic effects are related to the damage at DNA level in cells; however, it has been demonstrated that such effects can be eliminated if the concentrations used are appropriate to take care of the toxicological aspects in order to preserve the biological effects [1]. Furthermore, Lioglier [14] reported that the use of the seeds of the plant in traditional medicine is not recommended due to toxicity. One of the main medicinal effects is the effect against skin conditions, it has been demonstrated that *J. dioica* control wounds, skin infections, and inflammation.

Another important medicinal effect is the antiviral effect, mainly against influenza type A virus and simplex herpes virus [15]; this is important due to the fact that these two viral diseases are the most common throughout the world. There is no doubt that the anticancer effect is also the most important because it is a common and difficult condition to treat. *J. dioica* extracts have shown anticancer activity against melanoma cells, human hepatocellular carcinoma, and human pharynx carcinoma [16].

All these medicinal effects abovementioned are relevant, and this plant represents an option for treatment for different conditions on human health.

3. *Turnera diffusa* Willd (damiana)

The semiarid region of México has a great diversity of plant species that have been used in traditional medicine; this is the case of *Turnera diffusa* [17]. *T. diffusa* is commonly known as damiana, although it is also known by other names, such as "hierba de la postora," "hierba del venado," and "oreganillo." This plant is widely distributed in the semiarid region of México, mainly in the states of Baja California, Chihuahua, and Coahuila [18]. It is a small wild shrub that measures 60 cm–1 m and grows in rocky soil with dry climate and characteristics of the semiarid México [19]. This plant has been used in traditional Mexican medicine, such as infusions, teas, antiseptic solutions, for the treatment of various disorders. Damiana extracts have medicinal effects against digestive disorders (diarrhea), urinary (infections), and respiratory (expectorant). Damiana also has therapeutic effects against me nstrual and circulatory disorders because the plant has vasodilatory properties [9].

The compounds present in damiana extracts have other beneficial properties for human health; it has been shown that this plant has anxiolytic effects that reduce and prevent depression and its physiological effects [19]. The consumption of damiana infusions prevent diabetes because its hypoglycemic activity [20] and cutaneous application of damiana infusions control the process of inflammation in wounds [21] and prevent infections caused by microorganisms and parasites [22].

It has been demonstrated that damiana extracts have important medicinal properties. There are studies about the antiulcerogenic effects of this plant, it was demonstrated that due to the presence of damiana bioactive compounds, arbutina, it has an anti-inflammatory activity in tissue samples of cells from the stomach [23]. Other authors have reported that consumption of damiana infusions control and prevent diabetes mellitus and avoid dependence on insulin [24], and damiana infusions control polyuria, polydipsia, and glucosuria.

However, there is scarce information about the content of phytochemicals in this specie; however, it was reported that the specie has some important compounds in it. One of the groups that have been reported to damiana is terpenes; Alcaráz-Meléndez *et al.* [24] determined the proportion of compounds as cineole, alpha-pinene, beta-pinene, thymol, and p-Cymene (0.5–1%). Damiana also contains hydrolysable tannins (4%) [25], flavonoids (0.7%) [26], alkaloids, etc. Some reference compounds in damiana are ar arbutin (flavone) and apigenin (hydroquinone), and they have been reported to be the main bioactive compounds of this plant.

Zhao *et al.* [25] described the presence of uncharacterized compounds in damiana. These compounds were luteolin glycoside, apigenin glucopyranoside, apigenin coumaroylglucoside, syringetin glucopyranoside, and laricitin glucopyranoside. These compounds belong to the group of flavones and flavonoids that have biological activities such as anti-inflammatory, antibacterial, and antioxidant [27, 28].

The compounds identified in damiana possess biological activities that can improve the medicinal effects. Damiana has compounds such as flavonoids, polyphenols, and terpenes [25], and these compounds have antioxidant activity, which inhibits the activity of free radicals that cause damage to health by increasing the risk of cancer [29].

On the other hand, compounds of damiana have other activities that promote human health. These compounds have antimutagenic, antitumor, and anticancer activity [30, 31] against carcinogenic compounds such as pyrene-7,8-dio-9,10-epoxide (BPDE); therefore, damiana represents an option for prevention and treatment of cellular disorders.

The antiviral property of damiana compounds has been studied *in vitro*. Polyphenols and flavonoids inhibit the replication of human influenza type A virus [32], and these compounds inhibit the replication of human immunodeficiency virus (HIV) also, blocking the action of some specific enzymes.

The compounds that are present in damiana can also prevent infections caused by pathogenic microorganisms because these compounds have antimicrobial activity. Polyphenols and flavonoids have been evaluated against pathogens such as *Salmonella tiphy, Salmonella pyogenes, and Pseudomonas aeruginosa* [33, 34].

There is scarce information about the compounds present in damiana and its medicinal and pharmacological effects, this represents an opportunity to generate knowledge and expand the application field of the plant for the treatment of relevant conditions for human health.

4. *Larrea tridentata* (Creosote bush)

Larrea tridentata (Creosote bush) is known as "gobernadora," "hediondilla," or "guamis" in Mexico. It is abundant in the desert areas of the North Mexican states such as San Luis Potosi, Coahuila, Chihuahua, Durango, Sonora, and Zacatecas [35]. Creosote bush is a widespread perennial flowering bush thriving in the deserts of Mexico and is an important plant with a long history of medicinal use for different pathologies [36].

Creosote bush is widely distributed in nature, and it is a notable source of natural products with biological activities. The plant resin has been reported to contain a total of 19 flavonoid aglycones, some flavonoid glycosides, halogenic alkaloids, several lignans, and a large quantity of essential oils [35]. The leaves are shiny with a thick resinous coating and discharge a strong odor and have a sour flavor. Along with these compounds, Creosote bush extracts contain saponins, monoterpenes, sterols, tannins such as gallic acid (GA) and the antioxidant nordihydroguaiaretic acid (NDGA). All these compounds, especially NDGA and other phenols of the leaf surface, function as antimicrobial agents and as protection against herbivores, UV radiation, and water loss [37].

The medicinal use of Creosote bush is through extracts and preparations from this plant to treat a wide variety of disorders including skin sores, fungal and microbial infections, diabetes, kidney and gallbladder stones, arthritis, venereal diseases, cold virus infections, sinusitis, rheumatism, and cancer [38].

Particularly, NDGA and tannins has been identified to have a significant role in cancer therapy including different models of carcinogenesis such as lung, breast, skin, prostate, and esophageal cancers, demonstrated the capacity of these compounds to inhibit the growth and proliferation of several human cancer types [39]. In addition, NDGA has been found to be a potent antiviral and inhibitor of viruses such as herpes simplex virus (HSV), human papilloma virus (HPV), human immunodeficiency virus (HIV-1), and influenza virus [40]. NDGA suppresses regulated transcription DNA-binding site that plays an active role in the virus gene expression, leading to inhibition of gene expression from the early promoters and thus interferes with proteins function and transcription [41].

5. Cancer and bioactive compounds

Currently, some authors mention that the incidence of cancer is significantly lower in the people whose diet consists mainly of fruits, vegetables, and herbal teas, than people whose food consumption is mainly animal products. This has led researchers to search for natural anticancer compounds obtained from semidesert plants or foods with high phytochemicals and polyphenols [42].

Hopeful polyphenols are ellagic acid and gallic acid, among other polyphenols, that could be considered as alternative treatments against cancer. Some studies with GA obtained from various foods and plants have shown that this compound has anticancer activity against several types of cancer interfering in some stages of tumor growth, suppressing angiogenesis and metastasis in some tumor lines of lung, prostate, bladder, brain, kidney, and leukemia [43, 44]. Moreover, GA inhibits metastasis of P815 liver cells, induced apoptosis in DU145 and 22Rv1 cell prostate cancer in athymic mice, and reduced viability of U251n and U87 human cells glioma after 24 h of treatment [45, 46]. In contrast, for PWR-1E prostate epithelial cells that are not cancerous have no significant change, indicating that GA has a selective toxicity to cancer cells of prostate cancer. Besides, gallic acid treatment was found to diminish the cellular oxidative stress by decreasing ROS (Reactive Oxygen Species) production and hepatocarcinoma cell proliferation and also decrease hepatitis C virus (HCV) replication in Huh7 replicon cells decreasing the expression of nonstructural HCV proteins of the virus [47].

Moreover, the molecular mechanisms underlying the anticancer activities of Creosote bush lignans and antioxidants have been shown to involve wide cancer pathways. The specific inhibition of the Sp1 oncogenic factor (Sp1-dependent gene coding for cyclin-dependent kinase) promotes apoptosis by inhibiting expression of the surviving gene with these plant lignans and methylated NDGA derivatives and have been shown to induce a decrease in the proliferation of breast cancer cells [48, 49].

The mechanisms that Creosote bush compounds are antitumorigenic and antiproliferative are still being elucidated. Other authors carrying out *in vivo* studies revealed that NDGA suppresses tumor growth by inhibiting metabolic enzymes as well as RTK phosphorylation, which is overexpressed in certain cancer cells [50]. Also, several studies demonstrated that NDGA and some tannins have the property of inhibiting cancer cell growth *in vitro* in human tumor cell xenografts in mice [51].

Furthermore, the demonstration of the hypothesis that antioxidants from foods and plants can execute beneficial health effects, including acting as inducers of mechanisms relating to antioxidant defense [52], longevity [53], cell maintenance, and DNA repair [54].

Author details

Mayela Govea-Salas[1,2], Jésus Morlett-Chávez[1,2], Raúl Rodriguez-Herrera[3] and Juan Ascacio-Valdés[3*]

*Address all correspondence to: alberto_ascaciovaldes@uadec.edu.mx

1 Clinical Analysis and Molecular Biology Laboratory, School of Chemistry, Autonomous University of Coahuila, Saltillo, Coahuila, Mexico

2 Cellular Biology Laboratory, School of Chemistry, Autonomous University of Coahuila, Saltillo, Coahuila, Mexico

3 Food Science and Technology Department, School of Chemistry, Autonomous University of Coahuila, Saltillo, Coahuila, Mexico

References

[1] Martínez N, Almaguer G, Vázquez-Alvarado P, Figueroa A, Zuñiga C, Hernández-Cereulos A. Phytochemical analysis of *Jatropha dioica* and determination of its antioxidant and chemopreventive effect on the genotoxic potential of cyclophosphamide, daunorubicin and methyl methane-sulfonate evaluated by the comet assay. Boletin Latinoamericano y del Caribe de Plantas Medicinales y Aromaticas. 2014; 13, 437–457.

[2] Wong-Paz J, Castillo-Inungaray M, López-López L, Contreras-Esquivel J, Nevárez-Moorillon V, Aguilar C. *Jatropha dioica*: potential source of antimicrobial agents. Acta Química Mexicana. 2010; 2, 1–5.

[3] Manzanero-Medina G, Flores-Martinez A, Sandoval-Zapotitla E, Bye-Boettler R. Etnobotanic of seven medicinal plants from México. Polibotánica. 2009; 27, 191–228.

[4] Blanco M. Handbook of toxic plants from Chihuahua state. Centro Librero La Prensa, Plant records Geog. 1983; 4, 162–168.

[5] Fresnedo J, Orozco Q. Diversity and distribution of genus *Jatropha* in México.Genetic Resources and Crop Evolution. 2012; 60, 1087–1104.

[6] Martinez-Herrera J, Siddhuraju P, Francis G, Davila-Ortiz G, Becker K. Chemical composition, toxic/anti-metabolic constituents, and effect of different treatments on their levels, in four provenances of *Jatropha curcas* L. from Mexico. Food Chemistry. 2006; 96, 80–89.

[7] López-Ibarra J, Mendoza-Moreno R. Quantification of condensed tannins from sangre de drago (*Jatropha dioica*). Revista Chapingo: Serie Zonas Áridas. 2000; 1, 1–6.

[8] Pérez-Escandón B. Plants from Hidalgo State. Universidad Autónoma del Estado de Hidalgo, Pachuca, Hidalgo, México; 2003.

[9] Belmares R, Garza Y, Rodríguez R, Contreras J, Aguilar C. Composition and fungal degradation of tannins present in semiarid plants. Electronic Journal of Enviromental, Agricultural and Food Chemistry. 2009; 4, 312–318.

[10] Castillo F, Hernández D, Gallegos G, Méndez M, Rodríguez R, Reyes A, Aguilar C. *In vitro* antifungal of plant extracts obtained with alternative organic solvents against *Rhizoctonia solani* Kühn. Industrial Crops and Products. 2010; 32, 324–328.

[11] Montenegro G, Salas F, Pena R, Pizarro R. Antibacterial and antifungic activity of the unifloral honeys of Quillaja saponaria, an endemic Chilean species. International Journal of Experimental Botany. 2009; 78, 141–146.

[12] Aguilera A, Augur C, Prado L, Aguilar C, Favela E. Extraction and analysis of ellagic acid from novel complex sources. Chemical Papers. 2008; 62, 440–444.

[13] Sabandar C, Ahmat N, Mohd F, Sahidin I. Medicinal property, phytochemistry and pharmacology of several species (*Euphorbiaceae*): a review. Phytochemistry. 2003; 85, 7–29.

[14] Lioglier H. Medicinal Plants from Puerto Rico and Caribe. *Iberoamericana de Ediciones Inc.*, San Juan, Puerto Rico; 1990

[15] Mothana R, Mentel R, Reiss C, Lindequist U. Phytochemical screening and antiviral activity of some medicinal plants in the island Soqotra. Phytotherapy Research. 2006; 20, 298–302.

[16] Goel G, Makkar H, Francis G, Becker K. Phorbol esters: structure, biological activity and toxicity in animals. International Journal of Toxicology. 2007; 26, 279–288.

[17] Alcaráz L, Véliz M. Commercialization of desert plant: damiana *(Turnera diffusa)*. Revista Mexicana de Agronegocios. 2006; 19, 1–13.

[18] Roberts N. Baja California, plant field guide. Natural History Publ. Co., La Joya, California, E.U.A.; 1989.

[19] Suresh K, Saharma A. Apigenin: the anxiolytic constituent of *Turnera aphrodisiaca*. Pharmaceutical Biology. 2006; 44, 84–90.

[20] Kumar S, Sharma A. Anti-anxiety activity studies on homoeopathic formulations of *Turnera aphrodisiaca* ward. Evidence-Based Complementary and Alternative Medicine. 2005; 2, 117–119.

[21] Kumar S, Madaan R, Sharma A. Pharmacological evaluation of bioactive principle of *Turnera aphrodisiaca*. Indian Journal of Pharmaceutical Sciences. 2008; 70, 740–744.

[22] Quintero A, Pelcastre A, Solano J. Cytotoxic activity of crude extracts from Astragalus chrysochlorus (*Leguminosae*). Journal of Pharmacy and Pharmaceutical Science. 1999; 2, 108–112.

[23] Taha M, Salga M, Ali H, Abdulla M, Abdelwahab S, Hadi A. Gastroprotective activities of *Turnera diffusa* Willd. ex Schult. revisited: role of arbutin. Journal of Ethnopharmacology. 2012; 141, 273–281.

[24] Alcaráz-Meléndez L, Delgado-Rodríguez J, Real-Cosío S. Analysis of essential oils from wild and micropropagated plants of damiana (*Turnera diffusa*). Fitoterapia. 2004; 75, 696–701.

[25] Zhao J, Pawar R, Ali Z, Khan I. Phytochemical investigation of *Turnera diffusa*. Journal of Natural Products. 2007; 70, 289–292.

[26] Carr Z, Kleinerman R, Stovall M, Weinstock R, Griem M, Land C. Malignant neoplasms after radiation therapy for peptic ulcer. Radiation Research. 2009; 157, 668–677.

[27] Piacente S, Camargo E, Zampelli A, Gracioso J, Brito A, Pizza C, Vilegas W. Flavonoids and arbutin from *Turnera diffusa*. Zeitschrift für Naturforschung C. 2002; 57, 983–985.

[28] Umit H, Tezel A, Bukavaz S, Unsal G, Otkun M, Soylu A, Tucer D, Bilgi S. The relationship between virulence factors of *Helicobacter pylori* and severity of gastritis in infected patients. Digestive Diseases and Sciences. 2009; 54, 103–110.

[29] Cuzzocrea S. Role of nitric oxide and reactive oxygen species in arthritis. Current Pharmaceutical Design. 2006; 27, 3551–3570.

[30] Smith S, Tate P, Huang G, Magee J, Meepagala K, Wedge D, Larcom L. Antimutagenic activity of berry extracts. Journal of Medicinal Food. 2004; 7, 450–455.

[31] Huetz P, Mavaddat N, Mavri J. Reaction between ellagic acid and an ultimate carcinogen. Journal of Chemical Information and Modeling. 2005; 45, 1564–1570.

[32] Haidari M, Ali M, Casscells S, Madjid M. Pomegranate (*Punica granatum*) purified polyphenol extract inhibits influenza virus and has a synergistic effect with oseltamivir. Phytomedicine. 2009; 16, 1127–1136.

[33] Atta-Ur-Rahman, Ngounou N, Choudhary I, Malik S, Makhmoor T, Nur-E-Alam M, Zareen S, Lontsi D, Ayafor F, Sondengam L. New antioxidant and antimicrobial ellagic acid derivates from *Pteleopsis hylodendron*. Planta Medica. 2001; 67, 335–339.

[34] Nascimento G, Locatelli J, Freitas P, Silva G. Antibacterial activity of plant extracts and phytochemicals on antibiotic-resistant bacteria. Brazilian Journal of Microbiology. 2000; 31, 247–256.

[35] Arteaga S, Andrade-Cetto A, Cardenas R. Larrea tridentata (*Creosote bush*), an abundant plant of Mexican and US-American deserts and its metabolite nordihydroguaiaretic acid. Journal of Ethnopharmacology. 2005;98, 231–239.

[36] Jian-Ming L, Nurko J, Weakley S, Jiang J, Kougias P, Lin P, Yao Q, Chen C. Molecular mechanisms and clinical applications of nordihydroguaiaretic acid (NDGA) and its derivatives: an update. Medical Science Monitor. 2010; 16, 93–100.

[37] Anjaneyulu M, Chopra K. Nordihydroguairetic acid, a lignin, prevents oxidative stress and the development of diabetic nephropathy in rats. Pharmacology. 2004; 72, 42–50.

[38] Lia V, Confalonieri V, Comas C, Hunziker H. Molecular phylogeny of Larrea and its allies (*Zygophyllaceae*): reticulate evolution and the probable time of creosote bush arrival to North America. Molecular Phylogenetic Evolution. 2002; 21, 309–320.

[39] Gnabre J, Bates R, Huang C. Creosote bush lignans for human disease treatment and prevention: perspectives on combination therapy. Journal Traditional Complementary Medicine. 2015; 5(3), 119–126.

[40] Craigo J, Callahan M, Huang C, DeLucia A. Inhibition of human papillomavirus type 16 gene expression by nordihydroguaiaretic acid plant lignan derivatives. Antiviral Research. 2000; 47, 19–28.

[41] Noor R, Mittal S, Iqbal J. Superoxide dismutase—applications and relevance to human diseases. Medical Science Monitor. 2002; 8, 210–215.

[42] Nair S, Li W, Kong A. Natural dietary anticancer chemopreventive compounds: redox mediated differential signaling mechanisms in cytoprotection of normal cells versus in cytotoxicity in tumor cells. Acta Pharmacologica Sinica. 2007; 28, 459–472.

[43] Albini A. Molecular pathways for cancer angioprevention. Clinical Cancer Research. 2007; 13, 4320–4325.

[44] Chi A, Norden A, Wen P. Inhibition of angiogenesis and invasion in malignant gliomas. Expert Review Anticancer Therapy. 2007; 7, 1537–1560.

[45] Kawada M, Ohno Y, Ri Y. Anti-tumor effect of gallic acid on LL-2 lung cancer cells transplanted in mice. Anti-Cancer Drugs. 2001; 12, 847–852.

[46] Cai Y, Chopp M, Katakowski M, Jiang F, Jiang H, Lu Y, Shing-Shun T, Wu K, Zhen X. Gallic acid suppresses cell viability, proliferation, invasion and angiogenesis in human glioma cells. European Journal of Pharmacology. 2010; 641, 102–107.

[47] Govea-Salas M, Rivas-Estilla M, Rodríguez-Herrera R, Lozano-Sepúlpveda A, Aguilar-González C, Zugasti-Cruz A, Salas-Villalobos B, Morlett-Chávez J. Gallic acid decreases hepatitis C virus expression through its antioxidant capacity. Experimental and Therapeutic Medicine. 2015; 11, 619–624.

[48] Bailey-Dell K, Hassel B, Doyle A, Ross D. Promoter characterization and genomic organization of the human breast cancer resistance protein (ATP-binding cassette transporter G2) gene. Biochimica et Biophysica Acta. 2001; 1520, 234–241.

[49] Bongiovanni G, Cantero J, Eynard A, Goleniowski M. Organic extracts of *Larrea divaricata* Cav. induced apoptosis on tumoral MCF7 cells with an higher cytotoxicity than nordihydroguaiaretic acid or paclitaxel. Journal of Experimental Therapeutics and Oncology. 2008; 7, 1–7.

[50] Blecha E, Anderson O, Chow M, Guevarra C, Pender C, Penaranda C, Zavodovskaya M, Youngren F, Berkman E. Inhibition of IGF-1R and lipoxygenase by nordihydroguaiaretic acid (NDGA) analogs. Bioorganic and Medicinal Chemistry Letters. 2007; 17, 4026–4029.

[51] Park R, Chang C, Liang C, Chung Y, Henry A, Lin E. Systemic treatment with tetra-Omethyl nordihydroguaiaretic acid suppresses the growth of human xenograft tumors. Clinical Cancer Research. 2005; 11, 4601–4609.

[52] Hubbard P, Wolffram S, de Vos R, Bovy A, Gibbins M, Lovegrove A. Ingestion of onion soup high in quercetin inhibits platelet aggregation and essential components of the collagen-stimulated platelet activation pathway in man: a pilot study. British Journal of Nutrition. 2006; 96, 482–488.

[53] Ludwig A, Lorenz M, Grimbo N, Steinle F, Meiners S, Bartsch C, Stangl K, Baumann G, Stangl V. The tea flavonoid epigallocatechin-3-gallate reduces cytokine-induced VCAM-1 expression and monocyte adhesion to endothelial cells. Biochemical and Biophysical Research Communications. 2004; 316, 659–665.

[54] Vauzour D, Rodriguez-Mateos A, Corona G, Oruna-Concha J, Spencer J. Polyphenols and human health: prevention of disease and mechanisms of action. Nutrients. 2010; 2, 1106–1131.

3

Capsaicin: Aromatic Basis and Mechanism of Action—An Example of Positive Inhibition

Adebayo Taiwo Ezekiel Jolayemi

Abstract

This work will, in addition to describing the aromatic basis of capsaicin, elucidate its mechanism of action through a positive inhibition of the nerve conduction, which ultimately accounts for the various pharmacological effects of capsaicin on pain control, cardiovascular mechanisms, as well as its effects on genitourinary and gastrointestinal tracts.

Keywords: capsaicin, aromatics, desensitization, mechanism of action, positive inhibition

1. Introduction

The current study is a systemic review of the pharmacology and chemistry of capsaicin and capsaicinoids. The genus Capsicum is a member of the Solanaceae family that includes tomato, potato, tobacco, and petunia. The genus Capsicum consists of approximately 22 wild species and 5 domesticated species [1] including *C. annuum*, *C. baccatum*, *C. chinense*, *C. frutescens*, and *C. pubescens*.

Capsicum species have been used as medicinal plants to treat intestinal upsets and indigestion and also as stimulants, rubefacient, and tonic. They have also been used as folk remedies for dropsy, colic, diarrhea, asthma, arthritis, muscle cramps, and toothache. In addition, *Capsicum frutescens* L. has been reported to have hypoglycemic properties [2]. However, prolonged contact with the skin may cause dermatitis and blisters, while excessive consumption can cause gastroenteritis and/or kidney damage. Besides, paprika and cayenne pepper may be cytotoxic to mammalian cells, *in vitro*. Moreover, consumption of red pepper may aggravate symptoms of duodenal ulcers. It has also been shown that high levels of ground hot pepper have induced stomach ulcers and cirrhosis of the liver in laboratory animals. As a stimulant *Capsicum* species could stimulate body temperature, salivation, and increase gastric juices.

This study was undertaken to investigate the anti-inflammatory property of ***Capsicum frutescens*** ethyl acetate extract (CFE) and capsaicin (CPF) in rat model to provide a pharmacological rationale for the folklore medicine uses of capsaicin and capsaicinoids to treat arthritis, muscle sprain, and other inflammatory conditions in some communities. One of the main objectives of this study was to determine if *Capsicum frutescens* fruit extract in this study has similar efficacy on peripheral and central components of pain as so described for *Capsicum spp.* (Linn) [Solanaceae] from other parts of the world, such as from India, Mexico, Thailand, and South America [3].

2. Research methods

Following Ethics approval by the Animal Ethics Committee of the University of KwaZulu—Natal; Westville Campus, various parallel and comparative studies were carried out on crude extract ethyl acetate of *Capsicum frutescens* and synthetic capsaicin. The studies were to elucidate the analgesic, antiinflammatory, gastro-intestinal effects and the effects on coagulation of both compounds. The discussion that follows is a systemic review of the pharmacological effects of capsaicin. The "hot plate" and "acetic acid" analgesic tests methods were used for central and peripheral nervous system investigations on pain mechanisms, using the mean reaction time and inhibition of writhing, respectively. The effects of *Capsicum*-derived capsaicin on chick isolated parasympathetically innervated esophagus, rabbit duodenum, and guinea pig ileum were investigated in Ugo Basile organ baths, respectively. In all cases, concentration-response curves to standard agonists were investigated in the absence and in the presence of capsaicin (CPE), or standard antagonists. Following 2 weeks of treatment with capsaicin and capsicum extracts, the effects of capsaicin on coagulation was tested. The results of these studies show comparable analgesic to morphine and diclofenac on the peripheral analgesic mechanisms and more intense central analgesia compared to morphine ($p < 0.1$). Besides, capsaicin increased the INR by 1.25 times compared to control ($p < 0.01$) and has a dose-dependent relaxation of the gastro-intestinal smooth muscles ($p < 0.1$).

3. Data analysis

Experimental data obtained were analyzed and presented as means (+SEM). The data from "control" rats were used as baseline values while the mean reaction times to the pain stimulus or the writhing were recorded and subsequently analyzed, using a two-way ANOVA. Interobserver differences were assessed by Wilcoxon and Kruskal-Wallis tests. Student's t-test was used to test for the difference between the means when two groups were analyzed. Where the groups are more than two, ANOVA was used to test for differences between the groups.

Statistical significance was by using a double-tailed CI of 95% and a p-value of less than 0.05. Pearson correlation coefficient was used to assess the activity of *Capsicum frutescens*–derived capsaicin extract, compared to that of the synthetic capsaicin and to compare results from selected groups.

4. Discussion

Capsicum species occur worldwide, and has been used for more than 9000 years by the Chinese, Indians, and Africans for medicinal and nonmedicinal purposes [4], for example, for pain, among other things. Pain is perceived through both peripheral and central mechanisms. Peripheral mechanisms typically involve the nociceptors, while central mechanisms involve the process of central sensitization. Pain is sensed by nociceptors located in the sensory nerve endings. Messages are relayed through complex multisynaptic afferents to the dorsal column by means of transmission and transduction of chemical messages, which are relayed via the spinal mechanisms and processed for appropriate supranuclear interpretation. Finally, the motor effector organs are facilitated to respond according to the type of pain [5, 6].

The neural impulses, which originate from the nociceptors, relay through the primary afferent nerves (PAN), to the spinal cord, or via the cranial nerves to the brain stem, for those impulses that originate from the head and neck. The cell bodies of these ganglia are located in the dorsal root ganglia, or the respective cell bodies in the cases of cranial nerves V, VIII, IX, and X. By means of complex synapses, messages are relayed to ascending pathways.

There are several biochemical mediators (and neurotransmitters), which are involved in pain transmission and perception. Peripherally, the most important of these amines are the cyclo-oxygenase agonists and the leukotrienes. Others are catecholamines, acetylcholine, vasoactive intestinal polypeptides (VIP), neuropeptides Y (NPY), cholecystokinin, 5-hydroxytryptamine, neurotensin, tachykinin, and bradykinins [7, 8]. The opioid receptors act both centrally and peripherally. In addition, the central cyclo-oxygenase action has been found with acetaminophen [9]. Centrally acting neuromediators can be classified into "excitatory" and "inhibitory" neuromediators. Glutamate and aspartate are the examples of excitatory amino acids acting as neurotransmitters centrally, while substance P (SP), calcitonin gene-related peptide (CGRP) [10], and growth factors (e.g., brain-derived neurotrophic factors) are other examples. Inhibitory neuromediators include endogenous opioids, such as enkephalin and β-endorphins. Others are gamma-aminobutyric acid (GABA), glycine, and β-adrenergic agonists [11]. Conversely, any agent acting on these receptors and neuromediators have the ability to modulate pain. The aberration of inflammatory and neuropathic enhancement of pain perception as seen in allodynia (painful touch) and hyperalgesia are due to increased release of SP from *substantia gelatinosa.* This phenomenon is called "peripheral sensitization."

The memory of pain, neural plasticity, wide dynamic range activity, and the winding phenomenon are enhanced by *N*-methyl-D-aspartate receptor through an early expression of genetic coding through *c*-fos and *v*-fos oncogens [12–15]. This neural plasticity leads to the phenomenon of central sensitization as typified by stump and phantom pain. Both hyperalgesia and allodynia, which are known side effects of capsaicin [16], are results of peripheral and central sensitization. In addition, the repetitive C fiber stimulation produces the winding-up phenomenon.

Injury leads to nociception, transduction, receptor modification, uncoordinated sprouting, and growth of injured axons and ectopic epileptic firing of nerves [17]. Although the hypothalamus receives an enormous amount of stimuli, it is devoid of the ability to discriminate, since it is not somato-topically organized. It is also not able to localize pain. However, discrimination and localization are possible by the third-order neurons connecting to the prefrontal gyrus in the cerebral cortex. This is the basis for the use of secondary analgesia such as antidepressants and anticonvulsants.

The ascending order is not alone in pain modulation. There is enough evidence to suggest that the descending tracts have a role in the modulation of pain [18]. In the late 1960s, it was observed that neurons in the dorsal horn of decerebrated animals are more responsive to painful stimuli when the spinal cord is blocked [19]. Also in the late 1980s, electrical stimulation of the periaqueductal gyrus was found to produce profound relief of pain in animals [17]. These studies provided scientific basis for stimulation-produced analgesia. In addition, further studies showed that instillation of small doses of morphine in the regions such as periaqueductal system (PAG) produced significant analgesia.

Substance P is the active neurotransmitter that is released at the primary nerve endings of primary afferent neurons (PAN). It is usually synthesized at the *substantia gelatinosa* of the dorsal horn. On release from PAN, substance P from the dorsal horn of the spinal cord exhibits systemic actions. For example, the expression of substance P and vanilloid receptor (VR1) were found in the trigeminal sensory neurons projecting from PAN to the nasal mucosa in the mouse [20, 21]. The release of both substance P and neurokinin A (NKA) from PAN to various stimuli induced by capsaicin (vanilloid) receptor (VR1) results in potent proinflammatory effects on the airways [22, 23].

Expression of substance P was found to correlate with the severity of diarrhea in cryptosporidosis from the result in electrogenic chloride anion secretion [24,25] and found three kinds of current in response to substance P in bullfrog dorsal root ganglion neurons. They are either G-protein coupled channel, slow activating I (SP); or directly opened channel, fast activating I (SP); or both, moderately activating I (SP). All the three were inwardly directed currents with the ionic mechanism underlying slow activating I (SP) deduced as closure of K^+ channels. The fast-activating channel is due to the opening of sodium channels. These correlate with the three subtypes of SP receptor, immunoreactive interneurons described in the rat basolateral amygdala [26]. Furthermore, the secretion of HCO^-_3 through secretin was abolished by substance P [15, 24, 27].

Other systems affected by substance P include the cardiovascular system. Low dose systemic administration of substance P caused hypertension and tachycardia, while unilateral or bilateral injections into the rat's *nucleus tractus solitari* caused slow increase in blood pressure and heart rate, which peaked in 1.5–5 min after injection and lasted for 20–30 min. These effects are vagal mediated [28, 29].

Furthermore, the swellings that typically accompany complex regional pain syndrome have been found to be due to extravasation of substance P–induced protein [24, 30].

Capsaicin is the main pungent ingredient in "hot" chili peppers, and elicits a burning pain by selectively activating sensory neurons that convey information about noxious stimuli to the central nervous system [31, 32]. However, capsaicin-induced ion refluxes increase cyclic GMP and not cyclic AMP [33], capsaicin has selective action on unmyelinated C-fibers and thinly myelinated A primary sensory neurons [33].

Several sensory stimuli including noxious pressure, heat, and chemical irritation could affect capsaicin-sensitive fibers, which are polymodal in nature. These nociceptors are the most abundant class of nociceptive fibers. On stimulation by capsaicin, nociceptive neurons release glutamate, which are a rapidly acting central neurotransmitter and an excitatory amino acid. Likewise, the transient receptor potential (TRP) family of ion channels are activated by a diverse range of stimuli, including heat, protons, lipids, phorbols, phosphorylation, changes in extracellular osmolarity and/or pressure, and depletion of intracellular Ca^{2+} stores. In all, VR 1 remains the only channel activated by vanilloids such as capsaicin [34].

In addition, they also express neuropeptides, such as calcitonin-gene-related-peptide (CGRP), substance P, nerokinin A, and somatostantin, which, on release to the spinal cord, leads to intense stimulation. Noxious stimulation acting on peripheral nervous system results in a long-term increase in spinal excitability, which results in the central mechanisms of allodynia and hyperalgesia. There is neuronal cooperation and enhancement of activities by tachykinins (e.g., substance P and neurokinin A) and excitatory amino acids (EAAs) (e.g., glutamate), which ultimately increase synaptic activation of dorsal horn neurons via EAA receptors. Following synthesis at the dorsal root ganglia, most of the neuropeptides are exported peripherally and not centrally, to facilitate neurogenic inflammation. Capsaicin pretreatment in neonatal rats has been found to abolish the development of thermal hyperalgesia produced in a model of neuropathic pain in rats [35, 36].

An initial local application of capsaicin is algesic. However, its repeated application leads to desensitization, and its high concentration eventually blocks conduction of the C-fibers. This results in long-lasting sensory deficits. These properties give a logical basis for the use of capsaicin in treating pains that arise from cluster headache, complex regional pain syndrome, postmastectomy pain, postherpetic neuralgia, and diabetic neuropathy [16, 37, 38].

In his review, Caterina et al. [39] had shown that capsaicin has an expression-cloning strategy based on calcium influx to isolate a functional cDNA encoding of a capsaicin receptor from sensory neurons. Capsaicin receptor is a nonselective cation channel that is structurally related to members of the transient-receptor-potential V1 (TRPV1) family of ion channels [36, 40, 41]. The cloned-capsaicin receptor is also activated by increases in temperature in the noxious range, which suggests that it acts as a transducer of painful thermal stimuli *in vivo*.

In all, 28 mammalian transient receptor potential (TRP) cation channels have been identified and regrouped into six subfamilies [42]. These include TRPC ("canonical"), TRPV ("vanilloid"), TRPM ("melastatin"), TRPP ("polycystin"), TRPML ("mucolipin"), and TRPA ("ankyrin"). The TRPV subfamily (vanilloid receptors) comprises channels critically involved in nociception and thermo sensing. Moreover, the TRPV 1 receptors have been found in the brain, spinal cord, peripheral neurons, smooth and cardiac muscles, vascular tissues, bronchial muscles, GIT mucosa, and the urinary bladder.

The mechanism of action of capsaicin is based on neuronal desensitization to noxious stimuli. Two forms of desensitization are apparent. One is a capsaicin-induced loss of responsiveness. This is functional and it is reversible. On the other hand is a calcium-dependent desensitization involving the activation of phosphatase and leading to the inactivation of capsaicin channel.

High doses of capsaicin may lead to neurotoxicity. Axonal and terminal degeneration and impaired nociception appear to be irreversible. Both osmotic lysis and action of calcium-dependent proteases may be responsible for capsaicin-induced neurotoxicity [43–47].

In acute pain, studies in animals have shown that systemic capsaicin relieves pain in increasing doses from 0.5 to 10 mg/kg, but nerve degeneration was noted in doses of 50 mg/kg and greater. The relief was for mechano-thermal pain [48–51]. In human studies, it requires days to weeks before beneficial effects of capsaicin can be seen [52].

With an increase in the levels of substance P in inflammatory and neurogenic joint diseases (arthritis), topical or intra-articular injections of capsaicin have shown significant improvements, as well as reductions in the level of inflammatory mediators [53–57]. In the same vein, Perkins and Campbell [58] used 6 mg/kg of intra-articular capsaicin to reverse mechanical hyperalgesia for several hours [59, 60].

In rheumatoid arthritis, the effect of capsaicin is mixed. Whereas Deal et al. [48] showed significant reduction in the level of pain intensity in 31 patients with rheumatoid arthritis of the knee following treatment with zostrix (as 0.025%) for 4 weeks, McCarthy and McCarty [62] did not observe any improvement in 7 patients with rheumatoid hands, using 0.75% capsaicin. However, Weisman et al. [49, 61, 62] reported that application of capsaicin (0.75%) for 6 weeks produced a reduction in inflammatory mediators, including substance P, in the synovial fluid of patients with rheumatoid arthritis. In osteoarthritis, there is evidence to show increase in the level of substance P in patients, [4, 53]. Randomized, controlled trials have also shown significant improvement in pain relief following treatment with capsaicin cream [23, 34, 43, 53].

With neuropathic pain in mind, animal studies using intrathecal as well as subcutaneous or topical capsaicin have produced significant improvements in the relief of hyperalgesia and pain [37, 63–66, 72]. These studies show that capsaicin-sensitive nerves have a role in thermal hyperalgesia in the animals under study [66, 67].

Studies in humans with neuropathic pain include patients with postherpetic neuralgia [51, 68], diabetic neuropathy [69], and postmastectomy pain [44]. Others include the use of capsaicin in stump or phantom pain [70], complex regional pain syndrome type I [71], trigeminal neuralgia [72], and oral neuropathic pain [64]. Capsaicin was also studied in cluster headache, and fibromyalgia [17], as well as in acute or chronic conditions, such as osteoarthritis [48, 64]; and rheumatoid arthritis [37].

Notable among these studies are those by the Capsaicin Study Group [73] with a total of 277 patients (138 capsaicin 0.075%, 139 placebo) having diabetic neuropathy. The Group reported significant improvements in all measures (pain, walking, working, and sleeping) after administering capsaicin four times daily for up to 8 weeks. In their study, Jensen and Larson [74] found that capsaicin cream provides an alternative treatment option with a favorable outcome in painful diabetic neuropathy. Most of these studies were performed over similar periods of time, except the study by Watson et al. [75], which followed up 83 patients with postherpetic neuralgia for 2 years. The investigators found that in 86% of their patients, improvements in the pain scores were either maintained or further enhanced with no serious side effects. Furthermore, the efficacy of nasal application of capsaicin in the treatment of cluster headache had been confirmed following 7 days application of capsaicin with significant improvement when compared with placebo. The relief might have been produced through the effects of capsaicin on substance P–containing trigeminal nerve [76, 77].

Capsaicin has also been shown to relief pruritus in patients with psoriasis [28, 70, 78], brachioradial pruritus [79], aquagenic pruritus [80], notalgia parasthetica [24], nodular prurigo [79], and pruritus produced in patients on hemodialysis [81]. In human volunteers, capsaicin treatment was found to have inhibited itch after histamine and allergen challenge. Itch is mediated by a subset of capsaicin-sensitive nociceptive neurons through the inhibition of C fiber conduction [82, 83].

The wide systemic side effects have made topical capsaicin to be more acceptable in clinical state. The main side effects are neuronal, cardiovascular, mucocutaneous tissue, or open wounds. Electron microscopic observations have revealed degeneration and glial engulfment of buttons and unmyelinated axons in the dorsal horn, 2–6 hours after neonatal subcutaneous capsaicin injections in rats. There is increased latency of the nerves; convulsion and even death may follow with very high doses of capsaicin [84, 85]. Cannabinoids have been used to attenuate capsaicin-evoked hyperalgesia [78] and low-dose lidocaine was found to reduce capsaicin-evoked secondary analgesia by a central mechanism [34].

When capsaicin is in contact with mucocutaneous tissues, such as the conjunctiva, it produces intense inflammatory reaction [86]. This is consequent upon the initial release of substance P. Cardiovascular studies on blood vessels have shown that both capsaicinoids and capsaicin could inhibit vasoconstriction induced by norepinephrine [17], and the vasodilatation effect of capsaicinoids might be due to the action of capsaicin. The compounds also cause significant decreases in platelet aggregation induced by ADP and collagen and increase blood flow in volunteers. During their study in Thailand, Jaiarj et al. [67] first noticed that people who consume large amounts of red chili peppers experienced a lower incidence of thromboembolism, or potentially dangerous blood clots.

The alternative to the mixed actions of capsaicin is being looked into through the development of purer and more potent capsaicin analogs. Refs. [72, 79, 80, 62] reported significant thermal and mechanical analgesia and antiinflammatory activity following administration of olvanil oleamide, an analog, which lacked the acute toxicity of capsaicin. Nuvanil was found to be more soluble, thus allowing for oral administration, and also showed improved oral activity and significant analgesia [6,87]. The compounds were also found to show less pungency and reduced vagal-mediated blood pressure reflexes [6,79, 80, 83, 87]. In this regard, Lee et al. [88] and Lee and Gauci [27] discussed how acute toxicity of capsaicin can be prevented through structural modification. Moreover, Chen et al. [89] and Hua et al. [90] also reported that orally active capsaicin analog, civamide, showed a significant increase in response latency on the thermal withdrawal test that persisted for 3 days in adult rats.

5. Conclusion

From the synopsis above, it is obvious that capsaicin is a peripheral analgesic, which is cell specific. The opening of capsaicin-operated channels is required for efficacy and agonism. Improvement in the therapeutic window is required before the use of an orally active therapeutic drug. However, topical applications of capsaicin have been shown to be effective without side effect [34, 37]. There is also a growing body of evidence for the role of capsaicin in inflammation, coagulation, and gastro-intestinal function.

Author details

Adebayo Taiwo Ezekiel Jolayemi

Address all correspondence to: adebayoj@hotmail.com

Department of Anaesthetesia & ICU, Goulburn Base Hospital, Australia National University, Golburn City, Australia

References

[1] Bosland P.W. 22 Chilles: history, cultivation, and uses. Amsterdam: Elsevier Science B.V., 1994; 15: 764.

[2] Bosland P.W. Innovative uses of an ancient crop. In: Jannick, J. (ed.). Progress in new crops. ASHS Press, Arlington, 1996; 479–487.

[3] Hayes, A.G., Scadding, J.W., Skingle, M., and Tyers, M.B. Effects of neonatal administration of capsaicin on nociceptive thresholds in the mouse and rat. Journal of Pharmacy and Pharmacology 1981; 33: 183–185.

[4] Winter, J., Woolf, C., and Lynn, B. Degenerative and regenerative responses of sensory neurons to capsaicin-induced damage. In: Wood, J.N. (ed). Capsaicin in the Study of Pain. London: Academic Press 1993; 139–160.

[5] Sorkin, L.S. Basic pharmacology and physiology in acute pain process. Anaesthesiology Clinics of North America 1997; 15(2): 235–245.

[6] Walpole, C.S.J., Wrigglesworth, R., Bevan, S., Cambell, E.A., Dray, A., James, I.F., Perkins, M.N., Reid, D.J., and Winter J. Analogues of capsaicin with agonist activity as novel analgesic agents; structure-activity studies. 1. The amide bond "B-region". Journal of Medicinal Chemistry 1993; 36: 2373–2380.

[7] Miao, F.J., and Levine, J.D. Neural and endocrine mechanisms mediating noxious stimulus-induced inhibition of bradykinin plasma extravasations in the rat. Journal of Pharmacology and Experimental Therapeutics 1999; 291(3): 1028–1037.

[8] Mogil, J.S., Yu, L., and Basbaum, A.I. Pain genes? Natural variation and transgenic mutants. Annual Review of Neuroscience 2000; 23: 777–811.

[9] Sofowora, A. Proteins. In: Sofowora, A. (ed). Medicinal plants and traditional medicine in Africa, 2nd edition, Spectrum Books, Ibadan, Nigeria 1993; 218–220.

[10] Lou, Y.P., Franco-Cereceda, A., and Lundberg, J.M. Different ion channel mechanisms between low concentrations of capsaicin and nicotine regarding peptide release from pulmonary afferents. Acta Physiologica Scandinavica 1992; 146: 119–127.

[11] Olah, Z., Karai, L., and Iadarola, M.J. Anandemide activates vanilloid receptor 1 (VR1) at acidic p^H in dorsal root ganglia neurons and cells ectopically expressing VR1. Journal of Biological Chemistry 2001; 276(33): 31163–31170.

[12] Yang, Y.L., Yao, K.H., Gu, Y.Z., Guan, B.C., and Li, Z.W. Three kinds of current in response to Substance P in bullfrog DRG neurons. Brain Research 2003; 981(1-2): 70–77.

[13] Walpole, C.S.J., Wrigglesworth, R., Bevan, S., Cambell, E.A., Dray, A., James, I.F., Perkins, M.N., Reid, D.J., and Winter J. Analogues of capsaicin with agonist activity as novel analgesic agents; structure-activity studies. 1. The hydrophobic side chain "C-region". Journal of Medicinal Chemistry 1993; 36: 2381–2389.

[14] Chiang, C.Y., Hu, J.W., and Sessle, B.J. NMDA receptor involvement in neuroplastic changes induced by neonatal treatment in trigeminal nociceptive neurons. Journal of Neurophysiology 1997; 78(5): 2799–2803.

[15] Gronroos, M., Reunala, T., Kartamaa, M., and Pertovaara, A. Altered skin sensitivity in chronic itch: Role of peripheral and central mechanisms. Neurosciences Letters 1997; 228 (3): 199–202.

[16] Simone, D.A., Baumann, T.K., and Lamotte, R.H. Late effects of prolonged topical capsaicin on cutaneous sensibility and neurogenic vasodilation in humans. Pain 1989; 38: 99–107.

[17] Kim, K.J., Jeon, B.H., Kim, W.S., Park, K.R., and Choi S. Effect of capsaicin on causalgiform pain in the rat. Korean Journal of Physiology 1992; 26: 143–150.

[18] Szallasi, A., and Blumberg, P.M. Specific binding of resiniferatoxin: An ultrapotent capsaicin analog to dorsal root ganglion membranes. Brain Research 1990; 524: 106–111.

[19] Davis, J.B., Gray, J., Gunthorpe, M.J., Hatcher, J.P., Davey, P.T., Overend, P., Harries, M.H., Latcham, J., Clapham, C., Atkinson, K., Hughes, S.A., Rance, K., Grau, E., Harper,

A.J., Pugh, P.L., Rogers, D.C., Bingham, S., Randall, A., and Sheardown, S.A. Vanilloid receptor-1 is essential for inflammatory thermal hyperalgesia. Nature 2000; 40 (6783): 183–187.

[20] Liu, L., Oortgiesen, M., Li, L., and Simon, S.A. Capsaicin inhibits activation of voltage-gated sodium currents in capsaicin-sensitive trigeminal ganglion neurons. Journal of Neurophysiology 2001; 85(2): 745–758.

[21] Colpaert, F.C., Donnerer, J., and Lembeck, F. Effects of capsaicin in inflammation and on the Substance P content of nervous tissue in rats with adjuvant arthritis. Life Sciences 1983; 32: 1827–1834.

[22] Vasko, M.R. Prostagladin-induced neuropeptide release from spinal cord. Progress in Brain Research 1995; 104: 367–380.

[23] Roza, C., and Reeh, P.W. Substance P, calcitonin gene-related peptide and PGE2 co-released from the mouse colon: A new model to study nociceptive and inflammatory responses in viscera, in vitro. Pain 2001; 93(3): 213–219.

[24] Santicioli, P., Del Bianco, E., Geppetti, P., and Maggi, C.A. Release of calcitonin gene-related peptide-like (CRGP-LI) immunoreactivity from rat isolated isoleus muscle by low p^H, capsaicin and potassium. Neuroscience Letters 1992; 143: 19–22.

[25] Leibosohn, E. Treatment of nostalgia paresthetica with capsaicin. CUTIS 1992; 49: 335–336.

[26] Hajos, M., Svensson, K., Nissbrandt, H., Obal, F. Jr, and Carlsson, A. Effects of capsaicin on central monoaminergic mechanisms in the rat. Journal of Neural Transmission 1986; 66 (3-4): 221–242.

[27] Lee, J.J., and Gauci, C.A. Postherapeutic neuralgia: Current concepts and management. British Journal of Hospital Medicine 1994; 52 (11): 565–570.

[28] http://www.alternative-medicines.com/herbdesc/1capsicu.htm, Capsicum. In: Capsicum-Red Hot Chili Peppers 2002.

[29] Nakamura, A., and Shiomi, H. Recent advances in neuropharmacology of cutaneous nociceptors. Japan Journal of Pharmacology 1999; 79(4): 427–431.

[30] Robertson, B., Docherty, R.J., and Bevan S. Capsaicin inhibits voltage-activated calcium currents in a sub-population of adult rat dorsal root ganglion neurons. Society for Neurosciences Abstracts 1989; 15: 354.

[31] Sicuteri, F., Fusco, B.M., Marabini, S., Caimpagnolo, V., Maggi, C.A., Geppett, P., and Fanciullaci, M. Beneficial effect of capsaicin application to the nasal mucosa in cluster headache. Clinical Journal of Pain 1989; 5: 49–53.

[32] Wallace, M.S. Advances in pain research. Anaesthesiology Clinics of North America 1997; 15(2): 229–234.

[33] Dini, D., Bertelli, G., Gozza, A., and Forno, G.G. Treatment of post-mastectomy pain syndrome with topical capsaicin. Pain 1993; 4: 223–226.

[34] Kinnmann, E., Nygards, E.B., and Hansson, P. Peripheral alpha-adrenoreceptors are involved in the development of capsaicin induced on-going and stimulus evoked pain in humans. Pain 1997; 69 (1-2): 79–85.

[35] Simone, D.A., and Ochoa, J. Early and late effects of prolonged topical capsaicin on cutaneous sensibility and neurogenic vasodilatation in humans. Pain 1991; 47: 285–294.

[36] Caterina, M.J., Schumacher, M.A., Tominaga, M., Rosen, T.A., Levine, J.D., and Julius, D. The capsaicin receptor: A heat-activated ion channel in the pain pathway. Nature 1997; 389 (6653): 783–784.

[37] Caterina, M.J., and Julius, D. The vanilloid receptor: A molecular gateway to the pain pathway. Annual Review of Neuroscience 2001; 24: 487–517.

[38] Cesare, P., Moriondo, A., Vellani, V., and McNaughton, P.A. Ion channels gated by heat. Procedure of National Academy of Sciences of United States of America. 1999; 96 (14): 7658–7663.

[39] Chaudhary, P., Martenson, M.E., and Baumann, T.K. Vanilloid receptor expression and Capsaicin excitation of rat dental primary afferent neurons. Journal of Dental Research 2001; 80 (6): 1518–1523.

[40] McMahon, S.B., Lewin, G., and Bloom, S.R. The consequences of long-term topical capsaicin application in the rat. Pain 1991; 44: 301–310.

[41] Cervero, F., and McRitchie, H.A. Effect of neonatal administration of capsaicin in several nociceptive systems of the rat. In: Bonica, J.J., Liebeskind, J.C., and Albe-Fessard, D.G. (eds), Advances in Pain Research and Therapy. New York: Raven Press; 1997; 4: 87–94.

[42] Peikert, A., Henrich, M., and Ochs, G. Topical 0.025% capsaicin in chronic post-herpeutic neuralgia: Efficacy, predictors of response and long-term course. Journal of Neurology 1991; 238: 452–456.

[43] Rang, H.P., and Urban, L. New molecules in analgesia. British Journal of Anaesthesia 1995; 75: 145–156.

[44] Gamse, R. Capsaicin and nociception in the rat and mouse. Possible role of Substance P. Naunyn-Schmiedeberg's Archive of Pharmacology 1982; 320: 205–216.

[45] Vriens, J., Appendino, G., and Owsiank, G, Pharmacology of vanilloid transient receptor potential cation channels. Molecular Pharmacology 2009; 75 (6): 1262–1279.

[46] Carpenter, S.E., and Lynn, B. Vascular and sensory responses of human skin to mild injury after topical treatment with capsaicin. British Journal of Pharmacology 1981; 73: 755–758.

[47] Dray, A., Bettany, J., and Forster P. Actions of capsaicin on peripheral nociceptors of the neonatal rat spinal cord-tail in vitro: Dependence of extracellular ions and independence of second messengers. British Journal of Pharmacology 1990; 101: 727–733.

[48] Deal, C.L., Schnitzer, T.J., Lipstein, E., Seibold, J.R., Stevens, R.M., Levy, M.D., Albert, D., and Renold, F. Treatment of arthritis with topical capsaicin: A double-blind trial. Clinical Therapeutics 1991; 13: 383–395.

[49] McCarty, D.J., Csuka, M., McCarthy, G., and Trotter, D. Treatment of pain due to fibromyalgia with topical capsaicin: a pilot study. Seminars in Arthritis and Rheumatism 1994; 23 (Suppl 3): 41–47.

[50] Weisman, M.H., Hagaman, C., Yaksh, T.L., and Lotz, M. Preliminary findings in the role of neuropeptides suppression by topical agents in the management of rheumatoid arthritis. Seminars in Arthritis and Rheumatism 1994; 23 (suppl 3): 18–24.

[51] McCleskey, E.W., and Gold, M.S. Ion channels of nociception. Annual Review of Physiology 1996; 61: 835–856.

[52] Wood, J.N., Coote, P.R., Minhas, A., Mullaney, I., McNeill, M., and Burgess, G.M. Capsaicin-induced ion fluxes increase cyclic GMP but not cyclic AMP levels in rat sensory neurons in culture. Journal of Neurochemistry 1989; 53: 1203–1211.

[53] Watson, C.P.N., Evans, R.J., and Watt, V.R. The post-mastectomy pain syndrome and the effect of topical capsaicin. Pain 1989; 38: 177–186.

[54] Baron, R., Wasner, G., and Lindner, V. Optimal treatment for phantom limb pain in the elderly. Drugs and Aging 1998; 12(5): 361–376.

[55] Berring, P., Arendt-Nielsen, I., and Soderberg, U. Argon laser induced cutaneous sensory and pain thresholds in post-herpeutic neuralgia. Quantitative modulation by topical capsaicin. Acta Dermatology Venerology 1990; 70: 121–125.

[56] Woolf, C.J., Bennett, G.J., Doherty, M., Dubner, R., Kidd, B., Koltzenburg, M., Lipton, R., Loeser, J.D., Payne, R., and Torcbjork, E. Towards a mechanism-based classification of pain? Pain 1989; 77: 227–229.

[57] Kroll, F., Karlsson, J.A., Lundberg, J.M., and Persson, C.G. Capsaicin-induced bronchoconstriction and neuropeptide release in guinea-pig perfused lungs. Journal of Applied Physiology 1990; 68: 1679–1687.

[58] Perkins MN and Campbell EA. Capsezepine reversal of the antinociceptive action of capsaicin in vivo. British Journal of Pharmacology. 1992; 107 (2): 329–333.

[59] Petersen, K.L., and Rowbotham, M.C. A new human experimental pain model: The heat/capsaicin sensitization model. Neuroreport 1999; 10(7): 1511–1516.

[60] Leis, S., Weber, M., Isselmann, A., Schmelz, M., and Birklein, F. Substance P-induced protein extravasation is bilaterally increased in complex regional pain syndrome. Experimental Neurology 2003; 183 (1): 197–204.

[61] Campbell, E.A., Bevan, S., and Dray, A. Clinical applications of capsaicin and its analogues. In: Wood, J.N. (ed). Capsaicin in the Study of Pain. London Academic Press 1993; 255–272.

[62] McCarthy, G.M. and McCarthy, D.J. Effect of topical capsaicin in the painful osteoarthritis of the hands. Journal of Rheumatology 1992; 19: 604-607.

[63] Watt, J.M., and Breyer-Brandwijk, M.G. The medicinal and poisonous plants of Southern and East Africa. 1962; 862–942.

[64] Sinoff, S.E., and Hart, M.B. Topical capsaicin and burning pain. Clinical Journal of Pain 1993; 9: 70–73.

[65] Capsaicin Study Group. Treatment of painful diabetic neuropathy with topical capsaicin. A multi-centre, double blind, vehicle-controlled study. Archives of Internal Medicine 1999; 151: 2225–2229.

[66] Koppert, W., Ostermeier, N., Sittl, R., Weidner, C., and Schmelz, M. Low-dose lidocaine reduces secondary hyperalgesia by a central mode of action. Pain 2000; 85(1): 217–224.

[67] Jaiarj, P., Saichompoo, S., Wongkrajang, Y., Vongswan, N., Peungvicha, P., and Jiratchariyakul, W. Cardiovascular actions of capsaicinoids extract from Thai capsicum. Thai Journal of Phytopharmacy 1998; 5(2): 1–13.

[68] Docherty, R.J., Robertson, B., and Bevan, S. Capsaicin causes prolonged inhibition of voltage-activated calcium currents in adult rat dorsal root ganglion neurons in culture. Neuroscience 1991; 40: 513–521.

[69] Goodless, D.R., and Eaglstein, W.H. Brachioradial pruritus: Treatment with topical capsaicin. Journal of the American Academy of Dermatology 1993; 29: 783–784.

[70] Abdala, A.P., Haibara, A.S., and Colombari, E. Cardiovascular responses to Substance P in the nucleus tractus solitarii: Microinjection study in conscious rats. American Journal of Physiology of Heart and Circulation Physiology 2003; 285(2): 891–898.

[71] Levin, J.D., Clarke, R., Devor, M., Helms, M.A., Moskpwitz, M.A., and Basbaum, A.I. Intraneuronal Substance P contributes to the severity of experimental arthritis. Science 1984; 226: 547–549.

[72] Brand, L.L., Berman, E., Schwen, R., Loomans, M., Janusz, J., Bonne, R., Maddin, C., Gardner, J., LaHamn, T., Farmer, R., Jones, L., Chiaabrando, C., and Fanelli, R. NE-19950: A novel, orally active anti-inflammatory analgesic. Drugs in Experimental and Clinical Research 1987; 13: 259–265.

[73] Faulkner, D.C., and Growcott, J.W. Effects of neonatal capsaicin administration on the nociceptive response of the rat to mechanical and chemical stimuli. Journal of Pharmacy and Pharmacology 1980; 32: 657–658.

[74] Shir, Y., and Seltzer, Z. A-fibers mediate thermal mechanical hyperesthesia and allodynia and C-fibers mediate thermal hyperalgesia in a new model of causalgiform pain disorders in rats. Neuroscience Letters 1990; 115: 62–67.

[75] Maggi, C.A., Patacchini, R., Santiciolli, P., Giuliani, S., Delbianco, F., Geppetti, P., and Meli, A. Protective action of ruthenium red toward capsaicin desensitization of sensory fibers. Neuroscience Letters 1988; 88: 201–205.

[76] Menkes, C.J., Renoux, M., Loussadi, S., Mauborgne, A., Bruxelle, J., and Cesselin, F. Substance P (SP) levels in synovial tissue and synovial fluid from rheumatoid arthritis (RA) and osteoarthritis (OA) patients. Journal of Rheumatology 1993; 20: 714–717.

[77] Jensen, P.G., and Larson, J.R. Management of painful diabetic neuropathy. Drugs 2001; 18(10): 737–749.

[78] Kowalski, M.L., Dietrich-Milobedzi, A., Majkowska-Wojciechowska, B., and Jarzebska, M. Nasal reactivity to capsaicin in patients with seasonal allergic rhinitis during and after the pollen season. Allergy 1999; 54 (8): 804–810.

[79] Brand, L.M., Skare, K.L., Loomans, M.E., Reller, H.H., Schwen, R.J., Lade, D.A., Bohne, R.L., Maddin, C.S., Moorehead, D.P., Fanelli, R., Chiabrando, C., Castelli, M.G., and Tai, H.H. Anti-inflammatory pharmacology and mechanism of the orally active capsaicin analogs, NE-19950 and NE-28345. Agents and Clinical Research 1990; 31: 329–340.

[80] Breneman, D.L., Cardone, J.S., Blumack, R.F., Lather, R.M., Searle, E.A., and Pollack, V.E. Topical capsaicin treatment of hemodialysis-related pruritus. Journal of the American Academy of Dermatology 1992; 26: 91–94.

[81] Yakish, T.L. Spinal systems and pain processing: Development of novel analgesic drugs with mechanistically defined models. Trends in Pharmacological Science 1999; 20: 329–337.

[82] Yeats, J.C., Boddeke, H.W., and Docherty, R.J. Calcium dependent and independent desensitization in rat dorsal root ganglion neurons is due to activation of calcineurin. British Journal of Pharmacology 1992; 107: 238P.

[83] Johanek, L.M., Heitmiller, D.R., Turner, M., Nader, N., Hodges, J., and Simone, D.A. Cannabinoids attenuate capsaicin-evoked hyperalgesia through spinal and peripheral mechanisms. Pain 2001; 93(3): 303–315.

[84] Knight, T.E., and Hayashi, T. Solar (brachioradial pruritus)-response to capsaicin cream. International Journal of Dermatology 1994; 33: 206–209.

[85] Jancso, G.K., and Jancso-Gabor, A. Pharmacologically induced selective degeneration of chemo-sensitive primary sensory neurons. Nature 1977; 270: 741–743.

[86] The phytochemical collection, 2002 In molecular expressions: The phytochemical collection. http://micro.magnet.fsu.edu/phytochemicals/index.html

[87] Watson, C.P.N. Evans, R.J. and Watt, V.R. The post-mastectomy pain syndrome and the effect of topical capsaicin. 1989 Pain; 38: 177-186.

[88] Lee, S.S., Sohn, Y.W., Yoo, E.S., and Kim, K.H. Neurotoxicity and long lasting analgesia induced by capsacinoids. Journal of Toxicology Science 1991; 1: 3–20.

[89] Chen, I.J., Yang, J.M., Yeh, J.L., Wu, B.N., Lo, Y.C., and Chen, S.J. Hypotensive and antinociceptive effects of ether-linked and relatively non-pungent analogues of N-nonanoyl nanillylamide. European Journal of Medicinal Chemistry 1992; 27: 187–192.

[90] Hua, X.Y., Chen, P., Hwang, J., and Yaksh, T.L. Antinociception induced by civamide: An orally active capsaicin analogue. Pain 1997; 71(3): 313–322.

4

Education for Sustainable Development

Busisiwe Ndawonde, Sitwala Namwinji Imenda and

Humbulani Nancy Mutshaeni

Abstract

This chapter focuses on Education for Sustainable Development (ESD) for communities selling medicinal plants in northern KwaZulu-Natal, South Africa. The purpose is to equip the participating medicinal plant sellers with knowledge and skills related to the trade of medicinal plants. In particular, the study focuses on cultivating the participants' awareness of the importance of conducting their business based on principles of conservation, sustainable livelihoods and environmental sustainability. The study followed a case study design within a mixed methods research paradigm. Data collection involved the use of face-to-face questionnaire administration and follow-up focused group interviews. Phase 1 results revealed a number of challenges faced by the medicinal plant sellers. These included processing, storage and packaging, lack of business skills and the conservation of medicinal plants and their products. Following a capacity building intervention based on ESD and non-formal education principles, phase II results showed that the medicinal plant sellers had revised some of their business practices–such as pricing techniques and record keeping. However, processing of medicinal plant materials, storage, packaging and conservation remained a challenge that needed further attention. In particular, sustainable harvesting practices and cultivation of medicinal plants in home gardens still presented some difficulties.

Keywords: sustainability, indigenous knowledge, medicinal plants, storage, conservation, marketing and packaging

1. Introduction and background to the study

1.1. Introduction

This study is a multidisciplinary research involving various stakeholders various stakeholders. The stakeholders were, among others, medicinal plant sellers, author(s) (as the researcher) and nature reserve owners (where medicinal plant species are conserved).

In discussing IK [1], state that traditional indigenous knowledge developed through a close connectedness with the physical and social environment that people used to enjoy. Wolfensohn, (President of the World Bank) noted that, "Part of any society's past and cultural values are its Indigenous Knowledge where, as human beings, we are expected to learn from in order to enhance developmental issues." This way, knowledge transfer within and among communities creates an enabling environment for people to deal with social, political and economic issues that affect their lives.

Echoing the above, the ESD explains indigenous knowledge as, "An endless process of learning that produces creative thinking individuals who are able to scientifically tackle problems to the benefit of society, hence ensuring a fruitful and sustainable environmental future." [2] concurs with [1] in acknowledging that ESD prepares individual for ecologically sustainable future. It also empowers them on restoring the earth's natural resources, hence fosters support for the well-being of future generations by promoting sustainable lifestyles.

In this context, the concept of ESD is used to explore the sustainable development of medicinal plant sellers in light of the plants they sell. The idea is to conserve the indigenous medicinal plant species before they become extinct. Medicinal plant sellers were targeted because they are part of the medicinal plant market chain. By virtue of their trade, medicinal plant entrepreneurs harvest many plant species for their business. The following section is the background to the study.

Contained in this chapter is the section that deals with this study's background, followed by the rationale for the study, study objectives and method of investigation. The last section discusses the study's results, interpretation and discussion. Finally, the chapter concludes by highlighting significant issues that emerged from the results.

1.2. Background to the study

The findings reported here are based on an earlier case study on medicinal plant sellers concerning the types, uses, quantities, prices charged and conservation nature of medicinal plants [3]. The case study revealed, inter alia, that medicinal plants are harvested by medicinal plant sellers without any thought of conservation on their part, thereby threatening the long-term survival of the selected plant species. The following species (**Table 1**) were found to require urgent conservation if they were to survive uncontrolled harvesting. Worse still, literature identified these species as being at high risk due to over-harvesting [4-7].

The conservation status of the medicinal plants listed in **Table 1** was compared for authenticity using the scientific sources of Red Data Records [4]. It was observed that over time, there is danger that not all the 13 species may survive the current harvesting onslaught. For instance, medicinal plant species such as *Bauhinia bowker*, *Ocotea bullata* and *Warbugia salutaris* whose barks are harvested, take too long to mature, hence threat to their prolonged survival. For this study, the species mentioned were not propagated due to time constraint.

Family names	Scientific names	Zulu names	Conservation Status	Part used
Apiaceae	*Alepidia amatymbica* Ackl.& Zeyh.	i-Khathazo	Vulnerable	Root
Orchidaceae	*Ansellia africana* Lindl.	i-Mfeyenkawu	Vulnerable	Whole tree
Fabaceae	*Bauhinia bowkeri* Harv.	u-Mdlandlovu	Rare	Bark
Hycinthaceae	*Boweia volubilis* Harv.ex Hook.f.	u-Gibisila	Endangered	Bulb/tuber
	Merwilla plumbea (Lindl.) Speta	i-Nguduza	Vulnerable	Bulb
	Eucomis autumnalis(Mill.) Chitt.	u-Mathunga	Vulnerable	Tuber
Asphodelaceae	*Bulbine frutescens*(L.) Wild.	i-Bhucu	Endangered	Leaves
Zamiaceae	*Encephalartos natalensis* R. A. Dyer & I. Verd	i-Sigqiki somkhovu	Rare	Tuber
	Encephalartos villosus Lem	i-Mfingo	Rare	Root
Apolynaceae	*Haworthia limifolia N. E. Br.*	u-Mathithibala	Vulnerable	Whole plant
Apocynaceae	*Mondia whitei* (Hoof.f.) Skeels.	u-Mondi	Vulnerable	Root
Hypoxidaceae	*Ocotea bullata* (Burch.) Bill.	u-Nukani	Vulnerabled	Barks
Canellaceae	*Warbugia salutari* (G.Bertol.) Chiov.	i-Sibhaha	Critical endangered	Bark, stem, roots and leaves

Adopted with permission from Ref. [6].

Table 1. Priority species for conservation.

1.3. Rationale for the study

The rationale for this study was to identify ways by which medicinal plant sellers would conserve medicinal plant species since they are major stake holders in the medicinal plant selling business. Having realised that medicinal plant sellers harvested plant species in an unsustainable manner, it became necessary to bring to their attention the need to harvest plants in a sustainable manner. This involved various methods on plant conservation that ensured continued availability and future use of the said species. Thus, the study introduced the concept of sustainability, a concept described as a wise use of resources (medicinal plant species) for future generations [8]. Principles of sustainability include the recognition that the needs of future generations are not compromised as we seek to meet current demands. It was necessary for the author(s) to engage medicinal plant sellers to share ideas on how to sustain medicinal plant species that are dwindling. This was sought to be achieved by the following objectives:

1.4. Objectives of the study

The study's objectives were

- To establish challenges faced by medicinal plant sellers in their medicinal plant selling businesses.
- To identify the quantities of medicinal plants sold in northern KwaZulu-Natal.
- To establish the key role players in the medicinal plant selling businesses.
- To share information on scientific and indigenous methods of propagating medicinal plants during the intervention programme.
- To assess the effectiveness of the intervention.

1.5. Research methods

This study involved a survey and case study concerning medicinal plant sellers in northern KwaZulu-Natal, South Africa. The study was conducted in the Province's three biggest district municipalities namely, uThungulu, Zululand and uMkhanyakude. For the Zululand district municipality, the study locale was the Mona market in the Nongoma area. Mona market is the largest market in northern KwaZulu-Natal, and it operates once a month. At uThungulu, the survey took place in Richards Bay and Empangeni town markets. Mtubatuba town and uMhlabuyalingana were the research areas in uMkhanyakude District Municipality.

1.5.1. Population and sampling

The research targeted informal medicinal plant sellers. Medicinal plant sellers were targeted because they harvest and stock large quantities of traditional medicine for trade purposes. This is over and above what is harvested by traditional healers for healing purposes, although the later sometimes buy such products from the former. A sample of 56 medicinal plant sellers participated in the study, selected through purposive/judgmental sampling. Kumar [9] stated the major aspect for purposive sampling as enabling one to come up with suitable data so as to meet the research's purpose. Accordingly, one has to deal with prospective interviewees with regard to data for his/her study. Thus, the study's participants were purposively selected through informal household interviews with individuals who identified those with knowledge of medicinal plants, their willingness to share information and their experiences in selling medicinal plants. Participants also included those who volunteered to participate in the study within the confines of their medicinal plant shops. Other participants were the local authority employees from whom permission to conduct household interviews and field surveys were requested and subsequently granted.

1.5.2. The data collection process

ESD emphasises that people should enjoy their natural resources while not compromising future generational needs. In this study, the ESD programme served as a capacity-building intervention strategy, and it involved establishing trust between the researcher and community members who were medicinal plant sellers. The purpose was to address the issue of environmental awareness, conservation, marketing and storage of medicinal plant stocks. These aspects emerged as medicinal plant selling business's challenges that required attention. In addition the researcher roped in an expert resource person from the university to facilitate on economic and business management issues. Apart from the university-based resource persons and the community members, other stakeholders were the owners of the nature reserve (husband and wife) where the workshop was held. These two became resource persons during the workshop.

The first stage in data collection was preliminary research in public markets to identify resource persons for the study. Here, the researcher explained the purpose of the research. Subsequently, appointments were made with prospective participants for data collection. Market areas were chosen as initial sites for contacts. These provided important initial information about the medicinal plant sellers. Interviewing people at their business sites presented minor challenges such as possible interference from other respondents wanting to have an input where it was not required, in addition to direct interference with the flow of their business. In light of this, it became imperative to arrange for interviews at the participants' homes.

Interviews were followed by focus group discussions involving selected medicinal plant sellers from each market. This was to elicit, among other issues, challenges faced by the participants for which they needed capacitation. It is asserted by Borgatti [10] that focus group interviewing is particularly suited for obtaining several perspectives about the topic including gaining insights into people's shared experiences of daily life on the topic under discussion. The main purpose of focus group discussions in this study was to evaluate respondents' attitudes, feelings, beliefs, experiences and reactions concerning challenges they faced on daily basis in their business.

Furthermore, grey interview areas that needed further elucidation were followed up during the focus group discussions. There was one focus group per sampling site consisting of five individuals, except for the uMhlathuze Municipality which was represented by two members. These were the only medicinal plant sellers at that site. Altogether 12 people participated in the focus group discussions. The focus group discussions were audiotaped, transcribed, coded and analysed.

1.5.3. Nursery experiments

The experiments were conducted on vegetative propagation of the species highlighted in **Table 1**. The aim of doing these experiments was to replicate seedlings to supply to medicinal plant sellers. Vegetative propagation was chosen over sexual propagation in this regard since it yielded more seedlings at a faster rate than propagation of medicinal plants through seeds. The method of vegetative propagation and the plants appearances after propagation was demonstrated to medicinal plant sellers. As stated earlier, not all medicinal plant species were propagated due to time limit. These included species such as *Ansellia africana, Haworthia limofolia* and *Boweia volubilis.*

Another purpose for conducting experiments was to determine whether medicinal plants germinate in different environmental conditions, for example, temperature, growth substrate, water requirements and light intensity. The experiments were done without adding plant species seedlings with growth stimulants. That was so the medicinal plant sellers could conduct similar experiments without having to add fertilizers and hormones to plant seedlings at home. The plants were watered in the morning, once a day till their growth stabilised. All the experiments were conducted in a nursery. The detailed experimental procedure for the three plant species are given below.

1.5.4. Propagation of Ansellia africana Lindl.: Orchidaceae

The stems of the plant were marked at the base and strapped to the fork of a tree. Similarly, a semi-shaded deadwood trellis could be made to hold a number of plants in accessible positions. Vegetative propagation of *A. africana* was done by Zobolo et al. [11] using the stem cuttings. The aim of the experiments was to determine the effect of growth medium, that is, cow dung manure and river sand at the average temperature of 28°C. Sexual production of the plant species was conducted by Diederichs et al. [12]. The results of the experiments shown in this chapter were conducted by Ndawonde and Imenda [13] using river sand. It was found that river sand is a suitable medium for the plant species since it drains easily and this removes water logging, thereby allowing the plant to absorb water easily.

1.5.5. Propagation of Harworthia limifolia Harv.ex Hook.f.: Hycinthaceae

To plant *H. limifolia,* one has to cut offshoots from the stem and plant them separately. Roots would then develop from the part of the piece dug into the ground. A week later, roots also form from the upper part of the pieces, a sign that the cuts are stabilising. The adjustment would then lead to the expected growth of shoots after a month or so, but strictly under conditions from 23 to 30°C [12]. During experimentation, the top and bottom cuts were placed in river sand at the temperature range stated above.

1.5.6. Propagation of Boweia volubilis N. E. Br.: Apolynaceae

Bulb scales were broken off from large bulbs at the end of the growing season (that is, autumn or winter) and inserted upright into sand. Bulbs formed along the base were transplanted when large enough to handle.

Propagation through tubers was done by making two equal halves of the tubers, and then digging them into river sand. After a period of 2–3 weeks, the halves developed roots and become established.

2. The intervention

The Eurostat Adult Education Survey distinguishes four categories of non-formal education, namely classroom learning, distance learning, seminars and workshops and guided on-the-job training [14]. Practically, one finds a continuous interplay among formal, non-formal and informal education. As such, it is common to see non-formal and informal education dovetail in educational settings that are established to provide formal education. Certainly, within the notion of life-long learning, one has to be prepared to see continued interplays among these forms of learning. In this study, the dominant mode of non-formal education followed was a combination of seminar and workshop. Thus, the intervention was designed to address the challenges that emerged from the interviews and focus group discussions. Specifically, the workshop addressed conservation and marketing of medicinal plants, among other related issues.

Although the medicinal plant selling business is dominated by older women with minimal formal schooling [13], medicinal plant sellers were introduced to the concepts of balance sheet, record keeping and issues pertaining to banking. An accounting and business studies expert was invited to share with medicinal plant sellers viable business skills in terms of book keeping, marketing and pricing of their wares. As a scientist, the researcher handled issues of storage and conservation. Together with the nature reserve management team, they demonstrated how selected medicinal plant species could be properly cultivated and nurtured in order to capacitate the participants so that they could grow their own stock in their home gardens. The main purpose of conducting the demonstrations was to share with the participants' information on different environmental conditions under which different medicinal plants germinated and, therefore, how they could be cultivated. The demonstrations were carried out without any use of any growth stimulants. This way, it was envisaged that there would be an added desired outcome of creating space for social transformation among the plant selling communities, with the aim of taking them to a higher level of social responsibility.

This was done at a natural plant nursery chosen for its production of several plants regarded as now extinct due to over-harvesting in KwaZulu-Natal. The nature reserve was centrally located amongst the research sites. Its owners were part of resource persons who served as workshop facilitators. They understood and spoke iSiZulu, hence were able to communicate easily in participants' home language. The nature reserve owners facilitated on how to cultivate medicinal plant species. Discussions were carried out during the workshop, following various presentations in order to clarify issues raised during presentations and allow for the sharing of experiences and ideas.

3. Data analysis

Qualitative data involving the workshop results were analysed following qualitative methods of data analysis. Braun and Clarke [15] said qualitative analytic methods can be roughly divided into two camps: (a) those that are based on a particular theoretical or epistemological position and (b) those that "are essentially independent of theory and epistemology, and can be applied across a range of theoretical and epistemological approaches." Under the first category, for example, see Ref. [15] where conversation analysis and interpretative phenomenological analysis (which allow relatively limited variability in how the approach is applied within that framework) are placed.

4. Assessment of the intervention

The usefulness and effectiveness of the intervention was assessed through home visits by means of open-ended interviews, two months after the workshop (phase 1). The assessment focused on the areas directly addressed in the workshop, namely medicinal plant storage, marketing, sales and conservation. Assessment was done in phases so as to obtain near perfect results through constant monitoring.

5. Results

The results presented here are in line with the objectives of the chapter.

5.1. Challenges of the medicinal plant selling businesses

The study revealed that medicinal plant sellers were involved in the informal trade in traditional medicines. These results confirm findings by Botha et al. [16]. His/her findings were to the effect that traditional medicine vendors in South Africa traded under a shoe-string budget. Theirs was a case of surviving from hand to mouth, hence their failure to save enough to expand their vending ventures. In short, their income was spent on household needs.

This ESD study showed that the system of determining price units charged for the medicinal plants was determined by market leaders where medicinal plant sellers had shops. Neither banking nor record keeping of income versus expenditure was found to be commonly practised among medicinal plant sellers in this study. To further compound traditional medicine vendors' woes, they do not keep records of their business dealings, hence cannot keep track of the business trend as should be the norm.

In addition, their business is affected by their lack of knowledge in terms of proper tree harvesting. That is, traditional medicine plant sellers' methods of harvesting do not serve plants. Instead, their harvesting methods destroy the same plants they would need tomorrow to sustain their business. Positively, the medicinal plant sellers applauded the move to provide them with licences that would enable them to harvest their products in an environmentally acceptable manner.

The following subsection shows the quantities of medicinal plants sold at Mona Market, a wholesale of medicinal plants in northern KwaZulu-Natal.

The medicinal plant species in **Table 2** were also used in the Mona area. The wholesale has a variety of medicinal plant species, of which *Hypoxis hemerocallidae* was in highest demand (86–100%)

in all stalls. Although the plant cannot cure HIV/AIDS-related illnesses, it is believed to alleviate their symptoms [17]. Medicinal plant sellers were requested to reflect on this.

If transportation fee, time, work effort (in chopping up the plant material) and the risk of collecting plants in the fields is considered, a maximum price of R140.00 (14 dollars) per 50 kg reused maize bag would not be profitable enough to sustain the business.

Scientific name	Part used	Sub-sample (g)	Price (R)	25-kg and 50-kg size maize bags	Price (R)	Dollars
Acorus calamus	Rhizomes	207.09	5.00	25	60.00	6
Acridocarpus natalitus	Leaves	694.62	5.00	50	120.00	12
Aptenia cordifolia	Bark	65.72	5.00	25	30.00	3
Callilepis laureola	Bark	295.27	5.00	50	100.00	10
Calodendrum capense	Bark	235.52	5.00	25	60.00	6
Capparis tementosa	Bark	127.79	5.00	25	40.00	4
Chlorophytum modestum	Roots	562.40	5.00	25	50.00	5
Cliva minnata	Whole plant	194.49	5.00	50	70.00	7
Conia capensis	Whole plant	146.21	5.00	50	100.00	10
Drimia robusta	Bulb	207.09	5.00	25	60.00	6
Erythrophyleum lasianthum	Roots	350.94	5.00	50	100.00	10
Hypoxis hermellocallidae	Bulb	694.62	5.00	50	120.00	12
Mondia whitei	Bark/roots	14.10	5.00	50	140.00	14
Ocotea bullata	Bark	296.27	5.00	50	70.00	07
Olinia radifolia	Roots	146.11	5.00	50	80.00	8
Sarcophyte sanguinea	Roots	282.07	5.00	50	140.00	14
Urginea sanguinea	Roots	138.08	5.00	50	70.00	7

Table 2. Quantities of certain herbal medicines sold in Nongoma (Mona bulk sale), Northern KwaZulu-Natal region and, income generated by traders in standard 25-kg and 50-kg reused maize meal bags.

5.2. Role players in marketing and trade of medicinal plants in northern KwaZulu-Natal

There are no proper marketing strategies in place for medicinal plant sellers, be it national or worldwide. As a result any assessment of their customer base is hampered, inter alia, by demographic variances, different demands for different plants and the issue of those who do wholesale trade of medicinal plants (those responsible for the harvest when given orders). **Figure 1** provides an overview of the marketing chain of the plants harvested in KwaZulu-Natal.

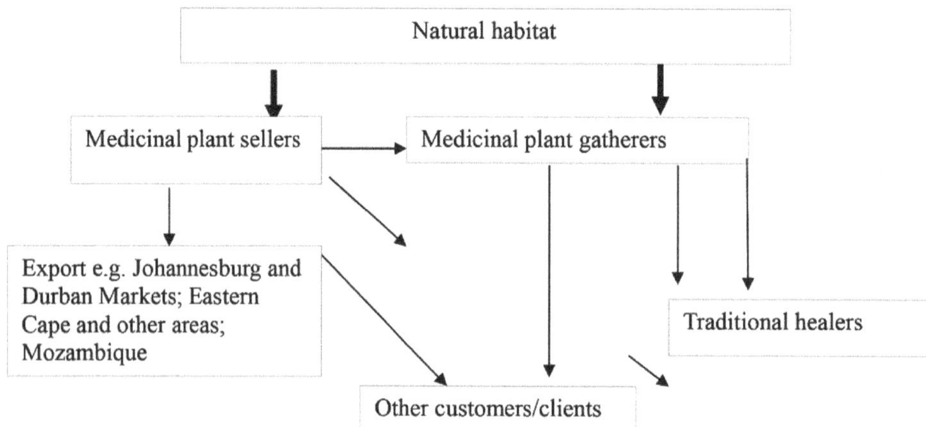

Figure 1. Marketing chain for medicinal plants harvested in Northern KwaZulu-Natal.

Figure 1 indicates a situation where prominent people in the medicinal plant business are wholesalers and retailers. But the majority are retailers as they also do plant harvesting as well.

The complicated market structure and inconsistences in prices charged for medicinal plants was seen as not viable for medicinal plant selling business. For this reason, an ESD in communities that harvest plant species was proposed. The idea was to empower medicinal plant sellers with skills for conservational cultivation of medicinal plants on their own. The following section shows plant propagation by authors and the results thereof. There was information sharing among authors, medicinal plant sellers and nature reserve owners about growth experiments of certain medicinal plants.

5.3. Information sharing during the intervention programme

The workshop started by demonstrating on how medicinal plants are propagated following scientific and indigenous methods.

The results from nursery experiments were demonstrated to the medicinal plant sellers during the workshop. The demonstrations began with the propagation of *A. africana.*

5.4. *Ansellia africana* Lindl.: Orchidaceae

The results showed that *A. africana* was able to strive in temperatures of 27–28°C in river sand. The following diagrams show the shoot formation of *A. africana* during experimentation.

5.5. Propagation of *Ansellia africana* using indigenous methods

Medicinal plant sellers reported that they propagated the plant species by attaching it to trees using cow dung. The same applied to the nature reserve.

For these indigenous ways of propagation, the time the plant takes to regenerate was not recorded by the propagators. The duration the plants take to grow, therefore, is not going to be reported on here.

When sharing information on vegetative production of *A. africana,* both the nature reserve manager and medicinal plant sellers wanted to try out propagation of the plant species in sand. The workshop participants confirmed that they did not know that *A. africana* could be propagated through cuttings and using sand as a growth medium. It was agreed that the issue of time the species take to form the shoots is important to consider. When using a traditional method, the success growth rate is 80%. It was reported, however, that the regeneration period is about 6–8 months. The second demonstration was on vegetative propagation of *H. limifolia.*

5.6. *Haworthia limifolia* Harv.ex Hook.f.: Hycinthaceae

It was interesting to note that the top cuttings developed roots seven days after the start of the propagation period. The cuttings at the bottom stimulated the growth of shoots. After a month, the plants appeared as shown below.

The medicinal plant sellers reported that they grew the medicinal plant species in old three-legged pots where the plants continued replicating themselves. They reported that they had not thought of propagating *H. limifolia* through cuttings. They said they grew the whole branch of the species and put it on top of their huts or on kraal poles. It was explained to them that it is possible to grow the plant species through cuttings. Participants were advised that the decision to propagate the species without the growth stimulants while exposing the other set of the experiments to the sun was done to get a cost-free propagation method. This could be easily done by medicinal plant sellers in their homes.

5.7. *Boweia volubilis* N. E. Br.: Apolynaceae

Results of vegetative propagation of *B. volubilis* were demonstrated to the medicinal plant sellers as well. Further, medicinal plant sellers were assisted on how to grow medicinal plants. This included the types of soil suitable for specific plant species and how to care for shoots. In addition, bookkeeping and banking strategies for small businesses such as medicinal plant selling were shared with them. At the end, participants were encouraged to adopt and adapt these to suit their specific business needs and requirements.

The sellers were made aware of how to calculate the unit prices of their medicinal plants. The facilitators presented the issue of considering labour, transportation, time spent and marketing of the products, as contributing towards pricing their commodities.

5.8. Assessment of the intervention programme

Phase I assessment results revealed a number of challenges faced by medicinal plant sellers. These included conservation and business skills (such as marketing, pricing, banking of profits–as well as record keeping of trading stock, income and expenditure) and conservation of medicinal plants and products. Following a capacity building intervention based on ESD and non-formal education principles, phase II results showed that the medicinal plant sellers had started revisiting some of their business practices–such as pricing techniques and record keeping. However, processing of medicinal plant materials, storage, packaging and conservation still persisted as challenges that needed further attention. In particular, sustainable harvesting practices and cultivation of medicinal plants in home gardens still presented some difficulties–including the non-availability of land and the lack of irrigation capacities to cultivate the various medicinal plant species. This was disturbing, especially given that most of the threatened and rare medicinal plant species exhibited very slow growth rates. The land issue appeared to be related to the matter of land ownership, particularly given that the majority of the medicinal plant sellers were women.

The second assessment revealed that medicinal plant sellers had diversified their businesses. That is, on top of their traditional merchandise they were observed selling a variety of small items such as edibles and none edibles. It goes without saying that this boosted their income. Given the new business trend, chances of medicinal plant sellers' businesses failing were thus reduced. Small business failures are attributed to small capital usually injected to that particular business [18]. At the same time, one should not lose sight of the need for proper management skills if one's business is to grow as well. Riddix [19] reiterated that diversification helps to protect business capital from wild swings of the market, while achieving long-term growth at the same time.

6. Conclusion

The study's educational intervention, which was aimed at equipping the participating medicinal plant sellers with knowledge and skills related to their trade, was recognised as an innovative way of sharing university knowledge and skills with indigenous communities. In particular, the focus of the study on cultivating the participants' awareness of the importance of conducting the medicinal plant selling business was based on principles of conservation, sustainable livelihoods and environmental friendliness. In addition, participants were equipped with life-long business skill to help them manage and development their informal ventures into sustainable business entities.

Author details

Busisiwe Ndawonde[1*], Sitwala Namwinji Imenda[2] and Humbulani Nancy Mutshaeni[3]

*Address all correspondence to: busisiwen@uj.ac.za

1 University of Johannesburg, Johannesburg, South Africa

2 University of Zululand, KwaDlangezwa, South Africa

3 University of Venda, Thohoyandou, South Africa

References

[1] Onwu G, Mosimege M: Indigenous Knowledge Systems and Science and Technology Education: A Dialogue. South Africa: University of Western Cape; 2004.

[2] Herremans GK, Reid S. Developing awareness of sustainability concept. The Journal of Environmental Education. 2000; 34 (1):16–20.

[3] Ndawonde BG. 2007. Medicinal Plant Sales: A Case Study in Northern Zululand [thesis]. South Africa: University of Zululand; 2007.

[4] Goldings JS. Southern African Plant Red Data Lists. South African Botanic Diversity Network Report Series No. 14. National Botanic Institute, Pretoria, South Africa; 2002.

[5] van Wyk B-E. Gericke, N. [editors]. Medicinal Plants of South Africa. South Africa, Pretoria: Briza Publications; 2009.

[6] Ndawonde BG, Zobolo AM, Dlamini ET, Siebert SJ. A survey of plants sold by traders at Zululand muthi markers with a view to selecting popular plant species for propagation in communal gardens. African Journal of Range and Forage Science. 2007; 24(2): 103–107.

[7] Williams VL, Victor JE, Crouch NR. Red listed medicinal plants of South Africa: Status, trends and assessment challenges. South African Journal of Botany. 2013; 86: 23–35.

[8] Ceschin F, Vezzoli C, Zhang J. Sustainability in design: now! Challenges and opportunities for design research, education and practice in the XXI century. In: Proceedings of the Learning Network on Sustainability (LeNS) Conference: 29 September–1 October 2010; Bangalore, India: Greenleaf Publishing.

[9] Kumar R. Research Methodology. A Step by Step Guide for Beginners. 2nd ed. London: SAGE Publications; 2005.

[10] Borgatti SP. Elements of research. Against U.S. militarism. In: Lois A. Lorentzen and Jennifer Turpin, editors. The Women and War Reader. 2**nd** ed., New York: New York University Press; 1999. pp. 308–322.

[11] Zobolo AM, Ndawonde BG, Dlamini ET. 2009. Propagation and growth of *Ansellia africana* and *Mondia whitei* from cuttings. South African Journal of Botany. 2009; 75: 428–442

[12] Diederichs N, Mander M, Crough N, Spring W, McKean S, Symmons R. Knowing and growing muthi. Scottvillle, South Africa: Institute of Natural Resources; 2009.

[13] Ndawonde BG, Imenda SN. Biographical characteristics of medicinal plant sellers. Studies on Ethno-Medicine. 2015; 9: 327–336.

[14] Boeren E. Gender differences in formal, non-formal and informal learning. Studies in Continuing Education. 2011; 33(3): 333–345.

[15] Braun V, Clarke V. Using thematic analysis in psychology. Qualitative Research in Psychology. 2006; 3(2): 77–101.

[16] Botha J, Witkowski ETF, Shackleton CM. Market profiles and trade in medicinal plants in the Lowveld, South Africa. Environmental Conservation. 2007; 31 (1): 38–46.

[17] Vermani K, Garg S. 2002. Herbal medicines for sexually transmitted diseases and AIDS. Journal of Ethnopharmacology. 2002; 80: 49–66.

[18] Baptista R, Karaöz M, Leitão J. Diversification by young, small firms. In: Procceedings of Summer Conference on 'Opening up Innovation: Strategy, Organisation and Technology'; 13–16 August 2010; London: Imperial Collage Business School.

[19] Riddix M. Three Advantages of Diversification as Part of Your Investment Strategy [Internet]. 2014. Available from. http://www.benzinga.com/economics/11/09/1897071/3-advantages-of-diversification-as-part-of-your-investment-strategy.pdf. [Accessed 2015-07-15].

5

Biological Properties of Essential Oils from the *Piper* Species of Brazil

Renata Takeara, Regiane Gonçalves,
Vanessa Farias dos Santos Ayres and
Anderson Cavalcante Guimarães

Abstract

Piperaceae, a Latin name derived from Greek, which in turn originates from the Arabic word *babary*—black pepper, is considered one of the largest families of basal dicots, found in tropical and subtropical regions of both hemispheres. The species that belong to this family have a primarily pantropical distribution, predominantly herbaceous members, occurring in tropical Africa, tropical Asia, Central America and the Amazon region. The Piperaceae family includes five genera: *Piper*, *Peperomia*, *Manekia*, *Zippelia* and *Verhuellia*. Brazil has about 500 species distributed in the *Piper*, *Peperomia* and *Manekia* genera. The *Piper* genus, the largest of the Piperaceae family, has about 4000 species. Within the *Piper* genus, about 260–450 species can be found in Brazil. *Piper* species have diverse biological activities and are used in pharmacopeia throughout the world. They are also used in folk medicine for treatment of many diseases in several countries including Brazil, China, India, Jamaica and Mexico. Pharmacological studies of *Piper* species point toward the vast potential of these plants to treat various diseases. Many of these species are biologically active and have shown antitumor, antimicrobial, antioxidant, insecticidal, anti-inflammatory, antinociceptive, enzyme inhibitor, antiparasitic, antiplatelet, piscicide, allelopathic, antiophidic, anxiolytic, antidepressant, antidiabetic, hepatoprotective, amebicide and diuretic possibilities.

Keywords: Piperaceae, *Piper*, essential oils, biological activities, chemical constituents

1. Introduction

Nature, in general, has produced most of the known organic substances. Among the various kingdoms of nature, the plant kingdom has contributed most significantly to the supply of secondary metabolites. For example, essential oils derived from plants have great value due to their applications as medicines, cosmetics, food and agrochemicals [1, 2].

Essential oils constitute a complex mixture of low molecular weight substances (usually less than 500 Da) obtained by hydrodistillation or by extraction with organic solvents [2, 3]. A single plant may contain between 20 and 100 secondary metabolites belonging to different chemical classes. Terpenoids, phenylpropanoids and aromatic compounds are metabolites present in essential oils [2]. Among the terpenoids, monoterpenes and sesquiterpenes make up the largest group of substances in essential oils [2, 4].

About 3000 essential oils are produced using less than 2000 plant species, among which 300 are important from a commercial point of view. Essential oil production is 40,000–60,000 tons/year with a market value estimated at $700 million, indicating an increase in production and essential oil consumption worldwide [2].

In Brazil, the production of essential oils began at the end of the second decade of the twentieth century based on the extraction of native species to meet the demands of the foreign market. Interest in essential oils is based not only on the possibility of obtaining aromatic compounds (pleasant odor) and the application of products such as perfumes, fragrances and cosmetics, but also on possessing therapeutic properties such as insecticides, fungicides, bactericides or a precursor compound of molecules with high added value [5].

2. Piperaceae family

Piperaceae is a Latin name derived from Greek, which in turn originates from the Arabic babary, which means black pepper. It is considered one of the largest families of basal dicots, present in tropical and subtropical regions of both hemispheres [5]. In this family, there are species with a primarily pantropical distribution, having mostly herbaceous representatives (vines, shrubs and even some trees) [5, 6].

This family includes five genera: *Piper*, *Peperomia*, *Manekia*, *Zippelia* and *Verhuellia* [7]. They are present in tropical Africa, tropical Asia, Central America and the Amazon region [6]. Brazil is represented by about 500 species distributed in the *Piper*, *Peperomia* and *Manekia* genera [8]. The family is very important as a source of substances with pharmacological activities [9]. Many chemical compounds such as amides, phenylpropanoids, chromone, lignans and neolignans have been found [10].

3. *Piper* genus

Piper is the largest genus of the Piperaceae family [7, 11]. The species of this genus have diverse biological activities and are used in pharmacopeia throughout the world. They are also used in folk medicine for treatment of many diseases in several countries including Brazil, China, India, Jamaica and Mexico [9–11].

In Brazil, *Piper* species are distributed throughout the national territory. Among the aromatic flora of the Amazon region, there are more than a dozen species that provide essential oils that are used by the population for therapeutic purposes [12]. The decoction of *Piper callosum* leaves is used to treat diseases of the gastrointestinal tract [5, 13, 14]. Moreover, the tea of the decoction of *Piper hispidum* leaves is useful for the treatment of malaria. *Piper marginatum* is used as a tonic, carminative, stimulant, diuretic and sudorific agent against stomach, liver and gallbladder pain, toothaches, and snake and insect bites [5, 15, 16]. *Piper cavalcantei* Yuncker is called "electric sky" or "electric oil". The decoction of its leaves is considered an excellent antipyretic and analgesic, especially for headaches. The infusion of the leaves is used as an antidiarrheal, to prevent dehydration and to combat menstrual cramps. Oil, extracted by soaking and heating, is used topically for earaches and other external pain [17].

The *Piper* species found in the Northeast of Brazil also have many uses in folk medicine, such as *Piper corcovadensis* used for toothaches [11]. The species found in the Atlantic rainforest are also used. For example, *Piper regnellii* (L.) Miq. is used as an anesthetic and anti-inflammatory agent. *Piper cernuum* Vell. is used as an analgesic (mainly for stomach aches) against liver and kidney diseases. Chewing the leaves of *Piper gaudichaudianum* Kunth. fights toothaches, while *Piper cf. lhostzkyanum* Kunth. is used to combat pain in the stomach, liver and kidney [17].

The decoction of *Piper umbellatum* leaves is used by those in the working class especially in the treatment of diseases in the digestive, urinary and respiratory tracts, and treatment of stomatitis, vaginitis and liver disorder [18, 19]. *Piper aduncum*, popularly known as pimenta-de-macaco and aperta-ruão, has been used in the treatment of gynecological diseases and intestinal disorders [14]. *Piper* sp, known as Jaborandi, is used to treat toothaches [19]. *Peperomia pellucida* H.B.K., popularly known as folha-de-vidro, is used against gastrointestinal ailments and high blood pressure and acts as a mild diuretic. The juice of the plant can be used to treat ocular diseases in general [20].

Many *Piper* species are biologically active and have shown antitumor [21], antimicrobial [22], antioxidant, insecticide, larvicide [5], anti-inflammatory, antinociceptive, enzyme inhibitor, trypanocidal, antiplatelet, piscicide, allelopathic, antiophidic, anti-malaria, antileishmania, ansiliotico/antidepressant, antituberculosis, antidiabetic, nematocide, herbicide, hepatoprotective, anti-*Helicobacter pylori* [23], amebicide [24] and diuretic [25] potential.

Piperaceae's contribution to scientific and technological knowledge is considered very significant. Chemistry studies of *Piper* species have led to the identification of a variety of new chemical compounds belonging to different classes, including alkaloids [26], amides [27], chromenes [28], derivatives of benzoic acids [29], lignans, neolignans, propenyl phenols, terpenes, steroids, chalcones, diidrochalcones, flavones, flavanones, kavalactones, piperolides, ceramides, fatty acids [5, 10] and flavonoids [23, 26].

4. Chemical composition of essential oils of the *Piper* species from Brazil

From a chemical point of view, essential oils are complex mixtures of volatile substances that are lipophilic and usually odoriferous and liquid. They are endowed with aromas that are almost always pleasant and colorless when recently extracted [29]. They can contain from 20 to 60 or more different compounds at various concentrations [30].

The composition of essential oils is constantly being transformed, according to seasonal variation and circadian rhythms. It may also be determined by genotype, environmental factors, and plant cultivation and collection procedures. It can vary according to geographical origin, drying, harvest time, type of fertilizer, but the main components responsible for the aroma seem to remain constant [31].

The *Piper* essential oils are characterized by the presence of monoterpenes, sesquiterpenes and phenylpropanoids with significant biological effects [10]. Essential oils of many *Piper* species in Brazil have been studied for their chemical composition (**Table 1**). We highlight the following species:

An analysis of the essential oil from the leaves and stem of a *P. marginatum* specimen collected in the city of Itacoatiara in the state of Amazonas showed the presence of the following: safrole (0.51 and 0.10%); 3,4-(methylenedioxy) propiophenone (8.01 and 8.92%); 2-methoxy-4,5-(methylenedioxy) propiophenone (1.10 and 1.35%); β-caryophyllene (4.01 and 5.57%); elemicin (1.32 and 1.53%); α-terpinene (0.73 and 0.45%); (*E*)-ocimene (2.31 and 0.68%); α-terpinolene (1.11 and 0.85%); myristicin (0.23 and 9.23%); α-pinene (0.84 and 0.68%); α-copaene (2.47 and 1.71%); γ-elemene (3.75% and trace) and α-humulene (1.34 and 0.59%) [47].

In Ref. [34], 35 constituents were identified in the essential oil from the leaves and stem of *Piper aleyreanum* collected in Porto Velho in the state of Rondônia and reported as the major components: caryophyllene oxide (11.5%), β-pinene (9%), spathulenol (6.7%), camphene (5.2%), β-elemene (4.7%), myrtenal (4.2%), verbenone (3.3%) and pinocarvone (3.1%).

In Ref. [48] mainly non-oxygenated sesquiterpenes were identified in the chemical composition of the essential oil of seven *Piper* species of the Brazilian Atlantic Forest, with *E*-caryophyllene and germacrene D being the most frequent. However, the non-oxygenated monoterpenes (*Z*)-β-ocimene, α-pinene and β-pinene were also present.

From the literature about the phytochemical study of the essential oil of *Piper tuberculatum* extracted from the fruit and fine stems from a specimen collected in Rondônia, the predominance of sesquiterpenes was demonstrated, with caryophyllene oxide (32.1 and 26.6%) and (*E*)-caryophyllene (17.7 and 12.3%) as the major compounds [48].

According to Ref. [49], the essential oil from the leaves of *P. aduncum* collected in the city of Bocaiuva, in the state of Minas Gerais, has as major constituents the compounds 1,8-cineole (55.8%), α-terpineol (5.9%), (*E*)-ocimene (4.8%), (*E*)-pinene (4.7%) and α-pinene (4.5%). The composition analysis of the essential oil from the leaves of *Piper hispidinervum* and *P. callosum* collected in the Amazon showed that both species have safrole (98.12 and 64%) as the major constituent [12].

The study of the essential oil of three *Piper* species collected in different areas of the Federal District revealed the predominance of sesquiterpenes in all species. In the essential oil of *Piper arboreum*, the only monoterpenes identified were δ-3-carene (0.9%) and linalool (1.1%). The constituents present in the highest concentrations were bicyclogermacrene (12.1%), 10-epi-γ-eudesmol (11.6%), spathulenol (8.4%), caryophyllene oxide (10.1%)

Species	Part of plant used	Main chemical compounds	Biological properties	References
Piper angustifolium	Leaves	Spathulenol; caryophyllene oxide	Anti-leishmania (*Leishmania infantum*)	[32]
P. anonifolium	Aerial parts	α-pinene; β-selinene; α-selinene; selin-11-en-4-α-ol	Cytotoxic; antifungal; antioxidant; anticholinesterase	[33]
P. aleyreanum	Leaves, stems, aerial parts	Caryophyllene oxide; spathulenol; β-pinene; camphene; δ-elemene; β-elemene; β-caryophyllene; germacrene D; bicyclogermacrene	Antinociceptive; anti-inflammatory; gastric antiulcer; cytotoxic; antifungal; antioxidant; anticholinesterase	[33, 34]
P. aduncum	Fruits, leaves	β-pinene; E- caryophyllene; β-cubebene; β-elemene; α-copaene; α-farnesene; 1,8-cineole; α-terpineol; dillapiole	Larvicidal (*A. aegypti* L.); osmotic and morphologic fragility of erythrocytes; antihelmintic (*Haemonchus contortus*); Antiacarid (*Rhipicephalus* (Boophilus) *microplus*)	[35–38]
P. callosum	Leaves		Antifungal (*C. perniciosa, P. palmivora* and *P. capsici*)	[39]
P. cernuum	Branches	Camphene	Antitumoral	[21]
P. corcovadensis	Leaves	1-butyl-3, 4-methylenedioxybenzene; terpinolene; *trans*-caryophyllene; α-pinene	Larvicidal (*A. aegypti* L.)	[11]
P. diospyrifolium	Leaves	(*E*)-eudesma-6,11-diene; (*E*)-caryophyllene; γ-muurolene; limonene; germacrene; (*E*)-β-ocimene	Antifungal	[40]
P. enckea	Leaves		Antifungal (*C. perniciosa, P. palmivora* and *P. capsici)*	[39]
P. gaudichaudianum	Leaves	*E*-caryophyllene; α-humulene; bicyclogermacrene; *E*-nerolidol; viridiflorol; aromadendrene; β-selinene	Cytotoxic (*Saccharomyces cerevisiae*); larvicidal (*A. aegypti* L.)	[41]
P. hispidum	Aerial parts	δ-3-carene; limonene; α-copaene; β-caryophyllene; α-humulene; β-selinene; caryophyllene oxide	Cytotoxic; antifungal; antioxidant; anticholinesterase	[33]
P. hispidinervum	Leaves	Safrol; α-terpinolene	Antifungal (*B. sorokiniana, F. oxysporum* and *C. gloeosporioides)*; insecticidal (*S. frugiperda*); amoebicidal (*A. polyphaga*)	[24, 42, 43]
P. hostmanianum	Leaves	Asaricin; myristicin	Larvicidal (*A. aegypti* L.)	[44]
P. humaytanum	Leaves	β-selinene; caryophyllene oxide	Larvicidal (*A. aegypti* L.)	[44]
P. malacophyllum	Leaves	α-pinene; camphene; camphor; *E*-nerolidol	Antimicrobial; antifungal	[45]
P. marginatum	Leaves	Isoelemicin; Apiol; δ-guaiene	Antifungal (*C. perniciosa, P. palmivora* and *P. capsici)*; larvicidal (*A. aegypti* L.)	[35, 39]
P. nigrum	Seeds	Limonene; *E* caryophyllene; caryophyllene oxide	Larvicidal (*A. aegypti* L.)	[35]
P. permucronatum	Leaves	Dillapiol; myristicin	Larvicidal (*A. aegypti* L.)	[45]
P. vicosanum	Leaves	α-Alaskene; Y-elemene; limonene	Anti-inflammatory	[46]

Table 1. *Piper* species of Brazil with biological properties.

and γ-eudesmol (6.7%). The constituents with the greatest quantities in the oil obtained from the leaves of *Piper dilatatum* were (*Z*)-β-ocimene (19.6%), β-caryophyllene (11.3%), sesquiterpene (8.8%), bicyclogermacrene (8.8%), spathulenol (6.5%) and caryophyllene oxide (5.3%). The analysis of the essential oil of *P. hispidum* leaves revealed the presence of β-pinene (19.7%), α-pinene (9.0%), δ-3-carene (7.4%), α-cadinol (6.9%) and spathulenol (6.2%) as major compounds [50].

The analysis of the essential oil of *Piper* species of the Amazon revealed the presence of the sesquiterpenes α-copaene, (*E*)-caryophyllene and spathulenol in all species analyzed. The major compounds identified in *Piper amapense* oil were (*E*)-caryophyllene (25.0%), β-selinene (15.0%) and caryophyllene oxide (17.0%). The oil of *Piper duckei* had a predominance of (*E*)-caryophyllene (23.5%), caryophyllene oxide (18.4%), β-eudesmol (9.4%) and α-eudesmol (9.1%). The major volatile compounds found in *Piper bartlingianum* were α-cadinol (11.2%), β-elemene (10.5%), α-muurolol (9.4%) and (*E*)-nerolidol [51].

Analyses of the essential oils from the leaves, stems and flowers of *P. regnellii* collected in Dourados in the state of Mato Grosso do Sul revealed the presence of myrcene and anethole, with the major constituent in the stem being dillapiole. In the leaves, the main compounds were myrcene (21.9%), anethole (*E*) (16.0%) and bicyclogermacrene (9.4%). In the stem, they were anethole (*E*) (13.4%), dillapiole (30.4%) and myrcene (14.9%). For the flowers, they were anethole (*E*) (28.2%), myrcene (23.0%) and bicyclogermacrene (9.6%) [52].

5. Biological activities of essential oils of the *Piper* species from Brazil

Due to their complex chemical composition, essential oils show a range of pharmacological actions, making them potential sources for the development of new drugs [53].

The antimicrobial activity of essential oils, both *in vitro* and *in vivo*, has justified research on traditional medicine focused on the characterization of their antimicrobial activity [54]. The search for more effective antimicrobial agents has become a challenge for the medical field and has gained increasing importance. According to studies by Ref. [45], the essential oil of *Piper malacophyllum* collected in Florianopolis in the state of Santa Catarina showed significant antimicrobial activity, especially antifungal activity shown to be moderate against the *Cryptococcus neoformans* yeast and the *Trichophyton mentagrophytes* filamentous fungus, both of clinical interest. This activity is attributed to the synergism of the chemical constituents present in the essential oil.

Work done with essential oils obtained from medicinal plants has shown activity on plant pathogen control that could replace the use of pesticides, which, in the long term, cause negative impacts on society and the environment due to pollution from their chemical waste [55]. The essential oils of *P. callosum*, *P. marginatum* and *Piper enckea* collected in the state of Pará showed inhibitory activity against several pathogens, including *Crinipellis perniciosa*, *Phytophthora palmivora* and *Phytophthora capsici*. *P. callosum* caused 100% mycelial inhibition of *P. capsici* at a concentration of 0.75 μL/mL, the best fungitoxic action on the three pathogens tested [39]. The essential oil of *P. hispidinervum* inhibited growth of the *Bipolaris sorokiniana*, *Fusarium oxysporum* and *Colletotrichum gloeosporioides* pathogens, attributing the fungicidal effect observed in the essential oil to the presence of safrole (89%), its major component [42].

Ref. [43] evaluated the insecticidal activity of the essential oil of *P. hispidinervum*, collected in Lavras in the state of Minas Gerais, on *Spodoptera frugiperda* (Fall armyworm), attributing the effect to safrole (82%), the major component of the essential oil being analyzed. The essential oil of *Piper betle* showed insecticidal activity by inhibiting the development of *Spodoptera litura* pupae without causing damage to the *Eudrilus eugeniae* organism [56].

Ref. [33] reported anticholinesterase activity for the essential oils of *Piper anonifolium* and *P. hispidum* collected in Bahia, while the oil of *P. aleyreanum* showed high cytotoxic activity against melanoma. The oils of the three species of *Piper* analyzed showed strong antifungal activity against *Cladosporium sphaerospermum* and *Cladosporium cladosporioides*.

Essential oils from the fruits of *P. aduncum*, leaves of *P. marginatum* and seeds of *Piper nigrum*, collected in Paraíba, were tested against dengue mosquito larvae and were shown to be active. The *P. marginatum* species had the greatest larvicidal effect [35]. The essential oil of *P. corcovadensis* revealed a potent larvicidal activity against the oviposition of *Aedes aegypti* [11].

In a study conducted by Girola et al. [21], the monoterpene camphene isolated from essential oil of *P. cernuum*, collected in Cubatão in the state of São Paulo, induced apoptosis in melanoma cells, and showed antitumor activity *in vivo*, thus showing itself to be a promising compound in cancer therapy.

The essential oil of *Piper vicosanum* collected in the city of Dourados, in the state of Mato Grosso do Sul, demonstrated anti-inflammatory activity in rodents and did not cause acute toxicity or mutagenicity [46]. The essential oil of *P. aleyreanum* extracted from a specimen from Porto Velho in the state of Rondônia, showed antinociceptive action, as well as anti-inflammatory and gastroprotective properties with great potential for the development of phytomedicines [34].

The literature reports a wide range of essential oils from the *Piper* genus with different biological properties. The essential oil of *P. hispidinervum* collected in Porto Alegre, in the state of Rio Grande do Sul, showed amebicide action against the trophozoites of *Acanthamoeba polyphaga*, preventing its encysting. This suggests that this essential oil has the potential to develop new drugs to treat keratitis. It also demonstrated little toxic effect against Vero cells (renal cells of the African green monkey) and is not toxic at concentrations less than 0.25 mg/mL [24]. The essential oil of *Piper diospyrifolium* collected in Maringa, in the state of Parana, showed antifungal activity against *Candida albicans*, *Candida parapsilosis* and *Candida tropicalis* isolated from catheter urine, blood culture and orotracheal tube samples donated by the University Hospital of Maringá, demonstrating effective activity as a possible new phytotherapy or natural fungicide [40].

6. Conclusions and future perspectives

According to the literature, we can say that the essential oils from the *Piper* species of Brazil have many uses. In addition, they are endowed with interesting biological activities and have a therapeutic potential. For example, they exhibit antimicrobial, anticholinesterase, antitumor, anti-inflammatory activities and may be useful as natural remedies and it seems that they can be used as a suitable therapy for many pathologies. Therefore, economic importance of essential oils from the *Piper* species of Brazil is indisputable. It appears therefore imperative to preserve our natural, diverse flora and support its protection in order to keep this inexhaustible source of molecules destined for multiple targets.

Author details

Renata Takeara*, Regiane Gonçalves, Vanessa Farias dos Santos Ayres and Anderson Cavalcante Guimarães

*Address all correspondence to: rtakeara@yahoo.com

Federal University of Amazonas, Institute of Science and Technology, Itacoatiara, AM, Brazil

References

[1] Pinto AC, Silva DHS, Bolzani V, Lopes N, Epifanio RA. Produtos Naturais: Atualidade, Desafios e Perspectivas. Química Nova. 2002;**25**:45–61. DOI: 10.1590/S0100-404220 02000800009

[2] Raut JS, Karuppayil SM. A status review on the medicinal properties of essential oils, Industrial Crops and Products. 2014;**62**:250–264. DOI:10.1016/j.indcrop.2014.05.055

[3] Nakatsu T, Lupo AT, Chinn JW, Kang RKL. Biological activity of essential oils and their constituents, Studies in Natural Products Chemistry. 2000;**21**:571–631. DOI: 10.1016/ S1572-5995(00)80014-9

[4] Carson CF, Hammer KA, Riley TV. *Melaleuca alternifolia* (Tea Tree) oil: a review of antimicrobial and other medicinal properties, Clinical Microbiology Reviews. 2006;**19**:50–62. DOI: 10.1128/CMR.19.1.50-62.2006

[5] Andrade EHA, Guimarães EF, Maia JGS. Variabilidade química em óleos essenciais de espécies de Piper da Amazônia. FEQ/UFPA: Belém; 2009. 448p.

[6] Jaramillo MA, Manos PS. Phylogeny and patterns of floral diversity in the Genus *Piper* (Piperaceae), American Journal of Botany. 2001;**88**:706–716. DOI: 10.2307/2657072

[7] Samain M, Vrijdaghs A, Hesse M, Goetghebeur P, Rodríguez FJ, Stoll A, Neinhuis C, Wanke S. Verhuellia is a segregate lineage in Piperaceae: more evidence from flower, fruit and pollen morphology, anatomy and development, Annals of Botany. 2010;1–12. DOI: 10.1093/aob/mcq031

[8] Guimarães EF, Carvalho-Silva M. Uma nova espécie e novos nomes em *Piper* seção *Ottonia* (Piperaceae) para o Sudeste do Brasil, Hoehnea. 2009;**36**: 431–435. DOI: 10.1590/ S2236-89062009000300004

[9] Di Stasi LC, Oliveira GP, Carvalhaes MA, Queiroz-Junior M, Tien OS, Kakiname, SH, Reis MS. Medicinal plants popularly used in the Brazilian Tropical Atlantic Forest, Fitoterapia. 2002;**73**:69–91. DOI: 10.1016/S0367-326X(01)00362-8

[10] Parmar VS, Jain SC, Bisht KS, Jain R, Taneja P, Jha A, Tyagi OD, Prasad AK, Wengel J, Olsen CE, Boll PM. Phytochemistry of the Genus *Piper*, Phytochemistry. 1997;**46**:591–673. DOI: 10.1016/S0031-9422(97)00328-2

[11] Silva MFR, Bezerra-Silva PC, Lira CS, Albuquerque BNL, Neto ACA, Pontual EV, Maciel JR, Paiva PMG, Navarro DMAF. Composition and biological activities of the essential oil of *Piper corcovadensis* (Miq.) C. DC (Piperaceae), Experimental Parasitology.2016;**165**:64–70. DOI: 10.1016/j.exppara.2016.03.017

[12] Maia JGS, Silva ML, Luz AIR, Zhogbi MGB, Ramos LS. Espécies de Piper da Amazônia Rica em Safrol, Química Nova. 1987;**10**:200–2004.

[13] Ritter RM, Monteiro MVB, Monteiro FOB, Rodrigues ST, Soares ML, Silva JCR, Palha, MDC, Biondi GF, Rahal SC, Tourinho MM. Ethnoveterinary knowledge and practices at Colares island, Pará state, eastern Amazon, Brazil, Journal of Ethnopharmacology. 2012;**144**:346–352. DOI: 10.1016/J.JEP.2012.09.018

[14] Van Den Berg ME. Plantas medicinais na Amazônia—contribuição ao seu conhecimento sistemático, 2nd ed. Museu Paraense Emílio Goeldi: Belém; 1993. 207p.

[15] Brú J, Guzman JD. Folk medicine, phytochemistry and pharmacological application of *Piper marginatum*, Revista Brasileira de Farmacognosia. DOI: 10.1016/j.bjp.2016.03.014

[16] D'angelo LCA, Chavier HS, Torres LMB, Lapa AJ, Souccar C. Pharmacology of *Piper marginatum* Jacq. a folk medicinal plant used as an analgesic, anti-inflammatory and hemostatic, Phytomedicine. 1997;**4**:33–40. DOI: 10.1016/S0944-7113(97)80025-6

[17] Di Stasi LC, Hiruma-Lima CA. Plantas medicinais na Amazônia e na Mata Atlântica, 2nd ed. Editora UNESP: São Paulo; 2002. 604p.

[18] Roesch CMFB. *Piper umbellatum* L.: a comparative cross-cultural analysis of its medicinal uses and an ethnopharmacological evaluation, Journal of Ethnopharmacology. 2010;**131**:522–537. DOI: 10.1016/j.jep.2010.07.045 2010

[19] Brandão MGL, Pignal M, Romaniuc S, Grael CFF, Fagg CW. Useful Brazilian plants listed in the field books of the French naturalist Auguste de Saint-Hilaire (1779–1853), Journal of Ethnopharmacology. 2012;**143**:488–500. DOI: 10.1016/j.jep.2012.06.052 2012

[20] Almeida MZ. Plantas medicinais, 3rd ed. EDUFBA: Salvador; 2011. 221p.

[21] Girola N, Figueiredo CR, Farias CF, Azevedo RA, Fereira AK, Texira SF, Capello TM, Martins EGA, Matsuo AL, Travessos LR, Lago JHG. Camphene isolated from essential oil of *P. cernuum* (Piperaceae) induces intrinsic apoptosis in melanoma cells and displays antitumor activity in vivo, Biochemical and Biophysical Research Communications. 2015;**467**:928–934. DOI: 10.1016/j.bbrc.2015.10.041

[22] Kitamura ROS, Romoff P, Young MCM, Kato MJ, Lago JHG. Chromenes from *Peperomia serpens* (Sw.) Loudon (Piperaceae), Phytochemistry. 2006;**67**:2398–2402. DOI: 10.1016/j.phytochem.2006.08.007

[23] Nascimento JC, Paula VF, David JM, David JP. Occurrence, biological activities and ^{13}C NMR data of amides from *Piper* (Piperaceae), Quimica Nova. 2012;**35**:2288–2311. DOI: 101590/S0100-40422012001100037

[24] Sauter IP, Rossa GE, Lucas AM, Cibulski SP, Roehe PM, Silva LAA, Rott MB, Vargas RMF, Cassel E, Poser GL. Chemical composition and amoebicidal activity of *Piper hispidinervum* (Piperaceae) essential oil, Industrial Crops and Products. 2012;**40**:292–295. DOI: 10.1016/j.indcrop.2012.03.025

[25] Novaes AS, Mota JS, Barison A, Veber CL, Negrão FJ, Kassuya CAL, Barros ME. Diuretic and antilithiasic activities of ethanolic extract from *Piper amalago* (Piperaceae), Phytomedicine. 2014;**21**:523–528. DOI: 10.1016/j.phymed.2013.10.014

[26] Facundo AV, Bálico LJ, Lima DKS, Santos ARS, Morais SM, Silva GVJ, Militão JLT. Non-substituted B-ring flavonoids and an indole alkaloid from *Piper aleyreanum* (Piperaceae), Biochemical Systematics and Ecology. 2012;**45**:206–208. DOI: 10.1016/j.bse.2012.07.010

[27] Kaou AM, Mahiou-Leddet V, Canlet C, Debrawer L, Hutter S, Azas N, Ollivier E. New amide alkaloid from the aerial part of *Piper capense* L.f. (Piperaceae), Fitoterapia. 2010;**81**:632–635. DOI: 10.1016/j.fitote.2010.03.006

[28] Parra JE, Delgado WA, Cuca LE. Cumanensic acid, a new chromene isolated from *Piper* cf. *cumanense* Kunth. (Piperaceae), Phytochemistry Letters. 2011;**4**:280–282. DOI: 10.1016/j.phytol.2011.04.015

[29] Parra JE, Patiño OJ, Pietro J, Delgado WA, Cuca LE. A new benzoic acid derivative isolated from *Piper* cf. *cumanense* Kunth (Piperaceae), Phytochemistry Letters. 2013;**6**:590–592. DOI: 10.1016/j.phytol.2013.07.014

[30] Simões CMO, Schenkel EP, Gosman G, Mello JCP, Mentz LA, Petrovick PR. Farmacognosia: da Planta ao medicamento, 6th ed. UFRGS: Porto Alegre; 2007. 1102p.

[31] Bakkali F, Averbeck S, Averbeck D, Idaomar M. Biological effects of essential oils—a review, Food and Chemical Toxicology. 2008;**46**:446–475. DOI: 10.1016/j.fct.2007.09.106

[32] Bosquiroli LSS, Demarque DP, Rizk YS, Cunha MC, Marques MCS, Matos MFC, Kadri MCT, Carollo CA, Arruda CCP. In vitro anti-Leishmania infantum activity of essential oil from Piper angustifolium, Revista Brasileira de Farmacognosia. 2015;**25**:124–128. DOI: 10.1016/j.bjp.2015.03.008

[33] Silva JKR, Pinto LC, Burbano RMR, Montenegro RC, Guimarães EF, Andrade EHA, Maia JGS. Essential oils of Amazon Piper species and their cytotoxic, antifungal, antioxidant and anti-cholinesterase activities, Industrial Crops and Products. 2014;**58**:55–60. DOI: 10.1016/j.indcrop.2014.04.006

[34] Lima DKS, Ballico LJ, Lapa FR, Gonçalves HP, Souza LM, Iacomini M, Werner MFP, Baggio CH, Pereira IT, Silva LM, Facundo VA, Santos RS. Avaliação da antinociceptivo

antiúlcera, anti-inflamatória e gástrica atividades do óleo essencial de *Piper aleyreanum* C.DC em roedores, Journal of Ethnopharmacology. 2012;**142**:274–282. DOI: 10.1016/j.jep.2012.05.016

[35] Costa JGM, Santos PF, Brito SA, Rodrigues FFG, Coutinho HDM, Botelho MA, Lima SG. Composição Quimica e Toxicidade de Oleos Essenciais de Especies de *Piper* Frente a Larvas de *Aedes aegypti* L. (Diptera: Culicidae), Latin American Journal of Pharmacy. 2010;**29**:463–467.

[36] Barros FJ, Costa RJO, Cesário FRAS, Rodrigues LB, Costa JGM, Coutinho HDM, Galvão HBF, Menezes IRA. Activity of essential oils of *Piper aduncum* anf and *Cinnamomum zeylanicum* by evaluating osmotic and morphologic fragility of erythrocytes. European Journal of Integrative Medicine. 2015. DOI: 10.1016/j.eujim.2016.02.011

[37] Oliveira GL, Vieira TM, Nunes VF, Ruas MO, Duarte ER, Moreira DL, Kaplan MAC, Martins ER. Chemical composition and efficacy in the egg-hatching inhibition of essential oil of *Piper aduncum* against *Haemonchus contortus* from sheep, Revista Brasileira de Farmacognosia. 2014;**24**:288–292. DOI: 10.1016/j.bjp.2014.07.004

[38] Silva WC, Martins JRS, Souza HEM, Heinzen H, Cesio MV, Mato M, Albrecht F, Azevedo JL, Barros NM. Toxicity of Piper aduncum L. (Piperales: Piperaceae) from the Amazon forest for the cattle tick Rhipicephalus (Boophilus) microplus (Acari: Ixodidae), Veterinary Parasitology. 2009;**164**:267–274. DOI:10.1016/j.vetpar.2009.06.006

[39] Silva DMH, Bastos CN. Atividade antifúngica de óleos essenciais de espécies de *Piper* sobre *Crinipellis perniciosa, Phytophthora palmivora* e *Phytophthora capsici,* FEBS Letters. 2007;**32**:143–145. DOI: 10.1590/S0100-41582007000200008

[40] Vieira SCH, Paulo LF, Svidzinski TIE, Dias-Filho BP, Nakamura CV, Young MCM, Cortez DAG. Antifungal activity of *Piper diospyrifolium* kunth (Piperaceae) essential oil, FEBS Letters. 2011;**42**:1001–1006. DOI: 10.1590/S1517-83822011000300020

[41] Sperotto ARM, Moura DJ, Péres VF, Damasceno FC, Caramão EB, Henriques JAP, Saffi J. Cytotoxic mechanism of *Piper gaudichaudianum* Kunth essential oil and its major compound nerolidol, Food and Chemical Toxicology. 2013;**57**:57–68. DOI: 10.1016/j.fct.2013.03.013

[42] Zacaroni LM, Cardoso MG, Souza PE, Pimentel FA, Guimarães LGL, Salgado APSP. Potencial fungitóxico do óleo essencial de *Piper hispidinervum* (pimenta longa) sobre os fungos fitopatogênicos *Bipolaris sorokiniana, Fusarium oxysporum* e *Colletotrichum gloeosporioides,* Acta Amazonica. 2009;**39**:193–198. DOI: 10.1590/S0044-59672009000100020

[43] Lima RK, Cardoso MG, Moraes JC, Melo BA, Rodrigues VG, Guimarães PL. Atividade inseticida do óleo essencial de pimenta longa (*Piper hispidinervum* C. DC.) sobre lagarta-do-cartucho do milho *Spodoptera frugiperda* (J. E. Smith, 1797) (Lepidoptera: Noctuidae), Acta Amazonica. 2009;**39**:377–378. DOI: 10.1590/S0044-59672009000200016

[44] Morais SM, Facundo VA, Bertimi LM, Cavalcanti ESB, Junior JFA, Ferreira SA, Brito ES, Neto MAS. Chemical composition and larvicidal activity of essential oils from Piper species, Biochemical Systematics and Ecology. 2007;**35**:670–675. DOI: 10.1016/j.bse.2007.05.002

[45] Santos TG, Rebelo RA, Dalmarco EM, Guedes A, Gasper AL, Cruz AB, Schmit AP, Cruz RCB, Steindel M, Nune RK. Composição química e avaliação da atividade antimicrobiana do óleo essencial das folhas de *Piper malacophyllum* (C. PRESL.) C. DC, FEBS Laters. 2012;**35**:477–481. DOI: 10.1590/S0100-40422012000300007

[46] Brait DRH, Vaz MSM, Arrigo JS, Carvalho NMB, Araújo FHS, Vani JM, Mota JS, Cardoso CAL, Oliveira RJ, Negrão FJ, Kassuya, CAL, Arena AC. Toxicological analysis and anti-inflammatory effects of essential oil from *Piper vicosanum* leaves, Regulatory Toxicology and Pharmacology. 2015;**73**:699–705. DOI: 10.1016/j.yrtph.2015.10.028

[47] Gobbo-Neto L, Lopes PN. Plantas medicinais: fatores de influência no conteúdo de metabólitos secundários, Química Nova. 2007;**30**:374–381. DOI: 10.1590/S0100-40422007000200026

[48] Santos PRD, Moreira DL, Guimarães EF, Kaplan MAC. Essential oil analysis of 10 Piperaceae species from the Brazilian Atlantic forest, Phytochemistry. 2001;**58**:547–551. DOI: 10.1016/S0031-9422(01)00290-4

[49] Facundo VA, Pollli AR, Rodrigues RV, Militão JSLT, Stabelli RG, Cardoso CT. Constituintes químicos fixos e voláteis dos talos e frutos de *Piper tuberculatum* Jacq. e das raízes de *P. hispidum* H. B. K, Acta Amazonica. 2008;**38**:733–742. DOI: 10.1590/S0044-59672008000400018

[50] Potzernheim CL, Bizzo HR, Vieira FV. Nálise dos óleos essenciais de três espécies de *Piper* coletadas na região do Distrito Federal (Cerrado) e comparação com óleos de plantas procedentes da região de Paraty, RJ (Mata Atlântica) Brazilian Journal of Pharmacognosy. 2006;**16**:246–251. DOI: 10.1590/S0102-695X2006000200019

[51] Santos AS, Andrade EHA, Zoghbi MGB, Luz AIR, Maia JGS. Sesquiterpenes of Amazonian *Piper species*, Acta Amazonica. 1998;**28**:127–130. DOI: 10.1590/1809-43921998282130

[52] Santos AL, Polidoro AS, Schneider JK, Cunha ME, Saucier C, Jacques RA, Cardoso CA, Mota JS, Camarão EB. Comprehensive two-dimensional gas chromatography time-of-flight mass spectrometry (GC × GC/TOFMS) for the analysis of volatile compounds in *Piper regnellii* (Miq.) C. DC, Microchemical Journal. 2015;**118**:242–251. DOI: 10.1016/j.micro214.07.007

[53] Amaral JFD. Atividade antiinflamatória, antinociceptiva, e gastroprotetora do óleo essencial de croton sonderianus muell.arg. [dissertação]. Fortaleza: Universidade Federal do Ceará; 2004.

[54] Agarwal V, Lal P, Pruthi V. Effect of plant oils on *Candida albicans*. Jounal of Microbiology, Immunology and Infection. 2010;**43**:447–451. DOI: 10.1016/S1684-1182(10)60069-2

[55] Moreira MR, Ponce AG, Del-Valle CE, Roura SI. Inhibitory parameters of essential oils to reduce a foodborne pathogen, LWT—Food Science and Technology. 2005;**38**:565–570. DOI: 10.1016/j.lwt.2004.07.012

[56] Vasantha-Srinivasan P, Senthil-Nathan S, Thanigaivel A, Edwin E-S, Ponsankar A, Selin-Rani S, Pradeepa V, Sakthi-Bhagavathy M, Kalaivani K, Hunter WB, Duraipandiyan V, Al-Dhabi NA. Developmental response of *Spodoptera litura* Fab. to treatments of crude volatile oil from *Piper betle* L. and evaluation of toxicity to earthworm, *Eudrilus eugeniae* Kinb, Chemosphere. 2016;**155**:336–347. DOI: 10.1016/j.chemosphere.2016.03.139

6

Phytochemistry, Antioxidant, Antibacterial Activity, and Medicinal Uses of Aromatic (Medicinal Plant *Rosmarinus officinalis*)

Imad Hadi Hameed and Ghaidaa Jihadi Mohammed

Abstract

Rosemary is a well-known aromatic and medicinal plant whose consumption serves to remedy the number of disorders. Its essential oil (EO) constitutes an important ingredient for well-being feeling improvement through beauty products such as soaps, perfumes, and deodorants. The identification of phytochemical compounds is based on the peak area, retention time molecular weight, molecular formula, chemical structure, and pharmacological actions. It contains chemical constitutions, which may be useful for various herbal formulations as anti-inflammatory, analgesic, antipyretic, cardiac tonic, and anti-asthmatic. Therefore, this chapter reviews the phytochemical compounds of *Rosmarinus officinalis*, using methanolic extraction. The phytochemical compound is screened by gas chromatography-mass spectrometry (GC-MS) method and the evaluation of antimicrobial and antioxidant activities of the essential oils.

Keywords: aromatic and medicinal plant, *Rosmarinus officinalis*, gas chromatography-mass spectrum analysis, essential oil, antibacterial activity, antioxidant activity

1. Introduction

Rosmarinus officinalis thrives well in dry and arid regions, hills and low mountains, calcareous, shale, clay, and rocky substrates. Its use since ancient times in traditional medicine is justified by its antiseptic [1, 2], antirheumatic [3], anti-inflammatory, antispasmodic [4, 5], antimicrobial, and anti-hepatotoxic properties [6]. Its appreciation as a spice for seasoning and food preservation [7] is supported by a very high antioxidant activity [8]. The potent antioxidant properties of rosemary extracts have been attributed to its phenolic compounds, mainly rosmarinic acid and diterpenes carnosic acid and carnosol [9, 10]. Rosemary extract relaxes smooth muscles and has choleretic, hepatoprotective, and antitumorigenic activity [11]. Recent research shows that rosemary extracts possess strong anticancer properties. In the last few years, gas chromatography-mass spectrometry (GC-MS) has become firmly established as a key technological platform for metabolite profiling in plant [12–16]. GC-MS-based metabolome analysis has profound applications in discovering the mode of action of drugs or herbicides and helps unravel the effect of altered gene expression on metabolism and organism performance in biotechnological applications.

2. History

Rosemary has been named the Herb of the Year in 2001 by the International Herb Association. Hippocrates, Galen, and dioscorides prescribed rosemary for liver problems. Rosemary is not a popular plant in India. It was introduced by the Europeans as a garden plant due to its pleasant fragrant-scented leaves.

3. Varieties

There are more than 20 varieties of rosemary plant. The different types of rosemary are as follows:

1. Upright rosemary: It measures between six and eight feet in diameter and two feet or more in height.
2. Creeping rosemary: It covers eight or 10 feet in diameter in a very short period of time. It can also trail down eight or 10 feet. It falls all the way to the ground and is covered with pale blue flowers.
3. Pine-scented rosemary: Pine-scented rosemary is a soft sea green that grows to about three to four feet high by about four or more feet wide.
4. Arp rosemary: This plant grows where winter temperatures are frequently in the teens or less.
5. Madalene hill rosemary: It is a cold hardy rosemary. It is rated to survive $-15°$ and is erect, growing to about three feet. Its flowers are light blue.
6. Pink rosemary: It has the thinnest leaves of all *R. officinalis* plants. The flower is pale in color and grows quickly to two feet.
7. Dancing waters rosemary: It is shorter, more mounding and has dark blue flowers.
8. Golden rain rosemary: It has weeping foliage. The golden hue of the plant turns darker green over summer and returns with cooler weather.
9. Blue boy rosemary: It is the smallest of all the rosemary varieties. It has small leaves and little light blue pearls for flowers. This plant grows out to cover about 12 inches but rarely gets over six inches tall.

4. Microscopic characteristics

The leaf is dorsiventral with upper epidermal cells polygonal in shape [17].

Serial no.	Phytochemical compound	Formula	Exact mass	Chemical structure	Pharmacological actions
1.	α-pinene	$C_{10}H_{16}$	136.1252	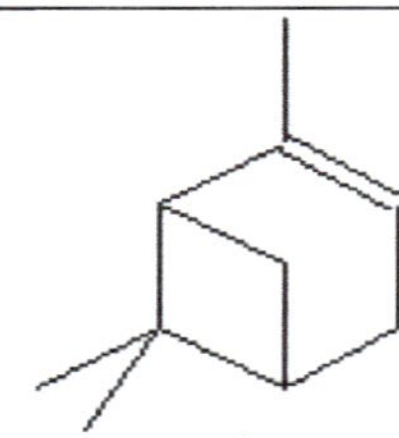	Antimicrobial against bacterial and fungal cells activities
2.	Camphene	$C_{10}H_{16}$	136.1252	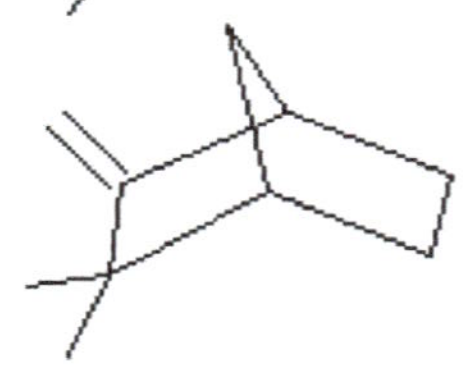	Antimicrobial against *Escherichia coli, Staphylococcus aureus*, and *Candida albicans*, but was not active against *Clostridium perfringens* up to the concentration of 100 g/ml. The significant antimicrobial and antioxidant activities of R. minima oil suggests that it could serve as a source for compounds with therapeutic potential
3.	Eucalyptol	$C_{10}H_{18}O$	154.13576	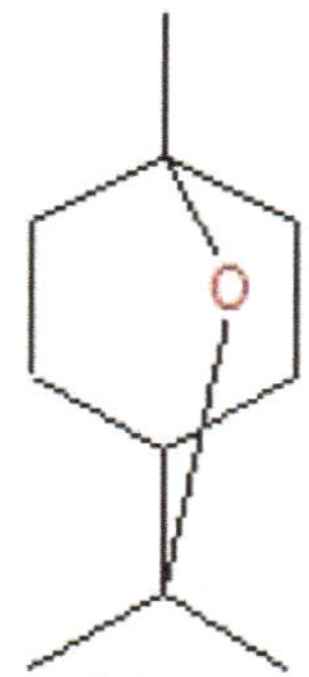	Eucalyptol, 1,8 cineole, is an essential oil present in large amounts in a variety of plants which is frequently used in the manufacture of cosmetics, to increase percutaneous penetration of drugs, as a nasal decongestant and anticough agent, in aromatherapy, and in dentistry (1-4). Eucalyptol has been used to treat bronchitis, sinusitis, and chronic rhinitis and also for the treatment of asthma
4.	2-Methoxy-4-vinylohenol	$C_9H_{10}O_2$	150.06808	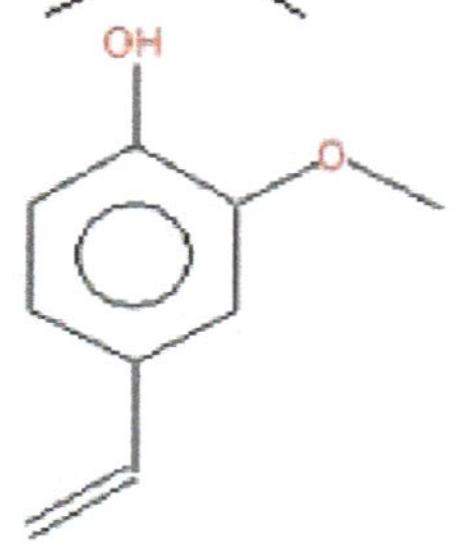	Antioxidant and anti-inflammatory

Serial no.	Phytochemical compound	Formula	Exact mass	Chemical structure	Pharmacological actions
5.	1-Oxaspiro[4, 5] deca-3,6-diene,2,6,10,10-tetramethyl	$C_{13}H_{20}O$	192.151415	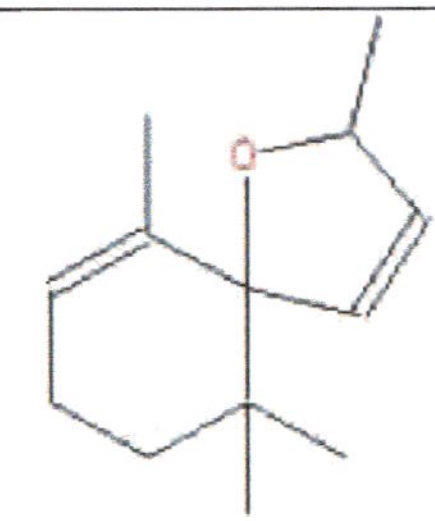	New chemical compound
6.	3-(*N,N*-Dimethyl lauryl ammonio) propanesulfate	$C_{17}H_{37}N_5O_3$	335.249414	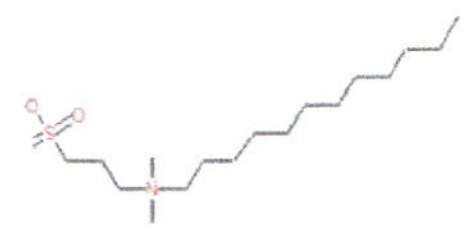	New chemical compound
7.	Neocurdione	$C_{15}H_{24}O_2$	236.17763	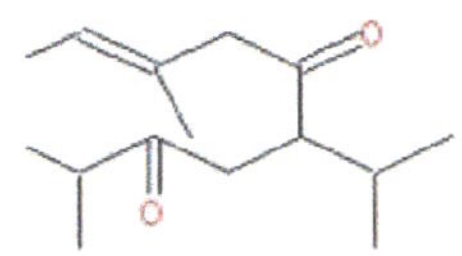	Anti-viral, anti-bacteria and anti-tumor activity
8.	Isoaromadendrene epoxide	$C_{15}H_{24}O$	220.182715	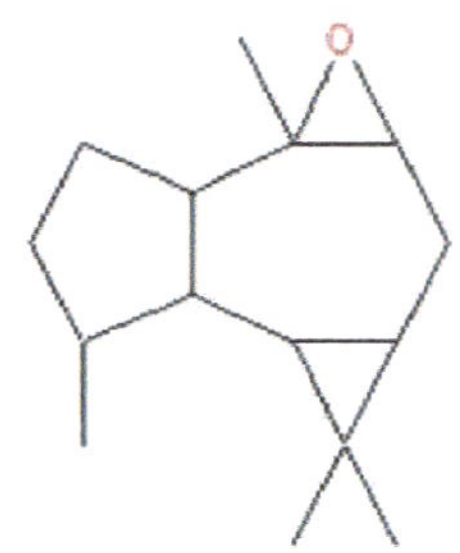	Antibacterial activity and antioxidant activity

Serial no.	Phytochemical compound	Formula	Exact mass	Chemical structure	Pharmacological actions
9.	1b,4a-Epoxy-2H-cyclopenta[3, 4] cyclopropa[8, 9]cycloundec.	$C_{22}H_{32}O_8$	424.209419	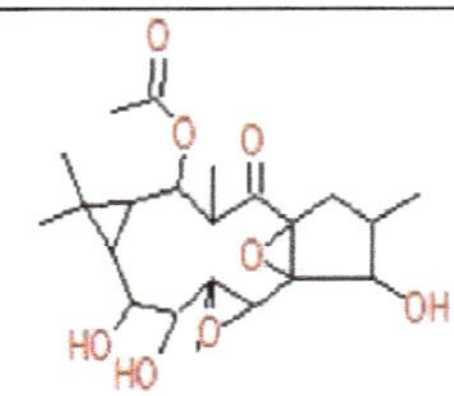	New chemical compound
10.	cis-Vaccenic acid	$C_{18}H_{34}O_2$	282.25588	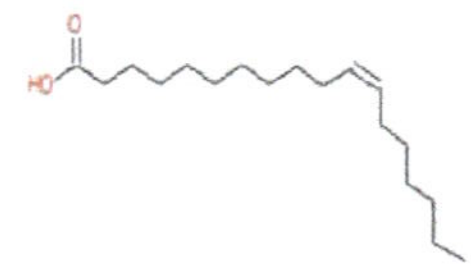	Anti-inflammatory
11.	2-Phenanthrenol,4b,5,6,7,8,8a,9,10-octahydro-4b,8,8-trimethyl-1	$C_{20}H_{30}O$	286.226999	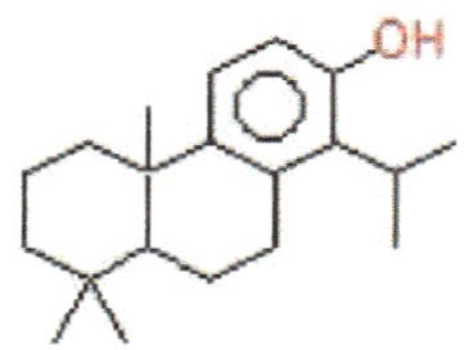	Antimicrobial activity
12.	Galanthamine	$C_{17}H_{21}NO_3$	287.152143	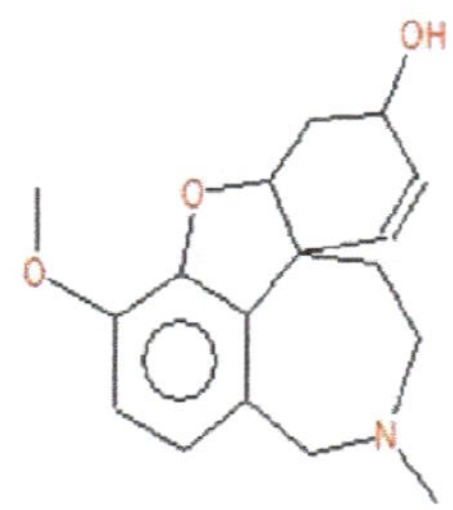	Galantamine hydrobromide is a tertiary alkaloid drug that has been developed and approved in a number of countries including the USA and several countries in Europe as a treatment for mild-to-moderate Alzheimer's disease (AD)

Serial no.	Phytochemical compound	Formula	Exact mass	Chemical structure	Pharmacological actions
13.	Dibenz[a,c] cyclohexane,2,4,7-trimethoxy	$C_{18}H_{20}O_3$	284.141245	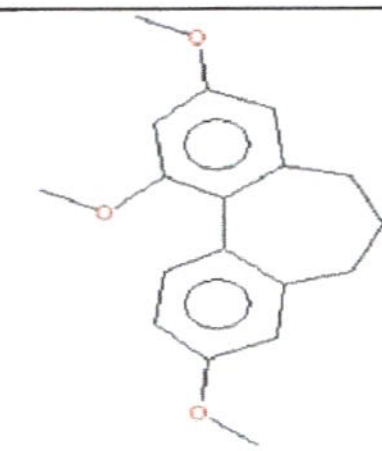	New chemical compound
14.	2,4a,7-Trihydroxy-1-methyl-8-methyleneqibb-3-ene. 1,10-carboxylic acid.	$C_{19}H_{22}O_6$	346.141623	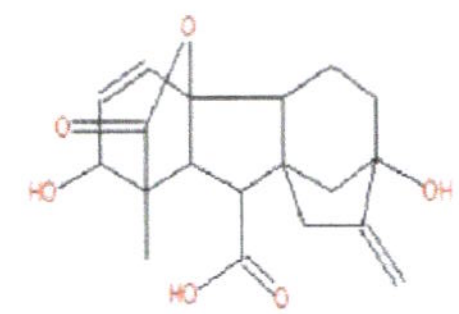	New chemical compound
15.	Retinoic acid	$C_{20}H_{22}O_2$	300.208931	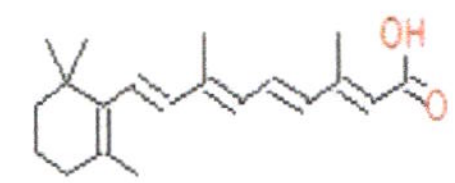	Antibacterial activity and antioxidant activity
16.	7,8,12-Tri-O-acetyl-3-desoxy-ingol-3-one	$C_{26}H_{34}O_9$	490.220284	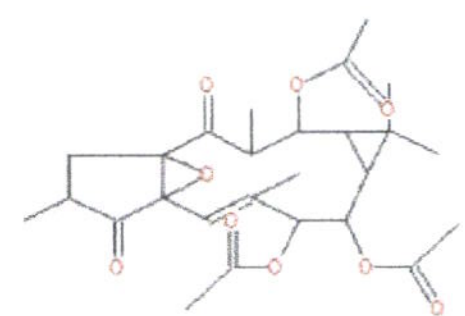	Antibacterial activity and antioxidant activity
17.	4,6-Androstadien-3β-ol-17-one,acetate	$C_{21}H_{28}O_3$	328.203844	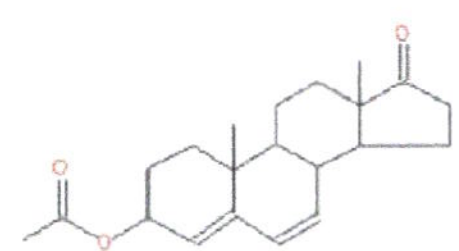	Antioxidant activity and antibacterial activity

Table 1. Phytochemical compounds identified in methanolic extract of *Rosmarinus officinalis*

5. Major chemical constituents of *R. officinalis* using gas chromatography-mass spectrum analysis

The GC-MS analysis of the plant extract was made in a (QP 2010 Plus SHIMADZU) instrument under computer control at 70 eV [18–36].

Gas chromatography and mass spectroscopy analysis of compounds was carried out in methanolic seed extract of *R. officinalis*, shown in **Table 1**. Among the identified phytocompounds have the property of antioxidant and antimicrobial activities. Plant-based antimicrobials have enormous therapeutic potential as they can serve the purpose with lesser side effects [37–41]. In addition, rosemary harvested in Portugal is rich in myrcene (25%), 1,8-cineole, and camphor [42] while rosemary from North East of Spain presents an essential oil (EO) containing camphor and α-pinene as main constituents [43]. Furthermore, the essential oil of Lebanese rosemary is characterized by 1,8-cineole (20%) and α-pinene (18.8–38.5%) [44]. The major compounds of *R. officinalis*' essential oil from Eastern Cape Province in South Africa are verbenone (17.43%), camphor (16.57%), 1,8-cineole (11.91%), α-pinene (11.47%), borneol (5.74%), and camphene (5.70%) [45]. Many factors affect yield and chemical composition of essential oils such as drying, harvest period, harvest region, extraction technique, and the age of the plant [46, 47].

6. Antioxidant activity

Antioxidant activity of *R. officinalis* is due to its phenolic compounds including carnosic acid, carnosol, rosmarinic acid, and hydroxycinnamic acid ester. Rosemary uptake improves memory, and it is sometimes used as an antidepressant. It is also useful against cough and digestive disorders such as diarrhea, spasms, and flatulence. Thanks to diuretic and antispasmodics properties, the aerial parts of rosemary are orally used to relieve renal colic and dysmenorrhea [48–52].

7. Antibacterial activity

R. officinalis and *R. eriocalyx* EOs are extremely active on *Pseudomonas aeruginosa* and *Klebsiella pneumoniae* strains. This result is very important especially for *P. aeruginosa*, which is known for its high resistance to all antibiotics. These results have some similarities with those of Taoufik Ouassil since he found that *R. officinalis* is active against the four species of bacteria (*Escherichia coli*: <14 mm, *Staphylococcus aureus*: <14 mm, *P. aeruginosa*: 14 mm, *K. pneumoniae*: 14 mm). Diameters of inhibition concerning *E. coli* and *S. aureus* are similar to ours but a great difference can be observed concerning *P. aeruginosa* and *K. pneumoniae*. Many researchers have highlighted sensitivity of Gram (+) bacteria compared to Gram (−) while testing natural extract but in our case it seems that Rosmarinus' essential oils are more active against Gram (−) bacteria. *R. officinalis* essential oil expressed a strong inhibitory activity against *K. pneumoniae* with an MIC of 2.08 mg/ml, and *S. aureus* with an MIC of 8.35 mg/ml. *E. coli* and

P. aeruginosa were inhibited with 16.7 mg/ml. *R. officinalis* EO has also a bactericidal power. Minimal bactericidal concentrations were 4.17 mg/ml for *K. pneumoniae* and 33.4 mg/ml for *E. coli, S. aureus*, and *P. aeruginosa*. According to our results, the MBC/MIC ratios are lower than four for all strains, so both essential oils have a bactericidal power against the tested strains. In Turkey (Izmir), Yesil Celiktas et al. (2007) worked on *R. officinalis* and found the following MIC: *E. coli* (20 mg/ml), *S. aureus* (10 mg/ml), *P. aeruginosa* (10 mg/ml), and *K. pneumoniae* (20 mg/ml). Okoh et al. [45] found that South African sample of *R. officinalis* (oriental region of the Cape) exhibited the following MIC: *E. coli* (7.5 mg/ml), *S. aureus* (3.75 mg/ml), and *K. pneumoniae* (0.94 mg/ml).

8. Brain, cardiovascular, gastrointestinal and other medicinal uses

It is used as carminative, rubifacient, and stimulant and as flavoring agent for liniments, hair lotions, inhaler, soaps, and cosmetics. Rosemary leaves have many traditional uses based on their antibacterial and spasmolytic actions. They are used orally for the treatment of dyspeptic complaints, and in external applications for supportive management of rheumatic complaints and circulatory disorders. *Aetheroleum Rosmarini* crude drug may enhance cognition. It is used as a cholagogue, diaphoretic, digestant, diuretic, emmenagogue, laxative, and tonic and also used in the management of headache, menstrual disorders, nervous menstrual complaints, tiredness, defective memory, sprains, and bruises:

1. Brain and nervous system conditions.
2. Cardiovascular conditions: It improves circulation, raises blood pressure, and stimulates the weak heart subject to palpitation when consumed in small doses.
3. Gastrointestinal circulatory systems: In conditions of bad breath, and stomach upset. Promotes proper digestion, toning, and calming effect on the digestion.
4. Reproductive system conditions: Stimulates the sexual organs.
5. Respiratory system: Colds and colic.
6. Other uses: The oil is used as perfume in ointments, shampoos, and soaps. The flowers are laid in clothes and cupboards to destroy moths. The leaves are crushed into meats, fish, potato salads, and so on.

9. Pharmacological properties

Singletary and Nelshoppen [53] studied the "Inhibition of 7, 12-dimethylbenz[c]anthracene (DMBA)-induced mammary tumorigenesis and of in vivo formation of mammary DMBA-DNA adducts by rosemary extract." Rosemary extract induces mammary tumorigenesis and in vivo formation of mammary dimethyl benz anthracene DNA adducts [54]. Hyperglycemic and insulin release inhibitory effects of *R. officinalis*. Krause et al. [55] studied the "Bioavailability of the antioxidative *R. officinalis* compound carnosic acid in eggs." Using this method, carnosic acid could be detected in 20 ng/g of egg yolk. Results showed that carnosic acid is bioavailable in egg yolk but not in albumen. Yen et al. [56] worked on the "Measurement of antioxidative activity in metal ion-induced lipid peroxidation systems." The antioxidant activity of α-tocopherol is less than that of rosemary extracts in the iron ion-induced peroxidation systems. Samman et al. [57] reported that "Green tea or rosemary extract added to foods reduces non-heme-iron absorption." The presence of the phenolic-rich extracts resulted in decreased non-heme-iron absorption [58]. Haloui et al. [59] studied the effects of aqueous extracts of the crude drug on the treatment of kidney function and diuresis in rats was determined. Jaswir et al. [60] studied "The synergistic effects of rosemary, sage, and citric acid on fatty acid retention of palm olein during deep-fat frying." A combination of 0.076% oleoresin rosemary extract, 0.066% sage extract, and 0.037% citric acid produced the optimal retention of the essential fatty acid [61]. Sotelo-Félix et al. [62] worked on the evaluation of the effectiveness of *R. officinalis* (Lamiaceae) in the alleviation of carbon tetrachloride-induced acute hepatotoxicity in the rat. Histological evaluation showed that *R. officinalis* partially prevented CCl4-induced inflammation, necrosis and vacuolation. Park et al. [63] reported the "Neuroprotective effect of *R. officinalis* extract on human dopaminergic cell line, SH-SY5Y. *R. officinalis* might potentially serve as an agent for the prevention of several human neurodegenerative diseases caused by oxidative stress and apoptosis. Sacchetti et al. [64] worked on the "Comparative evaluation of 11 essential oils of different origin as functional antioxidants, antiradicals and antimicrobials in foods." Antioxidant and radical-scavenging properties were tested by means of 1,1-diphenyl-2-picrylhydrazyl (DPPH) assay, b-carotene bleaching test, and luminol-photochemiluminescence (PCL) assay. Cavero et al. [65] reported the "*In vitro* antioxidant analysis of supercritical fluid extracts from rosemary (*R. officinalis* L.)." Using forward stepwise multiple linear regression, carnosic acid, methyl carnosate, and carnosol were the compounds selected to predict the mentioned activity, with a value of 0.95 for the coefficient of determination. Antioxidant, antibacterial, and antifungal activities of the extracts were confirmed [66]. Moghtader et al. [67] reported "The evaluation of antioxidant potential of *Veronica officinalis and R. officinalis* extracts by monitoring malondialdehyde and glutathione levels in rats." The reduced and total glutathione were quantified from rat plasma, after derivatization with o-phthalaldehyde, using a high-performance liquid chromatography (HPLC) method with florescence detection. Salido et al. [68] studied the "Oxidative stress modulation by *R. officinalis* in CCl4-induced liver cirrhosis." The effect produced by a methanolic extract of *R. officinalis* on CCl4-induced liver cirrhosis in rats was investigated using both prevention and reversion models.

10. Conclusion

R. officinalis is the native plant of Iraq. It contains chemical constitutions which may be useful for various herbal formulations as anti-inflammatory, analgesic, antipyretic, cardiac tonic, and antiasthmatic. The phytochemical screening of the species has highlighted that both plants contain flavonoids, tannins, sterols and triterpenes, saponins, free anthraquinones, mucilages, cardiac glycosides, and catechols. Preliminary results of antibacterial study showed in vitro efficiency of *R. officinalis* and *R. eriocalyx* on all tested bacteria with minimum inhibitory concentrations ranging from 1.04 to 16.7 mg/ml. The results presented here may contribute to the knowledge of antimicrobial potential of these species. Other studies on extracts activities of these species are needed to compare them with essential oils activity. Rosemary is an exotic evergreen shrub with multiple medicinal and cosmetic properties. It is a popular herb which serves as flavoring agent and spice. Although it is well renowned for all these potencies, the oil of the plant is adhered with many side effects and hence lacks safety data. Therefore, the use of rosemary in pediatrics, as well as in pregnant women, should be always dealt with utmost care. It could be concluded that *R. officinalis* displays a wide variation in essential oil chemical composition in correlation with the climatic conditions under which it is grown, as well as the genetic variation, thus generating different chemotypes.

Acknowledgements

I thank Dr. Abdul-Kareem Al-Bermani, Lecturer, Department of Biology, for valuable suggestions and encouragement.

Author details

Imad Hadi Hameed[1,*] and Ghaidaa Jihadi Mohammed[2]

*Address all correspondence to: imad_dna@yahoo.com

1 Department of Nursing, Babylon University, Hilla City, Hillah, Iraq

2 College of Science, Al-Qadisiya University, Al Diwaniyah, Iraq

References

[1] Atik F, Bousmaha L, Taleb Bendiab SA, Boti JB. Casanova. Chemical composition of the essential oil of *Rosmarinus officinalis* L growing in the spontaneous and cultivated state of the Tlemcen region. Biol. Santé. 2007;7:6–11.

[2] Bult H, Herman AG, Rampart M. Modification of endotoxin induced haemodynamic and hematological changes in the rabbit by methylprednisolone, F(ab_) fragments and rosmarinic acid. Br. J. Pharmacol. 1985;84:317–327.

[3] Makino T, Ono T, Muso E, Yoshida H, Honda G, Sasayama S. Inhibitory effects of rosmarinic acid on the proliferation of cultured murine mesangial cells. Nephrol. Dial. Transplant. 2000;15:1140–1145.

[4] Juhas S, Bukovska A, Cikos S, Czikkova S, Fabian D, Koppel J. Antiinflammatory effects of *Rosmarinus officinalis* essential oil in mice. Acta Vet. Brno. 2009;78:121–127.

[5] Beninca JP, Dalmarco JB, Pizzolatti MG, Frode TS. Analysis of the anti-inflammatory properties of *Rosmarinus officinalis* L. in mice. Food Chem. 2011;124:468–475.

[6] Stefanovits E, Tulok MH, Hegedus A, Renner C, Varga S. Acta Biologica Szegediensis. 2003;47(1–4):111–113.

[7] Arnold N, Valentini G, Bellomaria B, Laouer H. Comparative study of the essential oils from *Rosmarinus eriocalyx* Jordan & Fourr. from Algeria and *R. officinallis* L. from other countries. J. Essent. Oil Res. 1997;9:167–175.

[8] Wang W, Wu N, Zu G, Fu YJ. Antioxidative activity of *Rosmarinus officinalis* L. essential oil compared to its main components. Food Chem. 2008;108:1019–1022.

[9] Sergi M, Leonor A. Subcellular compartmentation of the diterpene carnosic acid and its derivatives in the leaves of rosemary. Plant. Physiol. 2002;125:1094–1102.

[10] Troncoso N, Sierra H, Carvajal L, Delpiano P, Gunther G. Fast high performance liquid chromatography and ultraviolet visible quantification of principle phenolic antioxidants in fresh rosemary. J. Chromatogr. 2005;1100:20–50.

[11] Al-Sereiti MR, Abu-Amer KM, Sen P. Pharmacology of rosemary (*Rosmarinus officinalis*) and its therapeutic potentials. Indian J. Exp. Biol. 1999;37(2):124–130.

[12] Fiehn O. Metabolomics – the link between genotypes and phenotypes. Plant Mol. Biol. 2002;48:155–171.

[13] Sumner LW, Mendes P, Dixon RA. Plant metabolomics: largescale phytochemistry in the functional genomics era. Phytochemistry. 2003;62(6):817–836.

[14] Fernie AR, Trethewey RN, Krotzky AJ, Willmitzer L. Innovation – Metabolite profiling: from diagnostics to systems biology. Nat. Rev. Mol. Cell Biol. 2004;5:763–769.

[15] Kell DB, Brown M, Davey HM, Dunn WB, Spasic I, Oliver SG. Metabolic footprinting and systems biology: The medium is the message. Nat. Rev. Microbiol. 2005;3:557–565.

[16] Robertson DG. Metabolomics in toxicology: A review. Toxicol. Sci. 2005;85:809–822.

[17] European Pharmacopoeia, 2005. Direct. Qual. Med. Counc. Eur. (EDQM), Strasbourg.

[18] Altameme HJ, Hameed IH, Abu-Serag NA. Analysis of bioactive phytochemical compounds of two medicinal plants, *Equisetum arvense* and *Alchemila valgaris* seed using gas chromatography-mass spectrometry and Fourier-transform infrared spectroscopy. Malays. Appl. Biol. 2015b; 44(4):47–58.

[19] Hamza LF, Kamal SA, Hameed IH. Determination of metabolites products by *Penicillium expansum* and evaluating antimicrobial activity. J. Pharmacogn. Phytother. 2015;7(9):194–220.

[20] Hameed IH, Altameme HJ, Idan SA. Artemisia annua: Biochemical products analysis of methanolic aerial parts extract and anti-microbial capacity. Res. J. Pharmaceut. Biol. Chem. Sci. 2016;7(2):1843–1868.

[21] Hameed IH, Hamza LF, Kamal SA. Analysis of bioactive chemical compounds of *Aspergillus niger* by using gas chromatography-mass spectrometry and Fourier-transform infrared spectroscopy. J. Pharmacog. Phytother. 2015b;7(8):132–163.

[22] Hameed IH, Hussein HJ, Kareem MA, Hamad NS. Identification of five newly described bioactive chemical compounds in methanolic extract of *Mentha viridis* by using gas chromatography-mass spectrometry (GC-MS). J. Pharmacog. Phytother. 2015c;7(7):107–125.

[23] Altameme HJ, Hadi MY, Hameed IH. Phytochemical analysis of *Urtica dioica* leaves by Fourier-transform infrared spectroscopy and gas chromatography-mass spectrometry. J. Pharmacog. Phytother. 2015a;7(10):238–252.

[24] Hameed IH, Ibraheam IA, Kadhim HJ. Gas chromatography mass spectrum and Fourier-transform infrared spectroscopy analysis of methanolic extract of *Rosmarinus officinalis* leaves. J. Pharmacog. Phytother. 2015d;7(6):90–106.

[25] Al-Marzoqi AH, Hadi MY, Hameed IH. Determination of metabolites products by *Cassia angustifolia* and evaluate antimicrobial activity. J. Pharmacog. Phytother. 2016;8(2):25–48.

[26] Al-Marzoqi AH, Hameed IH, Idan SA. Analysis of bioactive chemical components of two medicinal plants (*Coriandrum sativum* and *Melia azedarach*) leaves using gas chromatography-mass spectrometry (GC-MS). Afr. J. Biotechnol. 2015;14(40):2812–2830.

[27] Hussein AO, Mohammed GJ, Hadi MY, Hameed IH. Phytochemical screening of methanolic dried galls extract of *Quercus infectoria* using gas chromatography-mass spectrometry (GC-MS) and Fourier transform-infrared (FT-IR). J. Pharmacog. Phytother. 2016;8(3):49–59.

[28] Altameme HJ, Hameed IH, Idan SA, Hadi MY. Biochemical analysis of *Origanum vulgare* seeds by Fourier-transform infrared (FT-IR) spectroscopy and gas chromatography-mass spectrometry (GC-MS). J. Pharmacog. Phytother. 2015c;7(9):221–237.

[29] Jasim H, Hussein AO, Hameed IH, Kareem MA. Characterization of alkaloid constitution and evaluation of antimicrobial activity of *Solanum nigrum* using gas chromatography mass spectrometry (GC-MS). J. Pharmacog. Phytother. 2015;7(4):56–72.

[30] Hussein HJ, Hadi MY, Hameed IH. Study of chemical composition of *Foeniculum vulgare* using Fourier transform infrared spectrophotometer and gas chromatography - mass spectrometry. J. Pharmacog. Phytother. 2016;8(3):60–89.

[31] Hadi MY, Mohammed GJ, Hameed IH. Analysis of bioactive chemical compounds of *Nigella sativa* using gas chromatography-mass spectrometry. J. Pharmacog. Phytother. 2016; 8(2): 8–24.

[32] Mohammed GJ, Al-Jassani MJ, Hameed IH. Anti-bacterial, antifungal activity and chemical analysis of *Punica grantanum* (pomegranate peel) using GC-MS and FTIR spectroscopy. Int. J. Pharmacog. Phytochem. Res. 2016;8(3):480–494.

[33] Hussein HM, Hameed IH, Ibraheem OA. Antimicrobial activity and spectral chemical analysis of methanolic leaves extract of *Adiantum Capillus-Veneris* using GC-MS and FT-IR spectroscopy. Int. J. Pharmacog. Phytochem. Res. 2016;8(3):369–385.

[34] Kadhim MJ, Mohammed GJ, Hameed IH. In *vitro* antibacterial, antifungal and phytochemical analysis of methanolic fruit extract of *Cassia fistula*. Orient. J. Chem. 2016;32(2):10–30.

[35] Shareef HK, Muhammed HJ, Hussein HM, Hameed IH. Antibacterial effect of ginger (*Zingiber officinale*) roscoe and bioactive chemical analysis using gas chromatography mass spectrum. Orient. J. Chem. 2016; 32(2): 20–40.

[36] Al-Jassaci MJ, Mohammed GJ, Hameed IH. Secondary metabolites analysis of *Saccharomyces cerevisiae* and evaluation of antibacterial activity. Int. J. Pharmaceut. Clin. Res. 2016;8(5):304–315.

[37] Boutekedjiret C, Bentahar F, Belabbes R and Bessiere J. Extraction of rosemary essential oil by steam distillation and hydrodistillation. Flavour Fragr. J. 2003;18:481–484.

[38] Viuda M, Yolanda R, Juana F, José P. Chemical composition of the essential oils obtained from some spices widely used in Mediterranean Region. Acta Chim. Slov. 2007;54:921–926.

[39] Jamshidi R, Afzali Z, Afzali D. Chemical composition of hydrodistillation essential oil of rosemary in different origins in Iran and comparison with other countries. American-Eurasian J. Agric. Environ. Sci. 2009;5(1):78–81.

[40] Ram SV, Rahman L, Sunita M, Rajesh K V Amit C, Anand S. Changes in essential oil content and composition of leaf and leaf powder of *Rosmarinus officinalis*. CIM-Hariyali during storage. Maejo Int. J. Sci. Technol. 2011;5(02):181–19.

[41] Zaouali Y, Taroub B, Mohamed B. Essential oils composition in two *Rosmarinus officinalis* L. varieties and incidence for antimicrobial and antioxidant activities. Food Chem. Toxicol. 2010;48:3144–3152.

[42] Serrano E, Palma J, Tinocco T, Venencio F, Martins A. Evaluation of the essential oils of rosemary (*Rosmarinus officinalis* L.) from different zones of "Alentejo" (Portugal). J. Ess. Oil Res. 2002;14:87–92.

[43] Guillen M, Cabo NJ. Characterisation of the essential oils of some cultivated aromatic plants of industrial interest. J. Sci. Food Agric. 1995;70:359–363.

[44] Diab Y, L Auezova, H Chebib, JC Chalchat, G Figueredo. Chemical composition of Lebanese rosemary (*Rosmarinus officinalis* L.) essential oil as a function of the geographical region and the harvest time. J. Ess. Oil Res. 2002;14:449–452.

[45] Okoh O, Sadimenko AP, Afolayan AJ. Comparative evaluation of the antibacterial activities of the essential oils of *Rosmarinus officinalis* L. obtained by hydrodistillation and solvent free microwave extraction methods. Food Chem. 2010;120:308–312.

[46] Aberchane M, Fechtal M, Chaouch A, Bouayoune T. Influence of the duration and the extraction technique on the yield and the quality of the essential oils of the Atlas cedar (Cedrusatlantica manetti). Ann. Of Forest Research in Morocco. 2001;34:110–118.

[47] Bourkhiss M, Hnach M, Bourkhiss B, Ouhssine M, Chaouch A, Satrani B. Effet de séchage sur la teneur et la composition chimique des huiles essentielles de Tetraclinisarticulata (Vahl) Masters. Agrosolutions. 2009;20(1):44–48.

[48] Mizrzhi I, Juarez MA, Bandoni A. Essential oils of *Rosemarinus officinalis* growing in Argentina. J. Essent. Oil Res. 1991;3:11.

[49] Reverchon E, Senatore F. Isolation of rosemary oil: comparison between hydrodistillation and supercritical CO extraction. Flavor Frag. J. 1992;7:227.

[50] Chalchat JC, Carry RP, Michet A, Benjilali B, Chabart JL. Essential oils of rosemary, the chemical composition between hydrodistillation and supercritical CO extraction. J. Essent. Oil. Res. 1993;41:613.

[51] Pino JA, Estrarron M, Fuentes V. Essential oil of rosemary (*Rosemary officinalis* L.) from Cuba. J. Essent. Oil Res. 1998;10:111.

[52] Gonzalez-Trujano, ME, EI Pena, AL Martinez, J Moreno, P Guevara-Fefer, M Deciga-Campos, FJ Lopez-Munoz. Evaluation of the antinociceptive effect of *Rosmarinus officinalis* L. using three different experimental models in rodents. J. Ethnopharmacol. 2007;111:476–482.

[53] Singletary KW, Nelshoppen JM. Inhibition of 7,12-dimethylbenz[c]anthracene (DMBA)-induced mammary tumorigenesis and of *in vivo* formation of mammary DMBA-DNA adducts by rosemary extract. Cancer Lett. 1991;60:169–175.

[54] Al-Hader A, Hasan Z, Aqel M. Hyperglycemic and insulin release inhibitory effects of *Rosmarinus officinalis*. J. Ethnopharm. 1994;43:217–221.

[55] Krause EL, Ternes W. Bioavailability of the antioxidative *Rosmarinus officinalis* compound carnosic acid in eggs. Europ. Food Res. Technol. 1999;3,161–164.

[56] Yen GC, Chen HY, Lee CE. Measurement of antioxidative activity in metal ion-induced lipid peroxidation systems. J. Sci. Food Agric. 1999;79(9):1213–1217.

[57] Samman S, Sandström B, Toft MB, Bukhave K, Jensen M, Sørensen SS. Green tea or rosemary extract added to foods reduces nonheme-iron absorption. Am. J. Clin. Nutr. 2001;73:607–612.

[58] Dias PC, Foglio MA, Possenti A, Carvalho JE. Antiulcerogenic activity of crude hydroalcoholic extracts of *Rosmarinus officinalis* L. J. Ethnopharm. 2000;69:57–62.

[59] Haloui M, Louedec L, Michel JB, Lyoussi B. Experimental diuretic effects of *Rosmarinus officinalis* and *Centaurium erythraea*. J. Ethnopharm. 2007;71:465–472.

[60] Jaswir J, Che YB, Kitts DD. Synergistic effects of rosemary, sage, and citric acid on fatty acid retention of palm olein during deep-fat frying. JAOCS. 2000;77(5):527–533.

[61] Galobart J, Barroeta AC, Baucells MD, Codony R, Ternes W. Effect of dietary supplementation with rosemary extract and α-tocopheryl acetate on lipid oxidation in eggs enriched with ω3-fatty acids. Poultry Sci. 2001;80:460–467.

[62] Sotelo-Félix JI, Martinez-Fong D, Muriel P, Santillán RL, Castillo D, Yahuaca P. Evaluation of the effectiveness of *Rosmarinus officinalis* (Lamiaceae) in the alleviation of carbon tetrachloride-induced acute hepatotoxicity in the rat. J. Ethnopharmac. 2001;81:145–154.

[63] Park SE, Kim S, Sapkota K, Kim SJ. Neuroprotective effect of *Rosmarinus officinalis* extract on human dopaminergic cell line, SH-SY5Y. Cell. Molec. Neurobiol. 2001;30(5):759–767.

[64] Sacchetti G, Maietti S, Muzzoli M, Scaglianti M, Manfredini S, Radice M, Bruni R. Comparative evaluation of 11 essential oils of different origin as functional antioxidants, antiradicals and antimicrobials in foods. Food Chem. 2005;91:621–632.

[65] Cavero S, Jaime L, Martín-Alvarez PJ, Señoráns FJ, Reqlero G, Ibañez E. *In vitro* antioxidant analysis of supercritical fluid extracts from rosemary (*Rosmarinus officinalis* L.). Eur. Food Res. Technol. 2005;221:478–486.

[66] Aziza KG, Haiko H, Smānia AJ, Machado S. Rosemary (*Rosmarinus officinalis*) – a study of the composition, antioxidant and antimicrobial activities of extracts obtained with supercritical carbon dioxide. Cienc. Technol. Aliment., Campinas. 2008;28(2):463–469.

[67] Moghtader M, Salari H, Farahmand A. Evaluation of the antifungal effects of rosemary oil and comparison with synthetic borneol and fungicide on the growth of *Aspergillus flavus*. J. Ecol. Nat. Environ.2011;3(6):210–214.

[68] Salido S, Altarejos J, Nogueras M, Sanchez A, Lugue P. Chemical composition and seasonal variations of rosemary oil from southern Spain. J. Essen. Oil Res. 2003;15:10–14.

7

Lesser Known Aromatic Plants in Nigeria

Ngozichukwuka P. Igoli and John O. Igoli

Abstract

Herbs and spices are used in all cultures as natural foodstuffs and for medicinal purposes. *Siphonochilus aethiopicus*, *Monodora myristica* and *Crateva adansonii* are some of the spices which are not commonly used. They improve the taste of food, and through their anti-oxidant, anti-microbial and anti-fungal properties, they could act as food preservatives. There is an accumulation of evidence for the usage of these spices medicinally as anti-inflammatory, anti-plasmodial, anti-sickling, anti-oxidant and chemopreventive agents. There have also been investigations to identify the active constituents of these spices and to verify their pharmacological actions. This article aims at reviewing the available data on these investigations and the basis for usage in several diseases and conditions.

Keywords: *Siphonochilus aethiopicus*, *Monodora myristica*, *Crateva adansonii*, herbs, spices

1. Introduction

Aromatic herbs and spices are widely used in Nigeria for culinary and medicinal purposes. While some are quite common and used worldwide, others like: wild ginger (*Siphonochilus aethiopicus* (Schweinf) B.L Burtt), African nutmeg (*Monodora myristica* (Gaertn) Dunal) and sacred garlic pear (*Crateva adansonii* DC) are not. Herbs and spices make important contributions towards the odour and flavour of foods due to the presence of volatile (essential) oils and fixed oils. They confer new aromas to the foods, and their use for improving the taste of foods is a cultural achievement of all races which also led to cultural exchanges very early in history [1]. Moreover, there is an increasing interest in using the extracts of herbs and spices, for food preservation [2] since as natural foodstuffs, they appeal to many consumers who question the safety of synthetic food additives due to their carcinogenicity or other concerns [3, 4]. Indeed, since prehistoric times, herbs were the basis for nearly all medicinal therapy until synthetic drugs were developed, and even today, herbs are still found in 40% of prescription drugs [5].

Thus, in addition to imparting characteristic pleasant flavours, certain herbs and spices prolong the storage life of foods by preventing rancidity through their anti-oxidant activity or through bacteriostatic or bactericidal activity [6]. Consequently, herbs and spices have medicinal values, anti-oxidant and anti-microbial properties [7], and some do contain potent phytochemicals, which provide significant protection against cancer [8].

Wild ginger is an herb with perennial tuberous roots giving rise to annual leafy stems which grows in sub-Saharan Africa especially in savannah regions or regions with dry season [9]. It belongs to the family Zingiberaceae and has leafy shoots (pseudo-stem) which grow to about 35 cm high after flowering and is common throughout the West African region and elsewhere in tropical Africa [9]. The rhizomes which have a terrific scent of violets and ginger are spindle shaped and are about 5 cm by 1 cm, arranged radially on lateral roots that spread fairly readily underground [9]. The Nigerian variety flowers between April and May after the early rains and the flowers, which appear before the leaves, come up in considerable quantity followed by the leaves and the pseudo-stem [10]. The flowers, just borne above ground level in inflorescences separate from the leafy shoot, are purple with white corolla tube and a yellow flare on the central petal and are 7–10 cm long [9]. The leafy shoot dries up between September and December after which it falls off. The herb is found in the wild and could also be cultivated.

The South African variety is a deciduous aromatic plant, bisexual or female, up to 1 m high and sprout annually from the underground stem in spring [11]. The leaves are glabrous and 30–400 × 50–90 mm in size, light green, lance shaped and borne on the end of stem-like leaf bases [11, 12]. Between October and February, it gives faintly scented flowers that are white to bright pink with yellow markings on lip, white corolla tubes 30–40 mm long and tepal lobes 60–80 mm wide [12]. The tremendously attractive flowers often appear before the leaves in spring, perhaps to allow them to be more visible to pollinators [13]. They may also vary in colour from bright pink, purple-pink, yellow to white with a yellow centre and are delicately scented. About 15 flowers are produced per plant over the flowering season, each lasting a single day [14].

The roots, tubers and rhizomes of wild ginger are used for their aroma and medicinal properties in the West and South of Africa. While they are used as spice by the Igede people of Benue State of Nigeria [15], others mainly use them in traditional medicine for colds, coughs, influenza, hysteria, pain and malaria amongst other ailments [16, 17]. It is also used by Zulu people as a protection against lightning and snakes [18]. Infusions of the rhizome and roots are anti-inflammatory (prostaglandin synthetase inhibition), bronchodilatory, smooth muscle relaxant, mild sedative, anti-candidal and used to treat headache, influenza, mild asthma, sinusitis, sore throat, thrush, epilepsy, hysteria and relieve dysmenorrhoea [11] or administered to horses as prophylactics against horse sickness [19]. It is in such popular demand and coupled with the method of harvesting which involves removal of the entire rhizome that it has become extinct in certain areas [20]. The plant does not set much seed and splitting rhizomes is the best available option for plant propagation [14].

The seeds of *Monodora myristica* (Gaertn.) Dunal either fresh or roasted are used both as a spice in cuisine and medicinally in different parts of Africa and in the Caribbean [21, 22]. It is largely underutilized and has recently been used as popcorn flavouring in an attempt to increase its utilization [23]. It is also responsible for the distinct flavour of the Nigerian delicacy "isi ewu", and it is used in soups and peanut paste [23, 24]. Its aroma which is enhanced by mild roasting is similar to nutmeg; thus, the plant is commonly known as African nutmeg, calabash nutmeg or Jamaican nutmeg; and it is a large tropical tree which can reach 35 m height and 2 m in diameter [25]. It is native to tropical West Africa and further east to Uganda, Kenya and Tanzania where it grows naturally in evergreen forests but has been introduced to Jamaica, other parts of the Caribbean and elsewhere [26]. Its large leaves (35 cm long and 18 cm wide) are purple at first but turn a smooth deep green on the upper side with paler green underneath. They are prominently veined, and the petiole is purplish. The exotic, conspicuous and scented flowers hang down on long stalks and have three calyx lobes and three petals arranged in two whorls [27]. The flowers are followed by large woody fruits filled with brown seeds embedded in an aromatic pulp [25]. The medicinal uses of the seeds are to treat headaches, pains, toothaches, haemorrhoids, stomach ache, relieve constipation and control passive uterine haemorrhage in women immediately after child birth [24, 25, 28] and hypertension [25].

The leaves of sacred garlic pear (*Crateva adansonii*) which are eaten with soups or mixed with cereal are also used medicinally in different parts of Africa and Asia [29, 30]. It belongs to the family Capparaceae and is widely distributed as a small handsome tree of the galleried forest and savannah woodland often found on river banks across Africa [29]. The species is confined to Africa but bears very close affinity to the Asian *Crateva religiosa* G. Forst with which it has been equated by some authorities [29]. It attains a height of 7 m or more with an irregular trunk which is seldom straight and could be cultivated for ornamental purposes due to its dense masses of white flowers borne at the ends of all the shoots [29]. Where it survives bush burning and repeated stripping of its leaves, the tree is often stunted. The wood is strong-smelling when cut and is soft and yellow [29]. In Eastern Nigeria, *C. adansonii* is used medicinally, its leaves being in high demand for the treatment of ear and parasitic infections [31]. The leaves are applied externally to relieve joint pains; the fresh juice from the leaves is used for the relief of ear ache, eye infection and anodyne in toothache [32]. The leaves are also used in fumigations for treating jaundice and yellow fever, applied to the head as a mild counter-irritant for easing headaches, and a steam bath of over the face is used as a remedy for all troubles due to poor vision [29]. The bark is said to be rubefacient and tonic, widely used as a remedy for stomach-troubles and used both internally and externally for treating sterility. It is used in combination with *Flacourtia flavescens* as a treatment for leprosy [29]. Powdered and boiled in oil, it is used as an application for rheumatic condition, and a bark paste is used as a poultice on swellings [29]. The powdered bark is used in rheumatism, itch, epilepsy, stomach troubles and asthma [33]. The powdered leaves and bark are considered to be rubefacient and are used especially on cysts. The root is used as a febrifuge and in several treatments for syphilis. The dried, ground roots are used as an application to swollen parts of the body, while the seeds have unspecified medicinal uses [29].

This review identifies lesser known aromatic plants in Nigeria and current reports on their utilization, constituents and properties. The aim is to provide an insight into the health-promoting potentials of biologically active constituents of: wild ginger (*Siphonochilus aethiopicus* (Schweinf) B.L Burtt), African nutmeg (*Monodora myristica* (Gaertn) Dunal) and sacred garlic pear (*Crateva adansonii* DC). This is because diets rich in plant foods can provide biologically active phytochemicals that promote health [34].

2. Constituent phytochemicals

The sensory perception of wild ginger depends on a variety of odorants including esters, monoterpenes, sesquiterpenes, aldehydes, pyrazines and thiophenes which are important for the mild and pleasant aroma both in the fresh and in roasted spice as against the hot/pungent flavours of ginger and other Zingiberaceae [35]. Aroma extracts dilution analysis (AEDA) employing the gas chromatography/olfactometry (GC/O) technique was reported for the organoleptic evaluation of these odorants and their odour quality together with quantification from GC-FID/GC-MS profiles [35]. Thus, the sweet/fruity ester flavours, methyl-2-/-3-methyl butanoates and derivatives of the apple flavour were reported to be the most important odorants perceived at the highest dilution of the aroma extract of the fresh spice [35]. These were followed by the monoterpene β-phellandrene which has a terpenish/woody odour and is also important for the aroma of ginger and dill [35–37]. Another sweet/fruity flavour propyl-2-methylbutanoate also an apple flavour follows before the roasty/earthy smelling 2-isopropyl-3-methoxypyrazine and 2-isobutyl-3-methoxypyrazine which are known to have a hot/paprika taste and are also present in paprika pepper and chillies [35–38]. The sesquiterpene curzerenone (sweet/coconut-like) is perceived at the next significant dilution together with the roasty/potato-like methional [35]. In the roasted sample, terpenish/woody β-phellandrene is the most important odorant followed by the roasty/earthy smelling pyrazines before the sweet/fruity flavoured butanoates. The pungent smelling principle 2-acetyl thiophene, which is absent in the fresh sample, is next followed by the sesquiterpene curzerenone (sweet/coconut-like) together with the roasty/potato-like methional [35].

Principal component analysis using GC shows that the constituents of wild ginger are mostly sesquiterpenes as against monoterpenoids or diterpenoids [16, 35, 39]. Five eudesmane sesquiterpenoids as shown in **Figure 1**: 4aαH-3,5α,8aβ-trimethyl-4,4a,8a,9-tetrahydronaphtho[2, 3b]-furan-8-one; 2-hydroxy-4aαH-3,5α,8aβ-trimethyl-4,4a,8a,9-tetrahydro-naphtho[2, 3b]-furan-8(5H)-one; 4aαH-3,5α,8aβ-trimethyl-4,4a,8a,9-tetrahydronaphtho-([2, 3b]-dihydrofuran-2-one)-8-one; 9aβ-hydroxy-4aαH-3,5α,8aβ-trimethyl-4,4a,8a,9-tetrahydronaphtho-([2, 3b]-dihydrofuran-2-one)-8-one and 4aαH-3,5α,8aβ-trimethyl-4,4a,8a-trihydronaphtho-([2, 3b]-dihydrofuran-2-one)-8-one were isolated as the constituents of the South African variety [16, 17]. However, the elemane sesquiterpenoids: curzerenone and *epi*-curzerenone, the germacrane sesquiterpenoids: furanodiene (8,12-epoxy-1(10)E,4Z,7,11-germacratetraene); isofuranodiene (8,12-epoxy-1(10)E,4Z,7,11-germacratetraene) and furanodienone (8,12-epoxy-1(10)E,4Z,7,11-germacratetraen-6-one) together with the labdane diterpenoids: 8(17),12E-labdadiene-15,16-dial, 15-hydroxy-8(17),12E-labdadiene-16-al, and 16-oxo-8(17), 12E-labdadiene-15-oic acid (zerumin A) as also shown in **Figure 1** were isolated from the Nigerian variety [35, 39].

A yield of 45-6g kg^{-1} essential oils containing 75% monoterpene hydrocarbons; the major compounds being: α-phellandrene (50–4%), α-pinene (5–5%) and myrcene (4–35%) has been reported for the African nutmeg [40]. Few sesquiterpene hydrocarbons (3%) and oxygenated compounds such as germacrene-D-4-ol (9–5%) were also reported as against another report of 25.48% germacrene-D-4-ol [41]. Meanwhile, an essential oil yield of 6.2% (dry weight basis) has also been reported [42]. Prenylated indole alkaloids are considered a chemotaxonomic

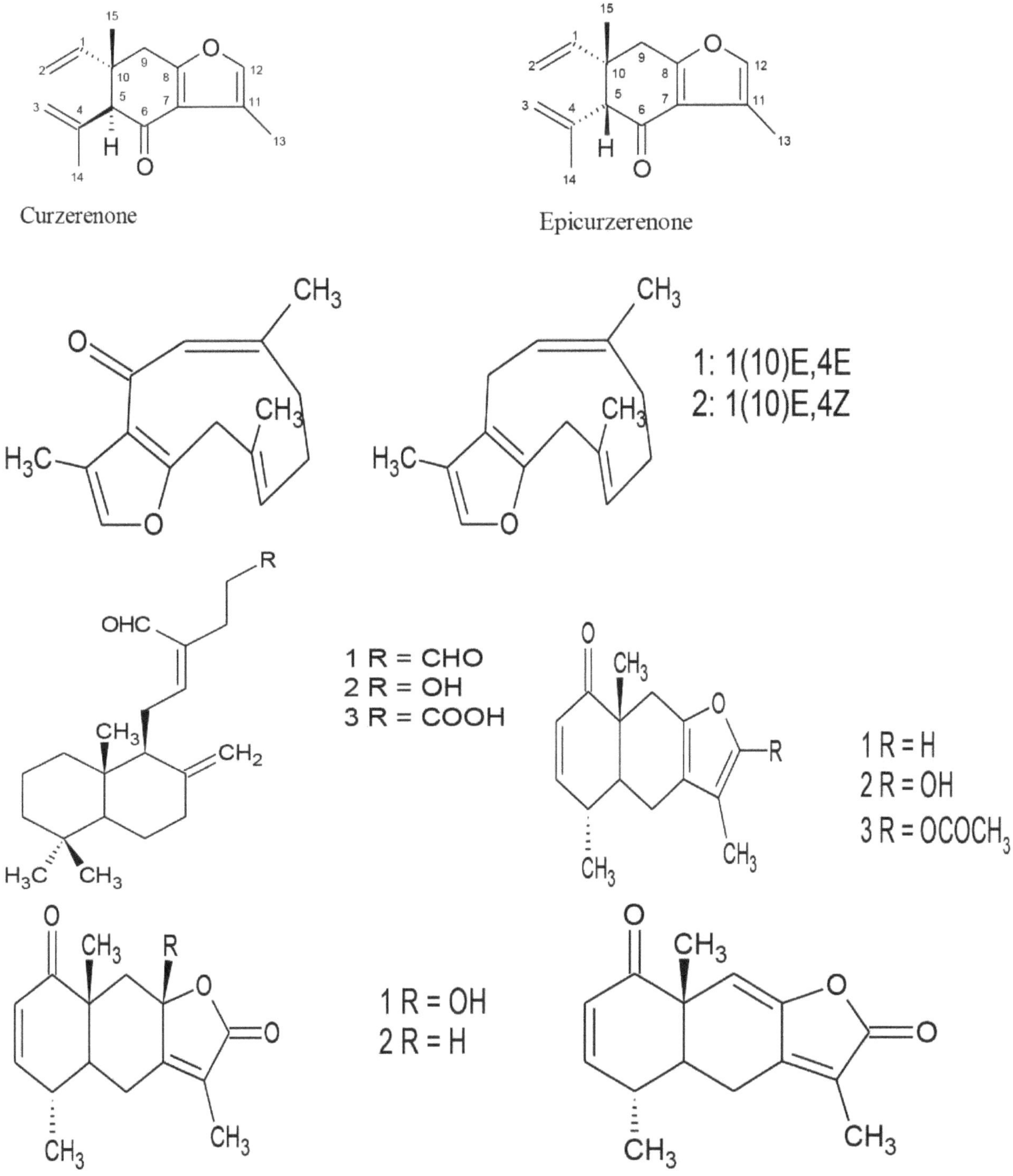

Figure 1. Isolated constituents of *Siphonochilus aethiopicus*.

marker of the genus, and 5-formyl indole and 5-(3-oxo-but-1-enyl) indole as shown in **Figure 2** have been reported from *Monodora myristica* and other species of *Monodora* [21, 43, 44].

The volatile oils of the sacred garlic pear whole plant reportedly show 43.5 and 41.1% oxygenated monoterpenes and aliphatic compounds, respectively. The major constituents are linalool (30.2%) and nonanal (17.2%), and it contains no sesquiterpene hydrocarbons [45]. The

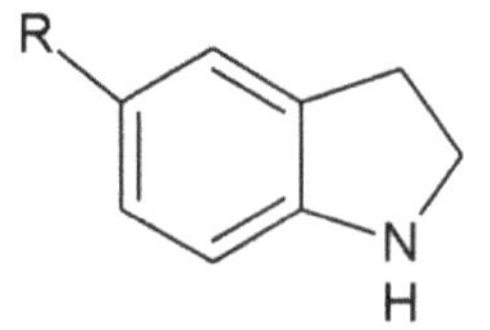

1 R = CHO
2 R = CH=CHCOCH$_3$

Figure 2. Isolated constituents of *Monodora myristica*

leaves are also known to have a disagreeable smell when crushed [29]. The triterpenes: oleanolic acid and 4-epi-hederagenin were isolated from the 1:1 C_2H_2:MeOH extract of its seed as shown in **Figure 3** [46]. Then, the hexane extract of the leaf yielded the antibiotic aurantiamide acetate while the ethyl acetate extract afforded ethyl pyropheophorbide A, purpurin-18 ethyl ester and pyropheophorbide A as also shown in **Figure 3** [31]. Additionally, the triterpene lupeol was also isolated from a 1:1 dichloromethane/methanol fraction of the leaf as illustrated in **Figure 3** [47].

It has been reported that the leaf and rhizome extracts of *S. aethiopicus* possess anti-microbial and anti-fungal properties [48]. However, the activities of the leaf extracts are much lower than those of the rhizome extracts which inhibited *Bacillus subtilis, Micrococcus kristinae, Bacillus cereus, Staphylococcus aureus, Staphylococcus epidermidis* and *Klebsiella pneumoniae* and showed anti-fungal properties against *Aspergillus flavus, Aspergillus glaucus, Candida albicans, Candida tropicalis, Trichophyton mentagrophytes* and *Trichophyton rubrum* [48, 49]. This is despite the similar chemical composition of the essential oils of the leaf and rhizome [20]. Again, the anti-fungal activities of some of the isolated constituents of the rhizomes and tubers: *epi*-curzerenone and furanodienone against *Candida albicans*, and 8(17),12E-labdadiene-15,16-dial against *Candida tropicalis* and *Candida guilliermondii* have been reported [50, 51]. Moderate activity of the crude rhizome extract and isolated diterpenes: 8(17),12E-labdadiene-15,16-dial and 15-hydroxy-8(17),12E-labdadiene-16-al against *Mycobacterium tuberculosis* has also been reported [39].

The in vitro anti-proliferative properties of the essential oils of wild ginger against MCF-7 cancer cells were reported [52]; indeed, it has been suggested that the presence of antiseptic monoterpenoids contributes to its bioactivity [11]. In vitro cytotoxicity determinations of the crude rhizome extract and isolated constituents using five cell lines: SH-SY5Y, Jurkat, L929, Hep G2 and Hs 27 were also carried out [39]. *Epi*-curzerenone and furanodienone were inactive against the five different cell lines tested, while two of the diterpenes reportedly showed specific cytotoxic effects. 8(17),12E-Labdadiene-15,16-dial had moderate effect on the normal cell line Hs 27 and was cytotoxic to SH-SY5Y, the cancerous Jurkat and L929. However, only Jurkat and SH-SY5Y were affected by 15-hydroxy-8(17),12E-labdadiene-16-al [39].

The in vitro and in vivo anti-inflammatory properties of *S. aethiopicus* have also been reported [53]. The rhizome extract and the isolated furanoterpenoid, 4aαH-3,5α,8aβ-trimethyl-4,4a,8a,9-tetrahydronaphtho[2, 3b]-furan-8-one, showed in vitro inhibition of glucocorticoid and histamine H1 receptor binding and phosphodiesterase IV activity [53]. OVA-sensitized and challenged mice showed significantly reduced lung inflammation and the percentage of eosinophils in bronchoalveolar lavage fluid after administration of *S. aethiopicus* extracts but airway hyper reactivity was not influenced supporting anecdotal accounts of effectiveness against asthma, sinusitis, colds and flu [53]. Another report on the anti-inflammatory properties of the extracts of various parts of *S. aethiopicus* showed that the in vitro cyclooxegenase-1 (COX-1) inhibition of the stem and leaf extracts was reportedly higher than that of the rhizome [54]. High

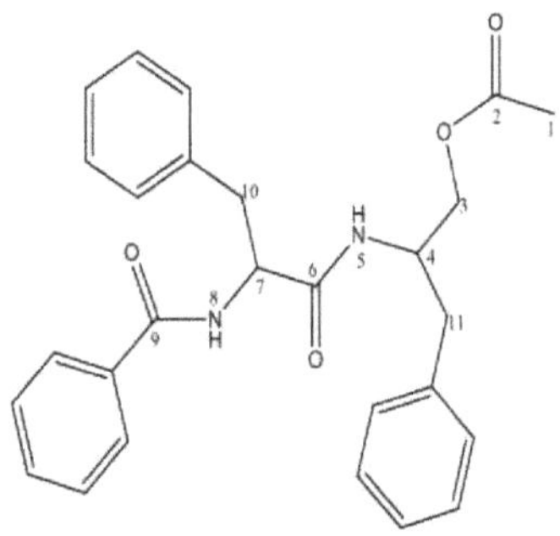

Aurantiamide acetate

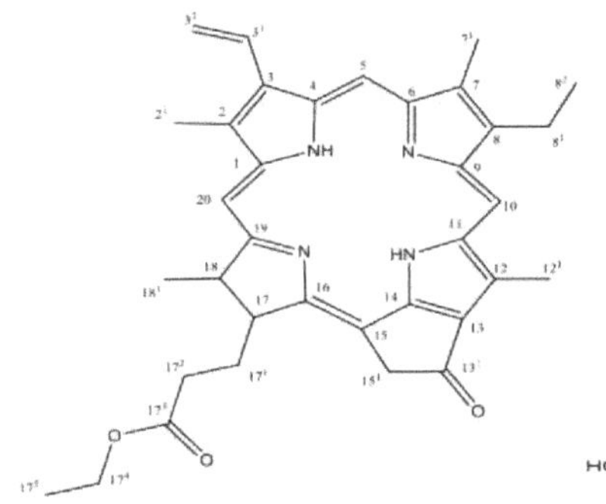

Ethyl Pyropheophorbide

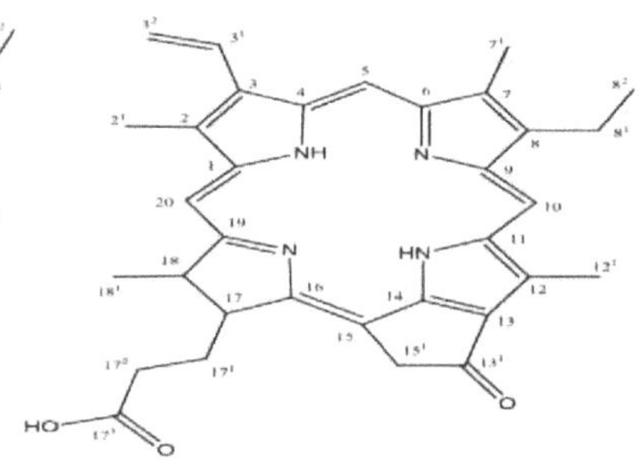

Pyropheophorbide A

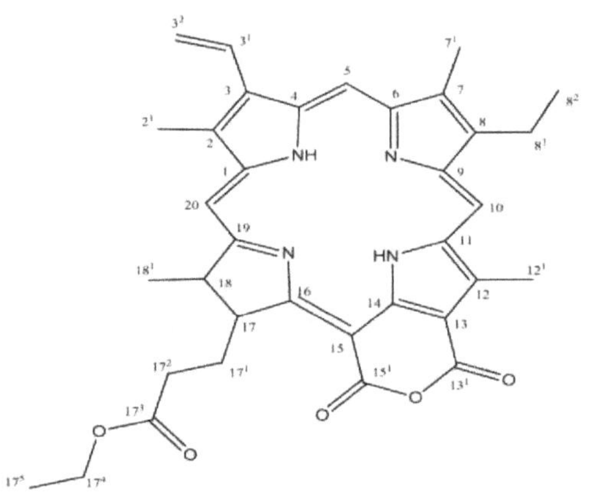

Purpurin-18 ethyl ester

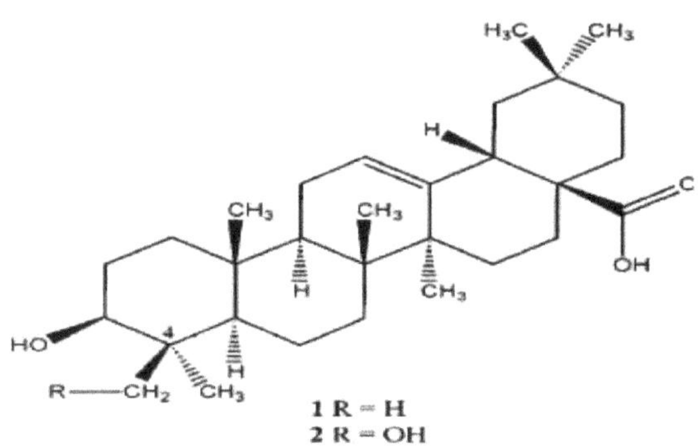

Oleanolic acid (1) and 4-epi-hederagenin (2)

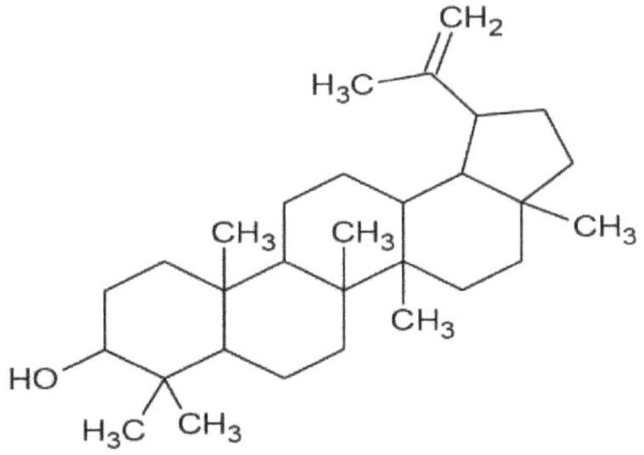

Lupeol

Figure 3. Isolated constituents from *Crateva adansonii* bioactivity.

inhibition of cyclooxygenase and hence the prostaglandin pathway which should prevent uterine contraction and relieve dysmenorrhoea was again reported for the leaves and tubers of wild ginger [55]. However, in vitro reduction of pre-contracted uterine muscle was not observed [55].

Additionally, the in vitro anti-plasmodial activity for the ethanolic extracts and isolated eudesmane sesquiterpenoids of *S. aethiopicus* rhizomes against the chloroquine-sensitive and chloroquine resistant strains of *Plasmodium falciparum* has also been reported [17]. The substitution of the OH group in the sesquiterpene structure with hydrogen resulted in a threefold increase in activity against the chloroquine-resistant strain and an introduction of a double bond further improved the activity [17]. It is suggested that the anti-plasmodial activity is due to the furan moiety [17, 56]. Further in vitro anti-protozoal property of *S. aethiopicus* was reported against T*rypanosoma brucei brucei* (S427) blood stream forms by the crude rhizome extract, and it increased with the pure components: 8(17),12E-labdadiene-15,16-dial, *epi*-curzerenone and furanodienone [39].

The crude seed extract of *Monodora myristica* and isolated 5-formyl indole and 5-(3-oxo-but-1-enyl)indole reportedly showed no in vitro cytotoxicity against normal PNT2A cells and no anti-trypanosomal activity against *Trypanosoma brucei brucei* (S427) blood stream forms [43]. There was also no in vitro cytotoxicity when the crude seed extract was tested against five different cancerous cell lines [57]. Similarly, no lethality against brine shrimp (*Artemia salina*) and low anti-microbial activity against the *Mycobacterium* species: *M. madagascariense* and *M. indicus pranii* were reported for the stem bark extract of *Monodora carolinae* and constituent 5-formyl indole [58]. However, some of these prenylated indole alkaloids reportedly show interesting in vitro anti-plasmodial properties against the multi-drug-resistant strain K1 of *Plasmodium falciparum* [59].

Again, there are reports on the in vitro anti-oxidant properties and protective potential against free radicals of *M. myristica* seeds which suggest usage in the management of diseases associated with oxidative stress [28, 59, 60]. In vivo studies on the aqueous extracts of the seed and fruit also suggest that anti-oxidant bio-constituents play an important role in the prevention of liver toxicity possibly by inhibiting bioaccumulation of free radicals in animal models and could also reverse liver toxicity induced by high cholesterol diets and exert hypocholesterolemic effects [25, 61].

Also, the crude seed extracts of *M. myristica* reportedly exhibit profound in vitro anti-sickling properties suggesting that the spice/extracts could be used in combination with other foods in the management and prophylactic control of sickle cell crisis [62].

In vitro anti-microbial properties have been reported for *C. adansonii* leaf extracts against *Pseudomonas aeruginosa, Escherichia coli, Salmonella typhii, Staphylococcus aureus, Klebsiella pneumoniae, Bacillus subtilis, Shigella sonei, Pasteurella pestis, Yersinia enterocolitica* and anti-fungal properties against two fungi: *Aspergillus niger* and *Candida albicans* [63–65]. It has also been suggested that the traditional use of the leaves against several inflammatory diseases such as rheumatism, arthritis and gout is due to xanthine oxidase inhibition [32].

In vitro anti-oxidant properties and in vivo analgesic properties have also been reported for the methanolic extracts of the stem bark [66]. The methanolic extracts of the leaves and constituent lupeol were also reported to show in vitro anti-oxidant properties [47].

Additionally, there is a report on the in vitro anti-trypanosomal activity of the leaf extracts and isolated aurantiamide acetate, ethyl pyropheophorbide A, purpurin-18 ethyl ester and pyropheophorbide A against the African trypanosome *Trypanosoma brucei brucei* (S427) blood stream forms [31]. *In silico* testing of these ligands with the potential biomolecular targets of *T. brucei*: riboflavin kinase, trypanothione reductase, sterol-14α-demethylase, rohedsain and glutathione synthetase revealed multi-functional scaffolds validating the possibility of anti-trypanosomal activity [31].

3. Conclusion

Overall, organoleptic studies encourage the increased utilization of wild ginger, African nutmeg and sacred garlic pear to flavour foods. Moreover, a significant number of in vitro and laboratory animal studies support and explain the folk medicinal usage of these herbs and spices. These spices have anti-microbial, anti-oxidant, anti-inflammatory and in some instances anti-plasmodial and anti-cancer actions. As several metabolic diseases and age-related degenerative disorders are closely associated with oxidative processes in the body, further clinical studies on the use of these spices or their constituents as sources of anti-oxidants and anti-inflammatory agents are needed.

Author details

Ngozichukwuka P. Igoli[1]* and John O. Igoli[2]

*Address all correspondence to: ngozi_igoli@yahoo.com

1 Centre for Food Technology and Research, Benue State University, Makurdi, Nigeria

2 University of Agriculture, Makurdi, Nigeria

References

[1] Alais C, Linden G. Food Biochemistry. 2nd ed. Maryland: Aspen; 1999. 213p.

[2] Smid EJ, Gorris LGM. Natural antimicrobials for food preservation. In: Rahman MS, editor. Handbook of Food Preservation. New York: Marcel Dekker; 1999. pp. 285–308.

[3] Ito N, Fukushima S, Hasegawa A, Shibata M, Ogiso T. Carcinogenicity of butylated hydroxy anisole in F344 rats. J. Natl. Cancer Inst. 1983; **70**: 343–347. doi:10.1093/jnci/70.2.343

[4] Shan B, Cai Y-Z, Brooks JD, Harold Corke H. The in vitro antibacterial activity of dietary spice and medicinal herb extracts. Int. J. Food Microbiol. 2007; **117**: 112–119. doi:10.1016/j.ijfoodmicro.2007.03.003

[5] Smith RJ, Winder ML. Medicinal Garden. In: Ober R, editor. The National Herb Garden Guidebook. Springfield: The Herb Society of America; 1996. pp. 61–71.

[6] Beuchat LR, Golden DA. Antimicrobials occurring naturally in foods. Food Technol. 1989; **43**: 134–142.

[7] Rehm S, Espig G. The Cultivated Plants of the Tropics and Subtropics. Berlin: Priese GmbH; 1991. pp. 277–321.

[8] Lai PK, Roy J. Antimicrobial and chemopreventive properties of herbs and spices. Curr. Med. Chem. 2004; **11**: 1451–1460. doi:10.2174/0929867043365107

[9] Burkill HM. The Useful Plants of West Tropical Africa. 2nd ed. vol. 5. Families S – Z. London: Crown Agents for Overseas Governments; 2000. 320–321p.

[10] Igoli NP. Identification of the flavour components of wild ginger (*Siphonochilus aethiopicus* (Schweinf) B.L. Burtt). [thesis]. Nsukka. University of Nigeria; 2009.

[11] Manzini TZ. Production of wild ginger (*Siphonochilus aethiopicus*) under protection and indigenous knowledge of the plant from traditional healers. [thesis]. Pretoria. University of Pretoria; 2005. [Internet] Available from: http://hdl.handle.net/2263/27497 [Accessed: 2016-09-06].

[12] Kiew KY. Taxonomic Studies in the genus *Kaempferia* (Zingiberaceae). Notes from the Royal Botanic Garden Edinburgh. 1980; **38**: 1–12.

[13] van Wyk B-E, Gericke N. People's Plants: A Guide to Useful Plants of Southern Africa. Pretoria: Briza Publications; 2007. 352pp.

[14] Nichols G. Some notes on the cultivation of Natal ginger (*Siphonochilus aethiopicus*). Veld Flora. 1989; **75**: 92–93.

[15] Igoli JO, Ogaji OG, Tor-Anyiin TA, Igoli NP. Traditional medicine practices amongst the igede people of nigeria. Part 11. Afr. J. Trad. CAM 2005; **2**: 134–152. doi:10.1.1.540.8653 &rep=rep1&type=pdf

[16] Holzapfel CW, Marais W, Wessels PL, Van Wyk BE. Furanoterpenoids from *Siphonochilus aethiopicus*. Phytochemistry. 2002; **59**: 405–407. doi:10.1016/S0031-9422(01)00402-2

[17] Lategan CA, Campbell WE, Seaman T, Smith PJ. The bioactivity of novel furanoterpenoids isolated from *Siphonochilus aethiopicus*. J. Ethnopharmacol. 2009; **121**: 92–97. doi:10.1016/j.jep.2008.10.007

[18] Hutchings A. A survey and analysis of traditional medicinal plants as used by the Zulu, Xhosa, and Sotho. Bothalia. 1989; **19**: 111–123. doi:10.4102/abc.v19i1.947

[19] Watt JM, Breyer-Brandwijk MG. The medicinal and poisonous plants of Southern and Eastern Africa. 2nd ed. London: Livingstone; 1962. 1467 p.

[20] Viljoen AM, Demirci B, Baser KH, van Wyk B-E. The essential oil composition of the roots and rhizomes of *Siphonochilus aethiopicus*. S. Afr. J. Bot. 2002; **68**: 115–116. doi:10.1016/S0254-6299(16)30467-7

[21] Nwaji MN, Onyiriuka SO, Taylor DA. 6-(3=Methylbuta-1 ,3=dienyl)indole from *Monodora tenuifolia*. J. Chem. Soc. Chem. Commun. 1972; 327–327. doi:10.1039/C39720000327

[22] Burkill HM, Dalziel JM. The Useful Plants of West Tropical Africa. vol. 1. Kew: Royal Botanic Gardens; 1985. 976 p.

[23] Enweruzoh RO, Okafor DC, Uzoukwu AE, Ukanwoke MO, Nwakaudu AA, Uyanwa CN. Flavour Extraction from *Monodora myristica* and Tetrapleura tetraptera and Production of Flavoured Popcorn from the Extract [Internet]. 2015. Available from: http://www.eajournals.org/wp-content/uploads/Flavour-Extraction-from-Monodora-myristica-And-Tetrapleura-tetraptera-and-Production-of-Flavored-Popcorn-from-the-Extract.pdf [Accessed: 2016-09-07].

[24] Eze-Steven PE, Ishiwu CN, Udedi SC, Ogeneh BO. Evaluation of antioxidant potential of *Monodora myristica* (African Nutmeg) [Internet]. 2013. Available from: http://www.ijcmas.com/vol-2-11/P.E.Eze-Steven, %20et %20al.pdf [Accessed: 2016-09-07].

[25] Nwozo SO, Kasumu TF, Oyinloye BE. African Nutmeg (*Monodora Myristica*) Lowers Cholesterol and Modulates Lipid Peroxidation in Experimentally Induced Hypercholesterolemic Male Wistar Rats [Internet]. 2015. Available from: https://www.ncbi.nlmnih.gov/pmc/articles/PMC4502738/ [Accessed: 2016-09-07].

[26] Keay RWJ. Trees of Nigeria. A revised version of Nigerian trees (1960, 1964) by Keay RWJ, Onochie CFA, Stanfield DP. Oxford: Clarendon; 1989. 5 p

[27] Kew Science. *Monodora myristica* (calabash nutmeg) Kew Science [Internet]. 2011? Avail–able from: http://www.kew.org/science-conservation/plants-fungi/monodora-myristica-calabash-nutmeg [Accessed: 2016-09-07].

[28] Feyisayo AK, Oluokun OO. Evaluation of antioxidant potentials of *Monodora myristica*(Gaertn) dunel seeds. Afr. J. Food Sci. 2013; **7**: 317–324. doi:10.5897/AJFS2013.1020

[29] Burkill HM. The Useful Plants of West Tropical Africa. vol. 1. Families A-D. Kew: Royal Botanic Gardens; 1985. 331–333p.

[30] Flowers of India. Garlic Pear Tree [Internet]. 2008? Available from: www.flowersofIndia.net/catalog/slides/Garlic%20Pear%20Tree.html [Accessed: 2016-09-13].

[31] Igoli NP, Clements CJ, Singla RK, Igoli JO, Nzekwe U, Gray AI. Anti-trypanosomal activity & docking studies of *Crateva adansonii* DC leaves: novel multifunctional scaffolds. Curr. Top. Med. Chem. 2014; **14**: 981–990.

[32] Abudullahi A, Hamzah RU, Jigam AA, Yahya A, Kabiru AY, Muhammad H, Sakpe S, Adefolalu FS, Isah MC, Kolo MZ. Inhibitory activity of xanthine oxidase by fractions *Crateva adansonii*. J. Acute Dis. 2012; **1**:126–129. doi:10.1016/S2221-6189(13)60029-3

[33] Sivarajan VV, Balachandran I. Ayurvedic Drugs and their Plant Sources. Delhi: Oxford and IBH Publishing; 1994. pp. 234–456.

[34] Shukla Y, Singh M. Cancer preventive properties of ginger: a brief review. Food Chem. Toxicol. 2007; **45**: 683–690. doi:10.1016/j.fct.2006.11.002

[35] Igoli NP, Obanu ZA. The volatile components of wild ginger (*Siphonochilus aethiopicus* (Schweinf) B.L. Burtt). Afr. J. Food Sci. 2011; **5**: 541–549.

[36] Belitz H-D, Grosch W. Food Chemistry. Berlin: Springer-Verlag; 1999. 319p.

[37] Kirk RS. Pearson's Composition and Analysis of Foods. Kirk RS, Sawyer R, editors. 9th ed. Essex: Longman; 1991. 393 p.

[38] Bruice PY. Organic Chemistry. 5th ed. New Jersey: Pearson; 2007. 732p.

[39] Igoli NP, Obanu ZA, Gray AI, Clements C. Bioactive diterpenes and sesquiterpenes from the rhizomes of wild ginger (*Siphonochilus aethiopicus* (Schweinf) B.L. Burtt). Afr. J. Trad. CAM. 2012; **9**: 88–93.

[40] Onyenekwe PC, Ogbadu GH, Deslauriers H, Gagnon M, Collin GJ. Volatile constituents of the essential oil of *Monodora myristica* (Gaertn) dunal. J. Sci. Food Agric. 1993; **61**: 379–381. doi:10.1002/jsfa.2740610317

[41] Owokotomo IA, Ekundayo O. Comparative study of the essential oils of *Monodora myristica* from Nigeria [Internet]. Available from: http://www.eurchembull.com/index.php/ecb/article/view/48/108 Accessed: 2016-09-14.

[42] Nguefack J, Letha V, Amvam Zollo PH, Mathur SB. Evaluation of five essential oils from aromatic plants of Cameroon for controlling food spoilage and mycotoxin producing fungi. Int. J. Food Microbiol. 2004; **94**: 329–334. doi:10.1016/j.ijfoodmicro.2004.02.017

[43] Igoli JO, Gray AI, Clements CJ, Mouad HA. Antitrypanosomal activity and Cytotoxicity of some Compounds and Extracts from Nigerian Medicinal Plants. In: Phytochemical-Bioactivities and impact on Health. Croatia: Intech; 2011. pp. 375–388.

[44] Nkunya MH, Makangara JJ, Jonker SA. Prenylindoles from Tanzanian *Monodora* and *Isolona* Species. Nat. Prod. Res. 2004; **18**: 253–258. doi:10.1080/14786410310001620529

[45] Ogunwade IA, Ogunbinu AO, Flamini G, Cioni PL, Okeniyi SO. Essential oil profiles of some Nigerian medicinal plants. J. Essent. Oil-Bearing Plant. 2009; **12**: 225–235.

[46] Cantrell CL, Berhow MA, Phillips BS, Duval SM, Weisleder D, Vaughn SF. Bioactive crude plant seed extracts from the NCAUR oilseed repository. Phytomedicine. 2003; **10**: 325–333. doi:10.1078/094471103322004820

[47] Tchimene MK, Nwaehujor CO, Ezenwali M, Okoli CC, Iwu MM. Free radical scavenging activity of lupeol isolated from the methanol leaf extract of *Crateva adansonii* Oliv. (Capparidaceae). Int. J. Pharmacogn. Phytochem. Res. 2016; **8**: 419–426.

[48] Coopoosamy RM, Naidoo KK, Buwa L, Mayekiso B. Screening of Siphonochilus aetiopicus (Schweinf.) B. L. Burtt for antibacterial and antifungal properties. J. Med. Plants Res. 2010; **4**: 1228–1231. doi:10.5897/JMPR10.240

[49] Stafford GI, Jäger AK, van Staden J. Effect of storage on the chemical composition and biological activity of several popular South African medicinal plants. J. Ethnopharmacol. 2005; **97**: 107–115. doi:10.1016/j.jep.2004.10.021

[50] Dolara P, Corte B, Ghelardini C, Pugliese AM, Cerbal E, Menichetti S, Lo Nostro A. Local anaesthetic, antibacterial and antifungal properties of sesquiterpenes from myrrh. Planta Med. 2000; **66**: 356–358. doi:10.1055/s-2000-8532

[51] Morita H, Itokawa H. Cytotoxic and antifungal diterpenes from the seeds of *Alpinia galanga*. Planta Med. 1988; **54**: 117–120. doi:10.1055/s-2006-962365

[52] Noudogbessi JP, Delort L, Chalard P, Billard H, Figueredo G, Ruiz N, Chalchat JC, Sohounhloue D, Chézetquée FC. Anti-proliferative activity of four aromatic plants of Benin. J. Nat. Prod. I. 2013; **6**: 123–131.

[53] Fouche G, Nieuwenhuizen N, Maharaj V, van Rooyen S, Harding N, Nthambeleni R, Jayakumar J, Kirstein F, Emedi B, Meoni P. Investigation of in vitro and in vivo anti-asthmatic properties of *Siphonochilus aethiopicus* [Internet]. 2011. Available from: <http://researchspace.csir.co.za/dspace/bitstream/10204/5647/1/Fouche_2011.pdf> [Accessed: 2016-09-14].

[54] Zschocke S, Rabe T, Taylor JL, Jäger AK, van Staden J. Plant part substitution—a way to conserve endangered medicinal plants? J. Ethnopharmacol. 2000; **71**: 281–292. doi:10.1016/S0378-8741(00)00186-0

[55] Lindsey K, Jäger AK, Raidoo DM, van Staden J. Screening of plants used by Southern African traditional healers in the treatment of dysmenorrhea for prostaglandin-synthesis inhibitors and uterine relaxing activity. J. Ethnopharmacol. 1999; **64**: 9–14. doi:10.1016/S0378-8741(98)00097-X

[56] Pillay P, Vleggar R, Maharaj VJ, Smith P, Lategan CA, Chouteau F, Chibale K. Antipla–smodial hirsutinolides from *Vernonia staehelinoides* and their utilization towards simplified pharmacophore. Phytochemistry. 2007; **68**: 1200–1205. doi:10.1016/j.phytochem.2007.02.019

[57] Iweala EEJ, Liu F-F, Cheng R-R, Li Y, Omonhinmin CA, Zhang Y-J. Anti-cancer and free radical scavenging activity of some Nigerian food plants in vitro. Int. J. Cancer Res. 2015; **11**: 41–51. doi:10.3923/ijcr.2015.41.51

[58] Magori N, Nyandoro SS, Munissi JJE, Heydenreich M. Antimycobacterial and cytotoxicity evaluation of the constituents of *Monodora carolinae* [Internet]. 2013. Available from: http://www.ajol.info/index.php/tjs/article/download/105696/95712

[59] Onguéné PA, Ntie-Kang F, Lifongo LL, Ndom JC, Sippl W, Mbaze LM. The potential of anti-malarial compounds derived from African medicinal plants. Part I: A pharmacological evaluation of alkaloids and terpenoids. Malaria J. 2013; **12**: 449. doi:10.1186/1475-2875-12-449

[60] Erukainure OL, Oke OV, Owolabi FO, Kayode FO, Umanhoulen EE, Aliyu M. Chemical properties of *Monodora myristica* and its protective potentials against free radicals in vitro. Oxid. Antioxid. Med. Sci. 2012; **1**:127–132. doi:10.5455/oams.080712.or.009

[61] Oyinloye BE, Adenowo AF, Osunsanmi FO, Ogunyinka BI, Nwozo SO, Kappo AP. Aqueous extract of *Monodora myristica* ameliorates cadmium-induced hepatotoxicity in male rats. Springerplus. 2016; **5**: 641. doi:10.1186/s40064-016-2228-z

[62] Uwakwe AA, Nwaoguikpe RN. *In-vitro* antisickling effects of *Xylopiaa ethiopica* and *Monodora myristica*. J. Med. Plant Res. 2008; **2**: 119–124.

[63] Igoli NP, Gray AI, Clements C, Igoli JO, Nzekwe U, Singla RK. Scientific Investigation of Anti-trypanosomal Activity of *Crateva adansonii* DC Leaves. Indo Global J. Pharm. Sci. 2012; **2**: 226–229.

[64] Agboke AA, Attama AA, Momoh MA. Evaluation of the antimicrobial activities of crude extract of *Cryptolepis sanguinolenta* and *Crateva adansonii* leaves and their interactions. J. Appl. Pharm. Sci. 2011; **1**: 85–89.

[65] Lagnika L, Anago E, Atindehou M, Adjahoutonon B, Dramane K, Sanni A. Antimicrobial activity of *Crataeva religiosa* Forst against bacteria isolated from *Thryonomys swinderianus* Temminck. Afr. J. Biotechnol. 2011; **10**: 10034–10039. doi:10.5897/AJB10.2435

[66] Udeh NE, Onoja SO. Analgesic and free radical scavenging activities of hydromethanolic extract of *Crateva adansonii* stem bark. J. Intercult. Ethnopharmacol. 2015; **4**: 224–227. doi:10.5455/jice.20150430010855

8

From Medicinal Plant Raw Material to Herbal Remedies

Sofija M. Djordjevic

Abstract

The use of medicinal plants is old as the existence of mankind. According to World Health Organization (WHO) data, about 80% of world population are using products based on medicinal herbs. Phytotherapy is based on the use of herbal drugs and medicinal products for the purpose of prevention and treatment. Rational phytotherapy is a modern concept of herbal medicines using, which are made of standardized herbal extracts. The quality of each final product is guaranteed by the use of raw materials of a standard quality, defined process of production, and validated equipment. Quality control of herbal drugs and herbal isolates (tinctures, extracts, and essential oils) is done according to the requirements of Pharmacopoeia and other relevant regulations. The scope of phytopreparation quality control depends on its pharmaceutical form. The formulation of a new phytopreparation is a process that has strictly defined phases: from analysis of literature and market, through defining recipes, validation of the production process, quality control of a final product to the preparation of technological and registration documents. The aim of this chapter is to present the process of herbal preparations production from selecting plant raw materials to herbal remedies (on the examples of making tea, tea mixture, drops, gels, and capsules).

Keywords: medicinal plants, medicinal plant raw material, quality control, formulation of phytopreparation, regulations

1. Introduction

Since ancient times, medical plants and simpler herbal remedies have been used in all parts of the world for the treatment and alleviation of various ailments. Although the use of medicinal plants is as old as mankind itself, their controlled application, the isolation and characterization of active substances, started only in the early nineteenth century. It is a known fact that the extractive plant isolates and isolated active substances played a major role in the development of modern pharmacotherapy. Many of the isolated compounds are still used today, or they have served as a model for the synthesis of a large number of drugs [1].

The use of plants as medicines has a long history in the treatment of various diseases. Plants especially those with ethnopharmacological uses have been the primary sources of medicine for early drug discovery.

Herbal remedies, from simple to complex forms, should be made of the raw materials required for quality, because only then they could be safe and effective for use. The Pharmacopoeia monographs, Monographs European Medicinal Evaluation Agency (EMEA), which encompasses monographs World Health Organization (WHO), European Scientific Cooperative on Phythotherapy (ESCOP), and Commission E (The German Commission E is a scientific advisory board of the "Bundesinstitut für Arzneimittel und Medizinprodukte" formed in 1978. The commission gives scientific expertise for the approval of substances and products previously used in traditional, folk, and herbal medicine) national regulations, precisely defined parameters of control quality.

The process of drafting a new herbal remedies is very complex and strictly defined phase. Each step in the process is important, from the initial idea, market analysis, selecting high-quality plant material and ancillary pharmaceutical raw materials, recipe formulation, production preparation, quality control of product, preparation of documentation, protection of intellectual property rights, to the introduction of herbal drug in regular production. The drafting process must be validated and secure documentation.

In modern pharmacotherapy, despite the widespread use of drugs obtained by chemical synthesis, the importance of herbal medicines in the treatment and prophylaxis is still large. According to the latest WHO researches, 11% of the 252 basic medicines are in fact herbal preparations [1].

2. Development and manufacturing of herbal preparations

2.1. Use of medicinal plants through history

The use of medicinal plants in the prevention and treatment of various diseases is known since ancient times. Documents of exquisite value show that herbs were extensively used by human population throughout the history. Since ancient times, people have sought safety and relief for their health problems in medicines from nature. Prehistoric men have dared to use particular medicinal plants, based on careful observation of the behavior of animals who have been using them [2, 3]. Over time, the use of herbal medicines and other natural products has developed on the basis of both positive and negative experiences. The collected rich experiences have gradually developed into folk medicine, such as traditional European medicine, traditional Chinese medicine, Indian Ayurveda, Japanese Kampo, or traditional Arabic and Islamic medicine. They consist, not only of herbal remedies but also of other types of drugs, for example, from minerals or animals, or physical procedures [3].

Material evidence on the use of medicinal plants in the distant past is kept by many ethnographic and archaeological sources. The oldest of these sources are clay tables, discovered in Mesopotamia (2600 BC), which in addition to the description showed also therapeutic application and galenical form in which the plants were to be used. In those ancient times, medical plants mentioned were castor oil, grapes, coffee, oils of cedar and cypress, licorice, myrrh, and poppy juice [4, 5]. The ancient Egyptian papyrus, Ebers Papyrus (1550 BC), represented some kind of first Pharmacopoeia. Egyptians were known for their skill of embalming, distilling scented water, and making perfume of aromatic plants, and for those they were using many medicinal plants that are still in use today (aloe, peppermint, plantain, poppy seeds, and coriander) [6]. The first written records about the use of medical herbs in Chinese traditional medicine date from the third millennium BC. Emperor Shen Nung made a collection of wild medicinal plants. He is credited with the discovery of tea and many of which are used nowadays: cinnamon, ephedra, rhubarb, camphor, and great yellow gentian [6, 7]. The Indian holy books provide many examples of the treatments using medical plants, widespread in that country. A large number of aromatic herbs and spices that are still in use nowadays throughout the world, such as pepper, cloves, nutmeg, originate from India. According to data from the Bible and the holy Jewish book, the Talmud, during various rituals accompanying a treatment, aromatic plants were utilized such as myrtle and incense [7].

With comprehensive development of science in ancient Greece, the pharmacy also receives a special place. The most famous doctor of ancient Greece, which is considered to be the "father of medicine," is Hippocrates (460–377 BC). He was the first to systematize overall medical and pharmaceutical experience and publish them in the capital work Corpus Hyppocraticum. The most ancient botanist Theophrastus (371–286 BC) together with his students founded the first botanical garden in Athens. He described more than 500 most important medicinal plants. Among others, he referred to cinnamon, iris rhizome, false hellebore, mint, pomegranate, cardamom, fragrant hellebore, monkshood, and so on. In the description of the plant, its toxic action was also stated [4, 7]. The founder of the European pharmacognosy, a Roman doctor of Greek origin, Dioscorides, who lived in the first century BC., described medicinal plants which were used in the ancient world, in his capital work De Materia Medica. Dioscorides' most appreciated domestic plants were as follows: willow, camomile, garlic, onion, marsh mallow, ivy, nettle, sage, common centaury, coriander, parsley, sea onion, and false hellebore. The strong influence of Hippocrates and Dioscorides was notable in the school of Alexandria, where some of the major breakthroughs in medicine were made. Unfortunately, a great fire has destroyed the vast library with approximately two million books, and at the same time all the knowledge of medicinal plants of that era [4, 7]. By the Roman conquest of Greece, Romans took over all the medical and pharmaceutical knowledge and certainly the most important mind in this area was the Roman statesman and military leader Pliny, the Elder (23–79). He is the writer of the capital work Historia naturalis. The most famous Roman doctor and a pharmacist is well-known Galenius-Galen, who lived from 131 to 201 and is considered to be the father of galenic pharmacy. In his writings on the development of complex preparations or galenic preparations, he described 304 drugs of plant origin [4].

The Arabs preserved a large amount of the Greco-Roman knowledge during the Dark and Middle ages (i.e., fifth to twelfth centuries), and complemented it with their own medicinal expertise, and with herbs from Chinese and Indian traditional medicines [8]. The treatments during the Middle Ages were conducted in the restricted environment of monasteries. Skills of cultivation and collection of herbal medicines, as well as making simple herbal remedies, were reserved for doctors-monks. They used the different herbs: mint, sage, tansy, anise, fenugreek, savory, and so on [7].

At the time of Charles V, the famous medical school of Salerno was founded and started its rise by introducing and applying experiences of Arab medicine and pharmacy. Benedictine monks played an important role in the preservation of the Greco-Roman tradition. Their legacy was large botanical gardens where mainly medicinal plants were grown [4]. The Arab world has promoted many sciences including medicine and pharmacy. Certainly, the most famous Arabic doctor was Abu Ali Ibn Sina (Avicenna) and his famous book, The Canon of Medical Science, has been translated into Latin and other languages, and has been used in Europe for many years.

In medieval Europe, the level of medical knowledge was quite low. Arab medicine, starting from the twelfth century, began to penetrate into Europe, through Spain and Sicily. The Arabic books were translated into Latin medicine, and in this sense also the Arabic translations of ancient Greek and Roman books. Paracelsus (during the late Middle Ages) argued that the salubrity of plant originates from chemical compounds that are represented in it [4]. In the eighteenth century, Swedish botanist Carl von Linné (1707–1778) created the Latin nomenclature for each plant (the name of the genus and species), and a botanical system for determining the species, which due to its transparency and convenience is used even nowadays. Scientific pharmacy began only after the French Revolution, and with it the development of the science of medicinal plants. In this area, the most distinguished pharmacists became Lavoisier in France, Scheele in Sweden, Priestley in England, and so on. [4]. The turning point in the approach and the use of herbal medicines is considered to be the beginning of the nineteenth century, when a German pharmacist Sertürner managed to isolate the alkaloid of morphine in its pure form, from poppy (1806). In the period from 1817 to 1820, French scientists isolated a whole series of alkaloids: caffeine, emetine, quinine, cinchonine, and strychnine. Improvements of instrumental analytical methods have allowed further detection of other groups and complexes of active substances, such as heterosides, saponosides, tannins, vitamins, and so on [7].

In the twentieth century, a large number of synthetic drugs were created and it represented the beginning of commercial production of a large number of allopathic medicines, which significantly led to neglect the use of herbs in pharmacotherapy.

2.2. Plants are valuable sources of drug discovery

As already mentioned, herbal medicines have been an extremely important source for the discovery of many drugs. Morphine, which was the first purely natural product to be isolated, was introduced in pharmacotherapy in 1826 (Merck). The first semisynthetic pure substance of aspirin, salicylic acid-based, was isolated from the bark of *Salix alba* willow and was produced in 1899 (Bayer). This was followed by the isolation of active compounds from old herbal drugs, such as digitoxin, codeine, pilocarpine, quinine, and many others, some of which are still in use today. Many herbal remedies, emerged after extensive scientific tests of "old and well-known" medicinal plants, were introduced in the therapy. Silymarin, extracted from the seeds of *Silibum marianum*, is used as a hepatoprotective, Paclitaxel from the bark of *Taxus brevifolia* in the treatment of lung, ovarian, and breast cancer, and Artemisinin from *Artemisia annua* herb to combat multiple-resistant malaria [1].

In recent years, many herbal medicines have found their way into the official medicine. Some of them are Dronabinol and Cannabidiol isolated from *Cannabis sativa*, Tiotropium derivative of atropine from *Atropa belladonna* for combating obstructive and chronic bronchitis, Galantamine, alkaloid from *Galanthus nivalis* which is used to relieve symptoms of Alzheimer's disease, and Apomorphine, which is a semisynthetic compound based on morphine from *Papaver somniferum* and is intended for people suffering from Parkinson's disease [1]. We can certainly say that a large number of medicinal plants, which in the past, were used and represent an important raw material for the production of herbal medicines, or have served as a model for similar synthesis of new molecules.

Given that man is an integral part of nature, the human body is compatible with medicines coming from nature. Nature, much like a flawless, perfect complex of laboratories, has created a variety of sophisticated active compounds contained in herbal medicines, which have a huge range of remedial action. Perhaps, this fact will speed up serious research of old manuscripts related to herbal medicines and brings out the "old drugs" of pure historical curiosity [8].

2.3. Basic terms related to herbal medicines

Phytotherapy, as a complementary part of pharmacotherapy, has an important place in many areas of modern medicine. It represents a system of treatments based on the use of natural medicinal resources (drugs) and herbal remedies (herbal remedies) in the purposes of prevention and treatment.

Herbal drug is the whole or grained, dried part of a plant, algae, fungi, or lichen, which is used for its medicinal properties. In addition to the plant organs (above-ground part of the blooming plant as flower, leaf, root, bark, fruit, and seed), plant exudates can also be considered as a drug (resins, balsams, and rubber). Herbal medicines, herbal remedies, or herbal medicinal products (HMPs) contain as active ingredients exclusively herbal drugs or herbal drug preparations. Herbal drug preparations are obtained from drugs, with the procedures of distillation, extraction, filtration, and so on. This concept does not include powdered forms of drugs, essential oils, fatty oils, tinctures, and extracts [9, 10].

Rational phytotherapy is a modern concept of use of herbal medicines, which was designed in Germany at the end of the last century and soon widely accepted in other European countries. It was created from the need to improve phytotherapy, in order for herbal preparations to be more efficient, safer, and their use based on the results of clinical trials. Herbal medicines, which are used in rational phytotherapy, are prepared from standardized herbal extracts, the chemical nature of their active principles is known, they exhibit dose-dependent therapeutic effect, their adverse effects and contraindications are known, and their pharmaceutical quality is well defined and standardized [11, 12].

Herbal medicines are used preventively, in the treatment of milder forms of a disease, or as adjunctive therapy for the treatment of chronic diseases. Most commonly, they are applied with the dysfunction of the respiratory, digestive, urogenital tract, mild, and medium forms of anxiety and depression, as well as of different lesions of the skin and mucous membranes. Their healing effects accrue gradually, so that the maximum effect manifested 2–3 weeks after the application.

2.4. Regulations

According to the WHO, preparations based on medicinal herbs are used by 80% of the world population. Medical use of medicinal plants has a long tradition in Europe, while in some parts of the world (e.g., China and India), herbal remedies still represent a central link in the chain of health services [13].

Extractive isolates of herbal medicines and herbal preparations are extremely complex multicomponent mixtures, as opposed to synthetic drugs that are most commonly a single pure compound. In the production of herbal remedies, certain actions and procedures are needed to be undertaken (collecting medicinal plants from spontaneous flora and plantation cultivation, obtaining extractive isolates, and their characterization), which do not precede the production of synthetic drugs. Fortunately, the procedures of making herbal medicines are largely modernized and defined in all segments. There are a number of guidelines that prescribe standards in all aspects of making herbal medicines: The European Medicines Agency guidelines for the quality of herbal medicines, the WHO guidelines provide standards and guidelines for good agricultural practices, good laboratory practices, and so on. The development of new, sophisticated analytical, and technological methods and procedures within the development and characterization of extractive isolate has greatly improved the quality of the final plant products. On the other hand, the process of harmonization of the quality system for the production and herbal drugs control is present in many countries. But globally speaking, more effort is yet to be made in order to revive the prescribed guidelines and regulations in practice [3]. The main goal of the Committee for herbal products (Herbal Medicinal Product Committee—HPMC) is to prepare a detailed list of monographs and processed herbal substances and preparations, which are in medical use for long enough time that their use is safe under normal conditions. The monograph contains the professional opinion of the Committee on a particular plant products based on scientific data or traditional use within the European Union (EU). For each plant, the substances are stated indications, speed, usage, and other relevant data concerning its safe use or composition that contains it. List and versions of monographs are available for public consultation [14]. In Europe, companies can apply for three different types of market authorization of an herbal medicinal products (HMPs):

- Full implementation. Manufacturer of a herbal drug must provide documentation proving its efficiency and safety, and studies are identical to those submitted for the registration of a synthetic drug.
- Well-established use. Manufacturer of a herbal drug may be permitted to register, on the basis of the submitted detailed scientific literature, stating that the herbal medicinal preparation

is in use for medical purposes not less than 10 years in Europe and has recognized efficiency and an acceptable level of safety.

- Traditional use. Efficiency and safety of a herbal drug can be accepted on the basis of long experience. Herbal remedies can be registered, if the documents prove their use in mitigating certain ailments, not less than 30 years, with at least 15 years in Europe.

The registration procedure for herbal medicines, at all levels of the European Union (EU), is done according to European Directive 2004/24/EC, which introduces simplified, but strictly defined procedures and affects the harmonization of existing national legislative regulations. Regarding the registration in the non-EU countries, despite the efforts made within the framework of national legislation and harmonization in larger systems, a limited number of herbal medicines have been registered. Therefore, the identification of problems and discrepancies and the systematic plan for overcoming them represent a major challenge for the presence of these herbal drugs on the market of EU countries [15].

In Republic of Serbia, legislation on plant products is harmonized with recommendations of The European Directive 2004/24/EC. Law on medicines and medical devices (Official Gazette of the Republic of Serbia No. 30/2010), Regulation on health safety of dietary products (Official Gazette of RS No. 45/2010), Guidelines of Good Manufacturing Practice, Annex 7- Manufacture of herbal medicines, are all in effect. According to the Law on medicines and medical devices, Herbal medicine, is each drug whose active ingredients are exclusively one or more substances of vegetable origin or one or more herbal preparations, or one or more substances of vegetable origin in combination with one or more herbal preparations. Traditional herbal medicine may be based on scientific principles and is the result of tradition or other traditional therapeutic approaches. The active components of a herbal medicine/ traditional herbal medicine are herbal drugs and herbal preparations and their combinations, and this is widely accepted in all European and national documents. In the context of food supplements (dietary supplements), a new the Regulation defines the notion of herbal dietary supplements. These are supplements that contain medicinal plants, their parts or preparations and their quantity in a daily dose of the product should not be less than 15% and greater than 65% compared to a known therapeutic dose of these plant materials or preparations.

2.5. Parameters of quality and quality control

The quality of each final product is ensured by the standard quality of raw materials, the application of validated production processes and procedures on validated equipment. It is similar with herbal remedies, which are made of high-quality herbal raw materials, extractive preparations (extracts and tinctures) and isolates (essential oil and fatty oil). The latest European Pharmacopoeia Ph Eur 8 comprises 270 Monographs on herbal drugs and herbal drug preparations [16]. Monographs define parameters of quality control.

2.5.1. Quality control of herbal drugs

The basis of high-quality herbal remedies is the plant material of a standard quality. Many factors affect the quality of plant material. Regardless of whether the medicinal plants are grown or collected from the wild, biogenetic factors are certainly important (species, variety, chemotype, and sorta). The following are the conditions in which a plant grows as air, climate, land, then agro-technical measures that are applied during the large-scale production (proper sowing, irrigation, fertilization, control against weed and pests), and then collection from the wild or harvest of the plantation, transport, proper storage, drying, and grinding. It is very important to educate people how to deal with the collection of herbal raw materials from spontaneous flora, as well as those who grow the plants, whether they are doing so in the conventional conditions or organic conditions of medicinal plants production. Quality control of herbal raw materials is strictly defined and traceable. First, the identification of plant raw materials is approached. Responsible and expert persons in laboratories for the pharmaceutical control or in other relevant institutions, conduct identification, and categorization under a certain number.

Table 1 gives a list of parameters of quality control of herbal drugs by Ph Eur 8.0, based on whose defined border values the quality of herbal drugs can be determined. For all the aforementioned

Parameters of quality control	
Herbal drugs	1. Definition: the name of the herbal drugs and content of active substances 2. Characters: appearance, taste, odor, solubility 3. Identification: macroscopic and microscopic examination, TLC 4. Tests: water, loss on drying, total ash, foreign matter, insoluble matter, extractable matter, swelling index, microbiological purity, bitterness value, broken drug 5. Assay: essential oils, tannins, declared active substances (GC, LC, UV-VIS)
Herbal drug preparations	**Dry extract** ***(Extractum siccum)*** 1. Definition: standardized dry extract prepared from..., content of active substances 2. Production: method of extraction and solvents 3. Characters: appearance 4. Identification: TLC 5. Tests: loss on drying, total ash, microbiological purity 6. Assay: declared active substances (LC) **Liquid extract (*Extractum fluidum*)** 1. Definition: liquid extract produced from …, and content of active substances 2. Production: method of extraction and solvents 3. Characters: appearance, taste, odor 4. Identification: TLC 5. Tests: ethanol, methanol and 2-propanol, loss on drying, microbiological purity 6. Assay: declared active substances (LC, UV-VIS) **Tincture (*Tinctura*)** 1. Definition: tincture produced from…, and content of active substances 2. Production: method of extraction and solvents 3. Characters: appearance, taste, odor 4. Identification: TLC 5. Tests: ethanol, methanol and 2-propanol, dry residue, microbiological purity 6. Assay: declared active substances (LC, UV-VIS) **Essential oil (*Aetheroleum*)** 1. Definition: essential oil obtained by …, and content of dominant components 2. Production: method of extraction and solvents 3. Characters: appearance, odor, solubility 4. Identification: TLC and chromatographic profile (GC and GC-MS) 5. Tests: relative density, refractive index, optical rotation, chromatographic profile

Table 1. Parameters of quality control of herbal drugs and herbal drug preparations (Ph Eur 8).

parameters, Pharmacopoeia prescribes the procedure. Any organization deals with herbs, forming his specs-attests that rely on the requirements of the applicable European Pharmacopoeia, standards, national regulations, and internal regulations. Definition includes biological source of drug, the Latin name of the genus and species, and the minimum amount of essential oil in the case of aromatic drugs or the minimum quantities of active substances to which the drug is declared. Characteristics define appearance, odor, taste, and solubility. Identification in addition to macroscopic analysis (organoleptic inspection), which includes appearance, color, odor, and microscopic analysis, is carried out for certain herbal drugs, followed by chemical analysis (specific chemical reactions and thin-layer chromatography (TLC)). Predicted tests include water, loss on drying, total ash, foreign matter, swelling index, microbiological purity, bitterness value, starch, and broken drug. Assay includes essential oils, tannins, declared active substance (gas chromatography (GC), GC/mass spectrometry (GC/MS), liquid chromatography (LC), and UV-VIS spectroscopy). For the evaluation of herbal raw materials quality, in addition to the determination of microbiological safety, complete analysis of the health safety is often performed, according to the current regulations (which includes not only the results of physical, physicochemical, and chemical tests but also organoleptic findings, preservatives, sweeteners, mycotoxins, metals and metalloids, pesticide residue, microbiological tests, and radioactivity).

2.5.2. Quality and quality control of extracts

The extracts are one of the most widely used herbal preparations. The extracts can be liquid, semi-solid, or solid consistency. They are most commonly made of dried and grained plant material. For the extract production various processes may be applied: maceration, percolation, extraction of the continuous, and so on. Nowadays, the procedure for extracting plant material by super critical fluids is increasingly in use [17–20]. Tinctures are extractive products which are usually obtained by the method of maceration.

The most often used extragents are ethanol, water, mixtures of water, and ethanol. The choice of solvent depends on the nature of ingredients that need to pass into the extract. In the product declaration, the ratio of components of the solvent mixture used for extraction must always be given. The quality of obtained extract depends on the plant material, the solvent, the drug/solvent ratio, and the extraction process technology. The process of extracts standardization is common. After the quantitative analysis, the extract is adjusted in order to contain a particular amount of an active compound or the group of compounds (or a marker compound) using an inert material or another extract [21]. Parameters of quality control of extracts are shown in **Table 1**. Qualitative and quantitative analyses of the essential oils are carried out by methods GC and GC-MS according to regulation Ph Eur or modified method [22].

2.5.3. Quality and quality control of phytopreparations

When it comes to *mono-components teas,* their quality matches the one defined for the individual drugs (**Table 2**). Quality control refers to the verification of the identity, the declared weight of packaging, and microbiological safety. In the case of *multi-component (mixtures) teas,* their control refers to the verification of the identity of each herbal drug on the recipe, checking the declared weight relationship of the components and microbiological purity.

Phytopreparations	Parameters of quality control
Mono-component tea and tea mixture	1. Identification 2. Appearance 3. Verification of components, declared mass ratio of components 4. Verification of package weight 5. microbiological purity
Liquid herbal preparations (liquid extracts, tinctures, and mixtures of extracts or tinctures), **herbal drops, solutions, syrups**	1. Identification 2. Appearance 3. Loss on drying 4. Content of ethanol 5. Relative density 6. Refractive index 7. Verification of package weight 8. Qualitative and quantitative analysis 9. microbiological safety and/or complete health safety control
Semi-solid forms (herbal gels, cream, and unguent)	1. Identification 2. Appearance 3. Verification of package weight 4. pH value 5. microbiological safety and/or complete health safety control
Solid-dosage forms (capsules, tablets, etc.)	1. Identification 2. Appearance 3. Declared mass of single-dose preparations 4. Disintegration 5. Qualitative and quantitative analysis of the declared active components 6. microbiological safety and/or complete health safety control

Table 2. Parameters of quality control of phytopreparation.

When a herbal remedy represents a *mixture of plant extracts or tinctures*, it is usually difficult to perform the quantitative analysis of active ingredients for each individual extract. For these preparations, the content analysis of active substances for which the preparation is declared is conducted (LC, UV-VIS spectroscopy, GC and GC-MS spectrometry, infrared (IR), nuclear magnetic resonance (NMR), etc.). Also, in principal, a manufacturer appends the typical fingerprint of chromatogram, spectrum, or some other physical parameter, of the preparation ingredient, which may be used by a control laboratory for identification. This approach can also be used for the quantitative analysis of the preparation.

Semi-solid forms (herbal gel, cream, and ointment) are checked for authentication, filling, pH, and microbiological purity. For *solid-dosage galenic forms* (capsules, tablets, etc.), a control is performed for each individual dose. Control for these forms of herbal remedies includes authentication, appearance, the declared weight of the package, or of the each individual dose of the preparation. Qualitative and quantitative analyses of the declared active components, or a marker compound, of the preparation, are obligatory. For this analysis, similar (or appropriately modified) methods to the analysis of herbal drugs or extractive preparations are applied (if not according to Pharmacopoeia, these methods must be validated by the CPMP/ICH/281/95)s.

2.5.4. Monitoring of phytopreparation stability

Medicinal herbs and products based on medicinal herbs are very sensitive to external influences—the presence of elevated temperatures, moisture, and direct light. They are prone to reactions of oxidation, degradation, hydrolysis, and evaporation, so during the preparation of herbal remedies special attention must be placed to a number of factors that can affect the quality of the final product. In order to determine the stability of a product, to define storage conditions, and durability, stability tests are carried out, which include the investigation of the environmental factors effect on the change in the final product quality. Stability tests are performed at different stages of development and production. During the period of investigation, the first stress test is carried out, in order to select the most optimal, compatible excipients, and the best formulation. All raw materials used, excipients, active ingredients, and extraction products, are subject to stability testing and durability defining, for appropriate packaging and under certain environmental conditions. Stability is defined as the period during which the product remains within the set quality limits of the prescribed specification. In accordance with the requirements of the EMEA, various specific stability tests are placed for different herbal [23].

2.6. Planning and development of new herbal preparation

The formulation of a new herbal products is a process that has strictly defined phases and includes the work of several sectors of the company that is developing products based on medicinal herbs. The dynamics of the process is divided into stages, and they are completed by performing a multitude of necessary activities. Of course, the scope of new product development depends on the complexity of the galenic form of the new herbal preparation. All steps are defined in the documents of quality standards and other regulations of the company (**Figure 1**).

Furthermore, the procedures of developing a new herbal preparation will be explained on the example of the development of herbal remedies in the Institute for Medicinal Plant Research "Dr Josif Pancic," Belgrade, Republic of Serbia (the Institute).

Stages in the development of new herbal products have their logical sequence. Administration, management, the sales department, and the demand of patients expressed through visits to our herbal pharmacies may suggest the need for a new preparation, to the department of pharmaceutical research and development. Management gives the order to the department of pharmaceutical research and development, to create a team that will be allocated to the project and appoint a project manager.

Project manager, who is usually a doctor of pharmaceutical sciences in the field of pharmacognosy, forms a team, writes, and presents a plan for a new product development. The plan, according to the system of quality management, must contain general information: project name, the subject of research, description of development activities, the aim of the research, the necessary equipment, an indication of the place of realization of activities, project duration, and start time of the applicability of the project results. The second segment is represented through dynamic activities (through phases) and the engagement of researchers

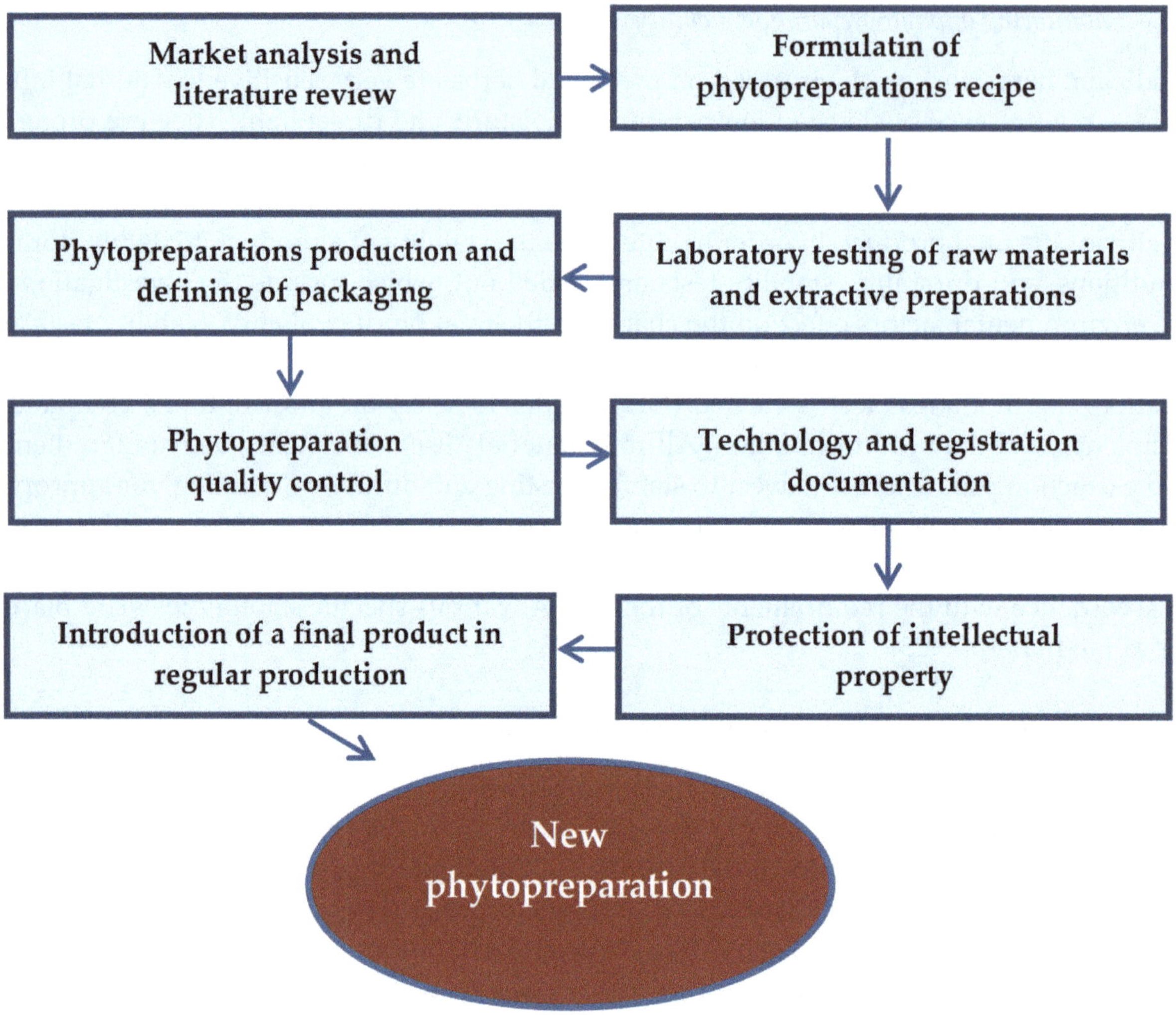

Figure 1. Schematic representation of the planning and development of new herbal preparation.

(throughout activities phases). The third segment is the planning of all material costs for the development of a new herbal remedy. When management of the Institute approves the presented plan for developing a new product, project manager starts with its execution.

The beginning phase represents preformulation studies. Market analysis and the review of relevant literature are very complex. It covers the activities of the Institution's herbal pharmacies that collect patients' requirements, commercial department, which collects data on herbal remedies from the observed therapeutic groups in the domestic and foreign markets. Analysis of relevant literature includes search for relevant directives and monographs, scientific, technical papers, patents, and so on.

When all relevant data are collected, an expert research team approaches the formulation of a recipe. The recipe for herbal remedies and the content of active substances, which will be declared in the preparation, depends on the plan for a herbal product registration. In addition to the selection of galenical form, auxiliary materials are also selected at this stage. Of course, the recipe is subject to small corrections during the production process.

Further on, laboratories are included in the process of preparations formulation. Analysis of active substances in the selected plant raw materials and quality control prescribed by Pharmacopoeia or other relevant document are performed. Then, the quality control of semi-final product is conducted. In the case of capsules, the analysis of the active substance in dry extract is performed, and also the analysis of other parameters that define its quality, and that is defined by Pharmacopoeia monographs or summarized in an internal specification or a certificate.

Afterwards, the preparation formulation is conducted (formulation of teas or herbal drops, herbal creams, capsules, etc.). In addition to the main plant raw materials, secondary raw materials are selected, which will synergistically facilitate the functioning of the dominant plant drugs, and auxiliary pharmaceutical raw materials are selected. Auxiliary raw materials are used as the basis for semi-solid galenic forms (creams, ointments, and gels), and capsule fillers (for the preparation of granules—mass for the capsule filling).

When the herbal remedy is designed, all laboratory examinations are carried out, as prescribed in specifications. The determination of the average capsule weight is performed, also the determination of active ingredients per capsule, stability testing for active substances per capsule, the capsule dissolution testing, and testing of complete health safety.

From the Intellectual Property Office, the search "recharge" is required and then the protection of the preparation name. The proposal for the primary and secondary packaging graphic layout is carried out. Technological documentation gets completed (processes specifications, recipes, and norms). After the test production of capsules, the production of capsules is introduced into regular production. The validation of technological processes, the validation of equipment, and the validation of laboratory methods are performed. Registration documentation, report writing, and the presentation of results are being prepared.

When the preparation is produced and packed in its primary and secondary packaging, quality testing of the final product is conducted (tea blends and herbal drops, ointments, and capsules). Quality testing is conducted according to the attest or the specification of the final product. It is necessary to examine the complete health safety of the preparation. The stability of the active substance is also monitored, to determine and define the expiration date.

Along with a new preparation production, the writing of technical documentation that represents the preparation file is carried out. The specifications of raw materials, semi-final products, and auxiliary materials are written. In order to define the dose for preparations, it is necessary to determine the range of content of the active substance. This is achieved by validation of the process, on the validated equipment.

Finally, the registration documents are prepared. The scope of the documentation is correlated with the desired herbal remedies group for registration (herbal medicine, traditional herbal medicine, or dietary supplement). If it is planned to register a new product as a herbal medicine or a traditional herbal medicine, then the instructions of the EMEA monographs need to be followed. If it is planned to register a new product as a dietary supplement, then the dose needs to be below 65% of the therapeutic dose.

Development of different galenic form of herbal remedies is presented in the following examples.

2.6.1. *Mono-component tea*

Herb yarrow *Achillea millefolium* L. is highly regarded medicinal and aromatic plant and has a long traditional use. According to WHO monograph, yarrow exhibits antibacterial, anti-convulsant, anti-inflammatory, antioxidant, antipyretic, antispasmodic, and antiviral activity. According to the Commission E monograph and the EMEA, yarrow is traditionally used only for temporary loss of appetite, mild spasmodic complaints of the digestive organs, bloating, flatulence, and externally as a bath with problems in the lower abdomen in women, and with superficial wounds [24].

The process of making mono-component tea from yarrow takes place in the following stages:

- Purchase of high-quality herbal material (overground top part of the blooming herb), which meets the quality parameters as prescribed by Pharmacopoeia.
- Grinding the herb up to a prescribed degree of fragmentation. Grinded herbal drug as a semi-final product is controlled on the microbiological safety, which is performed in accordance with the relevant regulations for tea and Pharmacopoeia requirements.
- Following the positive results obtained from the pharmaceutical and microbiological laboratories, chopped herbal drug is placed in packaging.
- Final product, mono-component yarrow tea, is sent for the control to pharmaceutical and microbiological laboratories. Pharmaceutical laboratory confirms the authentication and filling volume.
- When a controlled product receives the confirmation that corresponds to the standard quality, it is dispatched to the warehouse of final products and further distributed to pharmacies and other places.

The user manual is adapted to the prescribed use as a traditional herbal medicinal: as a means of relieving complaints of the digestive system, improve appetite, eliminate gases, regulating the secretion of bile, pains and cramps in the stomach, with the amenorrhea.

2.6.2. *Tea for weight loss in filter bags (1.5 g)*

For this indication, herbal drugs that have diuretic and laxative effect have been selected on one hand, and on the other hand, we have drugs that aid digestion and herbal drugs rich in polyphenols as potent antioxidants and vitamin C. The following herbal drugs are included in equal parts (ana partes) in the mixture composition: *Betulae folium, Frangulae cortex, Foeniculi fructus, Thea folium,* and *Cynosbati fructus*. The mixture of herbs whose active ingredients regulate digestion and excretion of urine, stimulate metabolism, and facilitate the breakdown of fat, and thus contribute to the cleansing and detoxification of body. Its is recommended as a supplement in weight loss diets and for helping to reduce and maintain a desired weight.

The process of making tea for weight loss in filter bags is as follows:

- Purchase of high-quality individual herbal material and quality control of parameters as prescribed by Pharmacopoeia.
- Grinding the herb up to a prescribed degree of fragmentation. Grinded herbal drugs are controlled on the microbiological safety and Pharmacopoeia requirements (appearance, moisture content, content of essential oils, impurities, and degree of fragmentation).
- Following the positive results obtained from the pharmaceutical and microbiological laboratories, homogeneous mixing of grinded herbal drugs is carried out, and then in the machine for tea bags, bags are filled with the contents. Afterwards, they are placed in special filter bags and packaging.
- Final product, herbal mixture in filter bags, is sent for the control to pharmaceutical and microbiological laboratories. Pharmaceutical laboratory confirms the authentication and filling volume of tea bags and the number of tea bags in a packaging.
- When a controlled product receives the confirmation that corresponds to the standard quality, it is dispatched to the warehouse of final products and further distributed to pharmacies and other places.

2.6.3. Herbal drops for weight loss

Herbal drops, meant to regulate body weight, represent a combination of tinctures and herbal extracts, whose active ingredients stimulate the metabolism, have a beneficial impact on digestion, and eliminate the excess fluids from the body. The composition of herbal drops includes *Betulae tinctura, Frangulae tinctura, Foeniculi tinctura* and *Cynosbati extractum fluidum.*

The process of making herbal drops at the Institute, takes place as follows:

- Purchase of high-quality individual herbal material and quality control of parameters as prescribed by Pharmacopoeia.
- Grinding the herb up to a prescribed degree of fragmentation. Grinded herbal drugs are controlled on the microbiological safety and pharmacopoeia requirements.
- Following the positive results obtained from the laboratories, homogeneous mixing tinctures and extract, filtered, and then filled into glass bottles.
- Final product is sent for the control to pharmaceutical and microbiological laboratories.
- When a controlled product receives the confirmation that corresponds to the standard quality, it is dispatched to the warehouse of final products and further distributed to pharmacies and other places.

2.6.4. Herbal cream with extract of comfrey: Comfrey gel

The root of comfrey *Symphyti radix* represents a very important medicinal herb raw material. According to the Commission E monograph, it is used for blunt injuries. According to EMEA, the traditional use of herbal preparations, it is used in semi-solid-dosage forms for cutaneous use. Traditional herbal medicinal remedy is also used for the symptomatic treatment of minor sprains and bruises. Gel with 10% propylene glycol extract of comfrey root (*Symphyti Extaractum fluidum* (1: 7)) containing mucus, tannins, saponosides, and allantoin improves epithelialization, drainage, and tissue regeneration. It has a beneficial effect with swellings, hematoma, fractures, sport injuries, and posttraumatic conditions. It should not be applied to open and infected wounds.

The production process of Comfrey gel is performed in the following stages:

- Purchase of high-quality herbal material *Symphyti radix* and quality control of parameters, as prescribed by Pharmacopeia selection of high-quality pharmaceutical raw materials according to the manufacturer attest.
- Grinding of comfrey root and producing the liquid extract with propylene glycol with a method of percolation. The resulting extract is controlled to authentication, relative density, and microbiological safety.
- Liquid extract of comfrey, after the processing procedure is incorporated into the semi-solid base, and then filled into tubes. The final product, herbal gel from the roots of comfrey, is sent to the control to laboratories.
- When a controlled product receives confirmation that corresponds to the standard quality, it is dispatched to the warehouse of final products and further distributed.

2.6.5. Herbal capsules ODOVAL S®, herbal sedative

Herbal product is used for the defense of organism against the effects of daily stress.

Valerian root (*Valerianae radix*) has a long traditional use. It is approved by Commission E to help combat restless states and difficulties falling asleep caused by nervousness. According to EMEA monograph, it has a well-established use as a herbal medicinal remedy for the relief of mild nervous tension and sleep disorders.

Melissa leaf (*Melissae folium*) is a favorite vegetable drug that is used as a mild sedative, carminative, antispasmodic, and aromatic. The EMEA monograph only credits *Melissae folium* with a traditional use: it is considered to be a traditional herbal medicinal remedy for relief of mild symptoms of mental stress and to aid sleep and for symptomatic treatment of mild gastrointestinal. Capsules of this herbal sedative are designed to have the *Valerianae extractum siccum* as a dominant component, with the synergistic effects of *Melissae extractum siccum*.

Odoval S® is a herbal remedy meant for maintaining mental balance. It contains extracts of valerian root and lemon balm leaf, medicinal plants traditionally used for their calming properties. The active ingredients of these extracts have a favorable effect on alleviating anxiety and irritability, facilitate sleep, and establishment of natural sleep patterns. Odoval S® can be used as a valuable help in alleviating various symptoms caused by chronic stress (mental tension and anxiety during the day, irritability, and feelings of worry).

In the Institute , the production process of capsules is carried out in the following stages:

- Purchase of high-quality herbal raw material of *Valerianae radix* and *Melissae folium* and quality control on parameters, as prescribed by Pharmacopeia.
- Production of dry extracts: *Valerianae extractum siccum* and *Melissae extractum siccum* in the circular extractor, according to the specifications of the process.
- The resulting dry extract is controlled as a semi-final product to authentication, moisture content, and microbiological safety.
- Controlled dry extracts, along with additional pharmaceutical materials, are used to produce granulate (mass for encapsulation). Granulate, as a semi-final product, also goes to the control to pharmaceutical and microbiological laboratories. Pharmacopoeial method is used to determine the content of valeric acid [2].
- Upon obtaining the results of quality control, encapsulation, that is, automatic filling of gelatin capsules with prepared granulate, is conducted. Capsules are forwarded in the glass jars, and then into the boxes.
- The final phytopreparation is sent to the control to laboratories. The following parameters are determined: properties, number of capsules in a package, the average weight of the capsule content, uniformity of mass capsule, identification of valeric acid LC and TLC for lemon balm, disintegration of capsules, and microbiological safety. The product is sent to the analysis of the complete health safety.
- When results confirm the quality according to certificates and specifications, the final product is dispatched to the warehouse of final products and afterwards distributed to pharmacies and other places.

3. Conclusions and perspectives

Natural products discovered so far have played a vital role in improving the human health and have been the drugs of choice despite facing a tough competition from compounds obtained by chemical procedures, due to their safety and efficacy. The most striking feature of natural products in connection to their long-lasting importance in drug discovery is their structural diversity that is still largely untapped [1].

Comprehensive development of science and technology, able to produce high-quality herbal medicines, is greatly improved in recent decades. The acceptance of herbal medicine as a natural and gentle alternative to synthetic drugs is very high in public in developed countries and, from a global perspective, unit sales of herbal medicines is constantly growing. However, we still face many problems in these areas [2].

A comprehensive approach to these problems, the state of the field of medicinal plants and herbal remedies, can be repaired. A better education of people is involved in the collection and cultivation of medicinal plants on the necessity of obtaining plant raw material of high quality. In particular, it should encourage the concept of organic production herbal products. Producers should be required to produce only quality-assured medicines.

Improved harmonization of regulatory classification of herbal preparations in the world would inevitably lead to greater transparency and consistency of the market.

Special attention should be paid to improving knowledge about the benefits of rational phytotherapy, particularly evidence-based phytotherapy, health workers, especially doctors.

The aim of all efforts would be to improve the overall awareness of the possibilities of choice in prevention and treatment and can judge the effectiveness of the use of medicinal herbs and herbal preparations.

Acknowledgements

Financial support of this work by the Serbian Ministry of Education, Science and Technological Development (Project III 46001) is gratefully acknowledged.

Author details

Sofija M. Djordjevic

Address all correspondence to: sdjordjevic@mocbilja.rs

Institute for Medicinal Plant Research "Dr Josif Pancic", Belgrade, Republic of Serbia

References

[1] Veeresham C. Natural products derived from plants as a source of drugs. Journal of Advanced Pharmaceutical Technology & Research. 2012;**3(4)**:200–201. DOI: 10.4103/2231-4040.104709

[2] Đorđević S, Dickov A, Pavkov S, Tadić V, Arsić I, Žugić A. Manufacturing process of high quality phytopreparation on example of herbal sedative. Medicinski Pregled. 2013;**66(3–4)**:170–176. DOI: 10.2298/MPNS1304170D

[3] Fürst R, Zündorf I. Evidence-based phytotherapy in Europe: where do we stand? Planta Medica. 2015;**81(12–13)**:962–967. DOI: 10.1055/s-0035-1545948

[4] Tasić S, Šavikin K, Menković N. Guide to Medicinal Herbs. 2nd ed. Belgrade: Alexandria; 2009. 6 p. ISBN: 978-86-6119-034-6

[5] Kišgeci J. Medicinal Plants. Belgrade: Partenon; 2002. 7 p. ISBN: 978-86-7157-188-6

[6] Cragg GM, Newman DJ. Natural products: A continuing source of novel drug leads. Biochimica et Biophysica Acta. 2013;**1830(6)**:3670–3695. DOI: 10.1016/j.bbagen.2013.02.008

[7] Petrovska BB. Historical review of medicinal plants' usage. Pharmacognosy Reviews. 2012;**6(11)**:1–5. DOI: 10.4103/0973-7847.95849

[8] Atanasov AG, Waltenberger B, Pferschy-Wenzig EM, Linder T, Wawrosch C, Uhrin P, Temml V, Wang L, Schwaiger S, Heiss EH, Rollinger JM, Schuster D, Breuss JM, Bochkov V, Mihovilovic MD, Kopp B, Bauer R, Dirsch VM, Stuppner H. Discovery and resupply of pharmacologically active plant-derived natural products: A review. Biotechnology Advances. 2015;**33(8)**:1582–1614. DOI: 10.1016/j.biotechadv.2015.08.001

[9] Blumenthal M, Hall T, Goldberg A, Kunz T, Dinda K. The ABC Clinical Guide to Herbs. Austin, TX: American Botanical Council; 2003. 19 p. ISBN: 3-13-132391-4

[10] Wichtl M. Herbal Drugs and Phytopharmaceuticals. Stuttgart: Medpharm; 2004. 17 p. ISBN 9780849319617.

[11] Schulz V, Hänsel R, Tyler V. Rational Phytotherapy. Berlin: Springer-Verlag; 2001. 326 p. DOT: 10.1007/978-3-642-98093-0

[12] Tadić V, Đorđević S, Arsić I. Herbal drugs in the treatment of nervous and cardiovascular disorders. HealthMED. 2011;**5(5)**:1206–1210. ISSN: 1840-2291

[13] Maridass M, John de Britto A. Origins of plant derived medicines. Ethnobotanical Leaflets. 2008;**12**:373–387. http://opensiuc.lib.siu.edu/ebl/vol2008/iss1/44

[14] Cupara S, Janković S. Significance of herbal drugs legislation for their rational use. Vojnosanitetski pregled. Vojnosanit Pregled. 2009;**66(1)**:53–56. UDC: 615.311:581.19

[15] Qu L, Zou W, Zhou Z, Zhang T, Greef J, Wang M. Non-European traditional herbal medicines in Europe: A community herbal monograph perspective. Journal of Ethnopharmacology. 2014;**156**:107–114. DOI: 10.1016/j.jep.2014.08.021

[16] European Pharmacopoeia. 8th ed. vol. 1. Ph Eur 8.1. Council of Europe (EDQM). Strasbourg. 2013. 1133 p. ISBN: 978-92-871-7525-0

[17] Žižović I, Stamenić M, Ivanović J, Orlović A, Ristić M, Đorđević S, Petrović DS, Skala D. Supercritical carbon dioxide extraction of sesquiterpenes from valerian root. Journal of Supercritical Fluids. 2007;**43(2)**:249–258. DOI:10.1016/j.supflu.2007.05.007

[18] Žižović I, Ivanović J, Mišić D, Stamenić M, Đorđević S, Kukić-Marković J, Petrović DS. SFE as a superior technique for isolation of extracts with strong antibacterial activities from lichen *Usnea barbata* L. Journal of Supercritical Fluids. 2012;**72**:7–14. DOI: 10.1016/j.supflu.2012.07.018

[19] Tadić V, Bojović D, Arsić I, Đorđević S, Aksentijević K, Stamenić M, Janković S. Chemical and antimicrobial evaluation of supercritical and conventional *Sideritis scardica* Griseb., Lamiaceae extracts. Molecules. 2012;**17(3)**:2683–2703. DOI: 10.3390/molecules17032683

[20] Ćujić N, Šavikin K, Janković T, Pljevljakušić D, Zdunić G, Ibrić S. Optimization of polyphenols extraction from dried chokeberry using maceration as traditional technique. Food Chemistry. 2016;**194**:135–142. DOI: 10.1016/j.foodchem.2015.08.008

[21] Kovačević N. Quality and quality control of herbal drugs, extracts and phytomedicines. Lekovite Sirovine. 2001;**20**:57–68. UDC: 615.322.07

[22] Đorđević S, Petrović S, Ristić M, Đoković D. Composition of *Carlina acanthifolia* root essential oil. Chemistry of Natural Compounds. 2005;**41(4)**:410–412. DOI: 10.1007/s10600-005-0163-2

[23] Huynh-Ba K (ed.). Handbook of Stability Testing in Pharmaceutical Development: Regulations, Methodologies, and Best Practices. Delaware: Pharmalytik Newark; 2009. 139 p. DOI: 10.1007/978-0-387-85627-8

[24] Arsić I, Tadić V, Đorđević S, Žugić A, Vujić Z, Petrović DS. Optimization of extraction of antioxidant components from Yarrow herb. Hemijska Industrija. 2014;**68(4)**:511–517. DOI: 10.2298/HEMIND130910076A

9

Meeting of the Minds: Traditional Herbal Medicine in Multiethnic Suriname

Dennis R.A. Mans, Deeksha Ganga and
Joëlle Kartopawiro

Abstract

The Republic of Suriname (South America) is located on the Guiana Shield, one of the regions with the highest biodiversity and the largest expanse of undisturbed tropical rain forest in the world. The population of almost 570,000 consists of a unique blend of ethnic groups and cultures from all continents. These include Indigenous Amerindians, the original inhabitants; Maroons, the descendants of runaway slaves who had been shipped from Africa between the seventeenth and the nineteenth century; Creoles, a generic term referring to mixed blacks and whites; the descendants from indentured workers from China, India, and Java (Indonesia) who arrived between the second half of the nineteenth and the first half of the twentieth century; as well as immigrants from various Middle Eastern, European, Caribbean, and South American countries. All these groups have made their own specific contribution to Suriname's traditional medicine, which has resulted in a myriad of remedies against many disorders, mainly employing a variety of plants. This chapter presents a brief history of Suriname, addresses the ethnopharmacological practices of Maroons and Creoles as well as Hindustanis and Javanese, and concludes with a few remarks on the previsions provided by the country's rich plant-based traditional medicine.

Keywords: Suriname, multiethnicity, Maroons and Creoles, Hindustanis, Javanese, traditional herbal medicine

1. Introduction

1.1. Suriname: general aspects

The Republic of Suriname is located on the northeast coast of South America, just north of the Amazon delta, and borders the Atlantic Ocean to the north, French Guiana to the east, Brazil to the south, and Guyana to the west (**Figure 1**) [1]. Despite its location in South America, Suriname is culturally considered a Caribbean rather than a Latin American country and is a member of the Caribbean Community (CARICOM) [1]. The climate is tropical with abundant rainfall, a uniform temperature of on average 27°C, and a relative high humidity of 81% in the capital city of Paramaribo [2]. There are four seasons, namely the long rainy season (April–July), the long dry season (August–November), the short rainy season (December–January), and the short dry season (February–March) [2].

Suriname's land area of roughly 165,000 km^2 can be distinguished into a northern urban-coastal and a rural-coastal area as well as a southern rural interior (**Figure 1**) [2]. The urban-coastal area comprises Paramaribo and the Wanica district (**Figure 1**) and harbors approximately 80% of the population of almost 570,000 [2, 3]. The rural-coastal area comprises the districts of Marowijne, Commewijne, Saramacca, Coronie, and Nickerie (**Figure 1**) and is, together with the southern-rural districts of Para, Brokopondo, and Sipaliwini (**Figure 1**), home to the remaining 20% of Suriname's inhabitants [2, 3]. The latter part of the country is referred to as the hinterland, encompasses more than three-quarters of its land surface, and consists largely

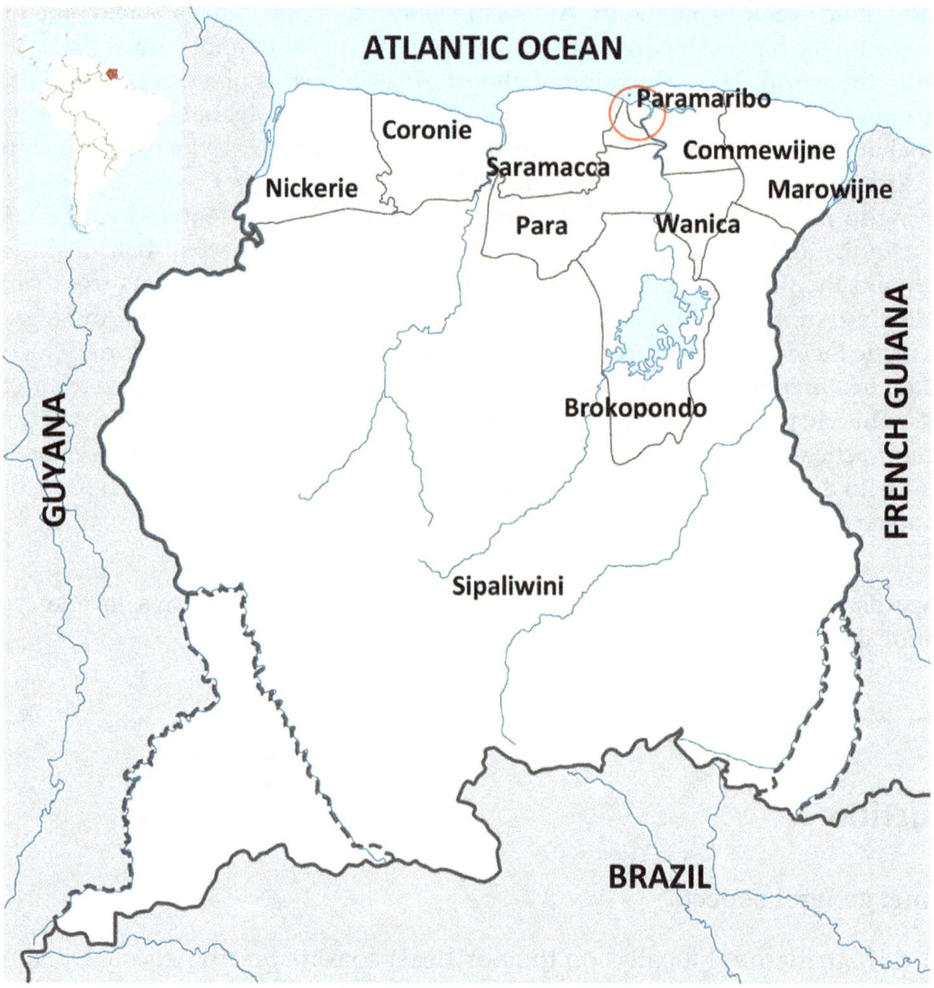

Figure 1. Map of Suriname depicting the 10 administrative districts. The insert indicates the location of Suriname in South America.

of sparsely inhabited savanna and dense, pristine, and highly biodiverse tropical rain forest [2]. This makes Suriname comparatively one of the most forested countries in the world [2, 4].

The urban areas are characterized by a "western" lifestyle, modern health-care facilities, and an economy that is mainly based on commerce, services, and industry [5]. The rural societies have a more traditional way of living, lack comprehensive public health services, and have agriculture, forestry, crude oil drilling, bauxite and gold mining, as well as ecotourism as major economic activities [5]. These activities have been growing in scale and economic importance in recent years and are, together with agriculture and fisheries, the country's most important means of support, contributing substantially to the gross domestic income in 2014 of U$ 5.297 billion and an average per-capita income of U$ 9583 [5, 6]. This positions Suriname on the World Bank's list of upper-middle income economies [5, 6].

1.2. Suriname: people

Suriname's population is among the most varied in the world, comprising the Indigenous Amerindians, the original inhabitants; descendants from enslaved Africans imported between the seventeenth and the nineteenth century (called Maroons and Creoles); descendants from contract workers from China, India (called Hindustanis), and the island of Java, Indonesia (called Javanese) attracted between the second half of the nineteenth century and the first half of the twentieth century; descendants from settlers from a number of European and Middle Eastern countries; and more recently, immigrants from various Latin American and Caribbean countries including Brazil, Guyana, French Guiana, Haiti, and Cuba [1, 3]. The largest ethnic groups are the Maroons and Creoles, as well as the Hindustanis and Javanese, comprising approximately 22 and 16%, and 27 and 14%, respectively, of the total population [3].

Although members of all ethnic groups are encountered throughout the country—particularly in Paramaribo—certain ethnic groups are clustered in relatively large numbers in certain areas of the country [2, 3]. For example, the district of Nickerie harbors predominantly Hindustanis, that of Para mostly Creoles, that of Commewijne mainly Javanese, while the Maroons and Indigenous peoples primarily populate the interior, living in villages along the major rivers [2, 3]. More importantly, the various ethnic groups have largely preserved their culture and identity, still practicing their original religion and speaking their original language in addition to Dutch, the official language of government, business, media, and education, as well as Surinamese or Sranan Tongo, the widely used English- and Portuguese-based lingua franca [1, 3].

The same holds true for their specific perceptions of health and disease and their ethnopharmacological traditions [7]. However, throughout time, considerable intercultural exchange has taken place about the knowledge and use of medicinal plants [7]. This paper first presents a brief historical overview of Suriname, then addresses the ethnopharmacological practices of the largest ethnic groups (the Maroons and the Creoles, as well as the Hindustanis and the Javanese), and concludes with a few remarks on the previsions provided by the various plant-based traditional medicinal practices.

2. Brief history of Suriname

2.1. The early days

Petroglyphs found at archeological sites in the western Corantijn basin and the eastern Marowijne basin of Suriname demonstrate that this region was inhabited by Indigenous peoples since at least 3000 BC, long before contact with Europeans [8]. The collection of 313 pre-Columbian pottery and charcoal fragments found in several caves at the Werephai site in the deep southwest of Suriname even dates human presence in Suriname as far back as 5000 before present [8]. It is possible that these peoples were nomadic tribes who roamed the Amazon area, and represent the ancestors of the present-day Akurio, Trio, Warrau, and Wayana, Indigenous tribes who still mainly populate the rainforest inland, but there is no documentation to support this assumption.

The Arawaks, a nomadic Indigenous tribe that lived at the coast from hunting and fishing, are generally believed to be Suriname's original inhabitants [9], but there are also no written documents to sustain this supposition. Around 1200 AD, the Caribs sailed to Suriname from their territory extending from the mouth of the Orinoco River in contemporary Venezuela to that of the Amazon River in present-day Brazil, and drove the Arawaks away from their lands [9]. The Arawaks moved to the savannas further land inward and the Caribs settled at the mouth of the Marowijne River in northeastern Suriname where they established, among others, the village of Galibi (from "Kupali Yumï," meaning "tree of the forefathers" in the Carib language) [9].

2.2. The first settlers

The first Europeans arrived in Suriname in the early 1600s. They were Spanish, English, French, and Dutch fortune hunters who were attracted by tales of a fantastical city of gold called El Dorado somewhere at South America's "Wild Coast" [10]. However, it were English settlers led by Captain John Marshall who first colonized the area in 1630 [10, 11]. They called the colony "Surinam" after the Surinen indigenous people who then inhabited the "land of many waters" in the fertile Guiana plains [11]. Encouraged by the successes in their colonies in Virginia and Barbados, the English established tobacco plantations at Marshall's Creek along the Suriname River, but this venture failed because of plummeting prices on the European market [11]. By 1645, Marshall's colony was abandoned [11], but "Marchallkreek" is marked on maps until today.

About 20 years later, in 1651, English troops commanded by Major Anthony Rowse succeeded in establishing the first permanent plantations in Suriname as well as a fort to defend the newly acquired asset [11]. The colony was named Willoughbyland in honor of their patron Lord Francis Willoughby, the then governor of Barbados [11]. Willoughby's intention was to establish a settlement for cultivating sugarcane, a cash crop that was fetching much higher prices in Europe than tobacco [11]. The much needed experience with sugarcane cultivation came from Dutch Jews who lived in Brazil and French Guiana but had to flee persecution by the Portuguese—the then owners of both regions—who were hostile to Protestantism and

Judaism [12]. The Jews mainly established sugarcane plantations in the savanna region which is still known today as the Jodensavanna (the "Jew's savanna") [12].

2.3. The plantation economy

Cheap labor was initially—in the 1650s—provided for by indentured servants from England, some Indigenous tribes people from the interior who had been captured by the coastal tribes and sold to the English colonists, as well as the relatively few black slaves who had directly been brought from Barbados by their owners or had been bought from the Dutch [11, 12]. However, because of the growing need of laborers on the sugarcane plantations, the British Royal Company of Adventurers occupied Dutch assets in Western Africa including centers for slave trading, initiating structured and government-sanctioned trans-Atlantic slave trade [11]. As a result, by 1663, most of the work on the approximately 50 plantations was done by over 3000 African slaves [11].

The victorious days of the British did not last long. In February 1667, Dutch ships from Zeeland led by Abraham Crijnssen invaded Willoughbyland, captured Fort Willoughby, and renamed it Fort Zeelandia [11, 13, 14]. Five months later, the English and Dutch signed the Treaty of Breda that assigned Suriname to The Netherlands in exchange for New Amsterdam, the main city of the former Dutch colony of New Netherlands in North America [11, 13, 14]. This arrangement was made official in the Treaty of Westminster of 1674, after the British had recaptured and again lost Suriname in 1667 and the Dutch regained the colony in 1668 [11, 13]. The Dutch renamed Willoughbyland Dutch Guiana and the English renamed New Amsterdam New York after the Duke of York [11, 13, 14].

2.4. Enslaved and indentured laborers

In 1683, the newly acquired colony was managed by the city of Amsterdam, the family Van Aerssen van Sommelsdijck, and the Dutch West Indies Company united in the Society of Suriname [13, 14]. In order to obtain maximum profits, the Society relied ever more on slave labor, dominating the trans-Atlantic slave trade for a long time [13–15]. All and all, around 300,000 Africans have been shipped to Suriname. In addition to sugar, the plantations produced cocoa, cotton, and indigo, which were exported to Amsterdam and returned enormous revenues [15]. However, treatment of the enslaved Africans was notoriously brutal, and many escaped to the interior from the start where they formed large communities—collectively called Maroons—with independent settlements and preservation of their culture that would last until today [15, 16].

The British again ruled Suriname from 1799 through 1816 during the occupation of The Netherlands by France and put an end to slave trade in 1807 [11], but it took the Dutch until 1863 to abolish slavery [13, 14]. However, the slaves who had remained on the plantations were obliged to conduct ill-paid work and were only fully released in 1873 [13, 14]. As soon as they became truly free, the majority abandoned the plantations and settled in Paramaribo [17]. Many of them mixed with other races, particularly Dutch, becoming a separate ethnic group from the Maroons called Creoles [17]. This is an important reason for the somewhat looser ties of Creoles with African traditions when compared to Maroons despite their common heritage [17]. Still, African-based traditional medicinal practices are deeply rooted in most Creoles [17].

In the meantime, as a plantation colony, Suriname still heavily depended on manual labor. To make up for the shortage after 1873, the Dutch arranged with the British to bring in indentured laborers from India [18, 19]. Around the turn of the twentieth century, in 1916, many workers were again imported, this time from the Dutch East Indies (modern Indonesia), especially from the island of Java [19, 20]. As mentioned above, these contract workers were the predecessors of the Hindustanis and Javanese, respectively, in Suriname. In addition, between 1850 and 1860, small numbers of (mostly male) laborers had been brought in from China and the Middle East [1, 21, 22].

2.5. The modern days

This history makes Suriname, notwithstanding its relatively small population, one of the ethnically most diverse countries in the world. It also provides an explanation for the large variety of traditional forms of medicine practiced in the country. Suriname received in 1954 the status of an autonomous constituent country of the Kingdom of The Netherlands, along with The Netherlands and the Netherlands Antilles [22]. In this construction, Suriname could elect its own government and manage its own administration, but The Netherlands retained control of its defense and foreign affairs [22]. Approximately 20 years later, in November 1975, the country became completely independent from The Netherlands [22].

However, fear of ethnic violence and disappointment about economic development led to massive migration of Surinamese to The Netherlands just before and after 1975, resulting in a Surinamese diaspora in that country of roughly 350,000 in 2008 [22]. To make matters worse, a group of soldiers led by Suriname's current president Desi Bouterse perpetrated a coup and took control of the country from February 25, 1980, on [22]. Absolute lows in that period were the execution on December 8, 1982, of 15 adversaries who were allegedly plotting a countercoup, and the Interior War between a group of mostly Maroon anti-government insurgents led by Ronnie Brunswijk and Bouterse's army between 1986 and 1992 [22].

Fortunately, since then, peace and democracy have been restored [22]. Currently, Suriname is a constitutional democracy with a president elected by the unicameral National Assembly or by the larger United People's Assembly [22]. Despite many economic and political problems, this young democracy continues to serve as a unique example of genuine unity in diversity.

3. Ethnopharmacological practices of Maroons and Creoles

3.1. The Maroon and Creole community in Suriname

The Maroons (from the Spanish expression "cimarrón" for "runaway") are the descendants from enslaved Africans who escaped from the plantations in coastal Suriname to the hinterland between the mid-seventeenth and the late eighteenth centuries [14, 15, 23, 24]. The slaves had mostly been imported from present-day Ghana, Benin, and Loango, but also from many other parts of West Africa such as Gambia, Guinea, Senegal, and Ivory Coast [14, 15]. The runaway slaves regrouped into small bands, settled in the forest, and established various small communities [23, 24]. Finding themselves in new and unfamiliar environments and in constant danger of recapture, they relied on the Indigenous peoples living in the adjoining rain forests to gradually develop means of subsistence and defense [25, 26].

They soon formed resistance groups in the interior and often raided the plantations to recruit new members and capture women as well as to acquire weapons, food, and supplies [16, 23, 24, 27]. The authorities retaliated, often with the help of militia consisting of the colonial army, mercenaries, and groups of urban slaves called Redi Musus ("those wearing red hats") and had occasional victories [16, 23, 24, 27]. However, accustomed to open-field army-to-army battle in Europe, they were no match for the Maroon guerilla warfare in the treacherous tropical jungle [16, 27]. After more than half a century of vicious combat, the Maroons' independence was recognized by the signing of a peace treaty with the Dutch colonial administration in the 1760s [16]. This allowed them to occupy a large part of the interior where they preserved much of their cultural concepts of health and illness and much of their traditional medicinal practices [28].

The new and unique Maroon culture was highly successful and several independent tribes developed [23, 24]. These currently include the Saramaka, the Paramaka, the Aukan, the Kwinti, the Aluku or Boni, and the Matawai, each with its own language and cultural characteristics [23, 24]. However, all groups maintain a strict hierarchical authority system organized along matriarchal lines, and all are headed by a paramount chief (the granman) who is chosen by a combination of descent and divination [23, 24]. The granman is assisted by several village captains (the kapitens) who are locally appointed. Important decisions about issues affecting the entire village are taken during lengthy gatherings called krutus [23, 24]. This system is acknowledged and respected by the central government in Paramaribo [23, 24].

The enslaved Africans who did not join the Maroons and continued to work on the plantations were granted their formal freedom on July 1, 1863, and their actual freedom on July 1, 1973 [13, 14, 17]. Many remained in Suriname's coastal area and mixed with Europeans, particularly Dutch but also members from other ethnic groups [17]. These Creoles were economically and politically highly successful and were the first non-Whites to hold public offices in Suriname from 1954 on, when the country received partial autonomy from The Netherlands [1, 17]. They widely adopted Christianity and Catholicism, but retained their affiliation with their African heritage and still adhere to various African traditions [17]. For instance, the generally appreciated call-and-response Creole kaseko and kawina songs supported by percussion can directly be traced to age-old African forms of music [1, 17]. This also holds true for many Creole perceptions of health and disease as well as the use of various plant-based medications which they refer to as oso dresis ("home-made medicines") [1, 17, 29].

3.2. Traditional African medicine

Many of the Maroon and Creole traditions have their roots in the early period of African dominance and Egyptian leadership before 3200 BC, when North Africa was home to many skilled practitioners who had developed a comprehensive medicinal system [30]. This holistic discipline was—and still is—mostly based on a large variety of medicinal plants and spirituality, spread throughout the continent, and was carried to Suriname by the enslaved Africans [28]. Traditional African medicine assumes that disease results from imbalances in social circumstances and spiritual perceptions. This would hold true for "physiological" diseases ranging from venereal diseases to cancer and even Ebola, but also for psychiatric disorders such as depression and anxiety [28]. The diagnosis is often reached through spiritual means, and the treatment is usually derived from the comprehensive herbal pharmacopeia and would accomplish both physical and spiritual healing [28]. Due to the relatively small number of university-trained physicians and the relatively high costs of allopathic medicines, as much as 86% of the inhabitants of Sub-Saharan Africa rely on traditional African medications [31]. For this reason, many African countries have expressed the commitment to develop safe, efficacious, quality, and affordable traditional medicines accessible to the majority of their inhabitants [32].

Based on these ancient African medicinal concepts, Afro-Surinamese have developed Winti ("wind" or "spirit"), a nature-oriented religion in which the spiritual world is consulted by music, singing, trances, and rituals in order to create and maintain a harmonious balance between humans and the visible and invisible powers of nature [29, 33, 34]. Winti is one of the most distinctive characteristics of Maroon and Creole culture and is mainly based on the abovementioned beliefs and magical rituals, the enslaved Africans had brought along [29, 33, 34] but has also been influenced by Indigenous traditions [25, 35]. The invisible powers are several gods called wintis, as well as the spirits of ancestors [29, 33, 34].

Specialized practitioners called Winti priests—either males or females—serve as intermediaries between man, specific wintis, and the spirits of ancestors, and can evoke the spirits by special rituals to solve physical, psychological, or social problems [29, 33, 34]. The condition may be diagnosed during a special Winti ritual and is treated by medicinal and spiritual therapies consisting of specific herbs, special rituals, or both [29, 33, 34]. The Winti priests are referred to as lukuman ("the one who looks", i.e., performs the diagnosis), dresiman ("the one who cures", i.e., prepares and administers the medication), or duman ("the one who accomplishes", i.e., treats and cures), to distinguish them from obiaman, bonuman, and wisiman who are in general associated with black magic practices [29, 33, 34].

Winti priests have a profound knowledge of the medicinal plants and the diseases and conditions they treat [29, 33, 34]. Some plants—such as the African rice *Oryza glaberrima* Steud. (Poaceae) and the Bambara groundnut *Vigna subterranea* (L.) Verdc. (Fabaceae), but also crops that originated from Asia such as the taro *Colocasia esculenta* (L.) Schott (Araceae) and the banana Musa sp. L. (Musaceae)—were grown in Suriname from leftovers of the food provided to the slaves or from seeds they had smuggled during their trans-Atlantic journey [35]. Others such as the cassava *Manihot esculenta* Crantz (Euphorbiaceae) and several yam species (*Dioscorea* spp.) have been adopted from the Indigenous [25, 26, 36]. And still others—particularly members of the plant families Fabaceae, Euphorbiaceae, and Asteraceae—were deemed useful because of their resemblance with species known from Africa or by trial and error [35].

3.3. Medicinal and ritual plants used by Maroons and Creoles

One of the first traditional medicinal healers of Suriname was the freedman Quassie van Timotibo, also known as Kwasi, who popularized one of the earliest and most popular Surinamese traditional medicines, kwasibita ("Kwasi's bitter") [37]. Suspected to be a member of the Redi Musus and held responsible for the fall of Fort Buku headed by Boni—one of the most revered Maroon rebel generals [16, 24, 27]—Kwasi was considered a traitor among a large part of the slave population [37]. However, he was respected by many Whites as the most proficient dresi- and lukuman of eighteenth-century Suriname [37]. Kwasi had obtained much of his medicinal knowledge from the Indigenous peoples and discovered around 1730 the remarkable qualities of the bitterwood or kwasibita *Quassia amara* L. (Simaroubaceae) for treating malaria fevers and stomach troubles [37, 38]. This owed him the reputation of "the most honorable and most learned gentleman, master Phillipus of Quassy, professor of Herbology in Surinam" [37]. Today, kwasibita preparations are among the most consumed oso dresis for promoting general health [38].

Maroons and Creoles use many other plants for treating a variety of disease conditions including, among others, parasitic infections, hypertension, diabetes mellitus, bone fractures, and psychological conditions [33, 34, 38–44]. Spiritual herbal baths and ritual washing are often part of the treatment, as they would have a medicinal and magical effect on the body, calming the nervous system [33, 34, 38, 39]. The washings would also provide spiritual purification, protect against injury, repair broken relationships, and exorcise evil forces [33, 34, 38–44]. A few popular plant-based medicinal applications are the so-called kowru dresis, genital steam baths for females, and remedies for children's ailments [35, 38].

Kowru dresis ("medicines against a cold") are prepared from several plants including the leaves from *Senna* spp. (Fabaceae), the seeds from the aniseed *Pimpinella anisum* L. (Apiaceae), the aerial parts from the stonebreaker *Phyllanthus niruri* L. (Phyllanthaceae), the leaves from the birthwort *Aristolochia* spp. L. (Aristolochiaceae), the roots from the liquorice *Glycyrrhiza glabra* L. (Fabaceae), and/or the roots from the Chinese rhubarb *Rheum palmatum* L. (Polygonaceae) [28, 33, 34, 38]. These preparations are used to remove obstructions in bowels, airways, blood circulation, and genitourinary system, but also for mental well-being [28, 33, 34, 38]. The latter use is presumably based on the ancient African belief that even psychological conditions result from an imbalance between "hot" and "cold" and can be reversed by removing the "cold" [30]. Notably, in various communities *Senna* spp. and *R. palmatum* are traditionally used as a laxative and a purgative, respectively [45, 46]; *P. anisum* as a carminative and for colics [47]; *P. niruri* for stomach, genitourinary, liver, and spleen problems [48]; *Aristolochia* spp. for their antihelminthic activity [49]; and *G. glabra* for rejuvenation [50].

Genital steam baths are abundantly used by females for their personal hygiene [28, 33–35, 38] but also—as indicated by their suggestive vernacular names—to improve the appearance of the vagina in order to enhance sensation during intercourse, securing the relationship with and economic support by the male partner [28, 33–35, 38]. A few of the dozens of plants used in genital steam baths are the broko pipi ("broken penis") *Bellucia grossularioides* (L.) Triana 1871 (Melastomataceae); the Paranamklem ("Paranam grip") *Ludwigia nervosa* (Poir.) H. Hare (Onagraceae); the musude baasa ("early-morning hug") *Miconia tomentosa* (Rich.)

D. Don ex DC. (Melastomataceae); and the kunami ("come to me") *Clibadium surinamense* L. (Asteraceae). Leaves from the shy plant *Mimosa pudica* L. (Fabaceae) that fold inward and droop when touched, and aromatic plants such as the pêpë uwíi *Guatteria schomburgkiana* Mart. (Annonaceae) may be added to the bath [28, 33–35, 38].

Important childhood conditions requiring traditional treatment include atita and evil eye. Atita, commonly known in Suriname as zuurte or suri ("sourness"), is an ill-described condition in newborns that is characterized by stomach ache, cramps, diaper rash, yellow, sour-smelling feces, and diarrhea with small grains resembling okra seeds [28, 33–35, 38]. Atita may be caused by the baby's intestinal flora which must adapt to the uptake of proteins from breast milk [35]. This condition is treated by bathing the baby with a decoction of the leaves and/or flowers from the ingiwiri ("Indian herb") *Nepsera aquatica* (Aubl.) Naudin. (Melastomataceae), the yorkapesi ("demon pea") *S. occidentalis* (L.) Link. (Fabaceae), or the busipesi ("bush pea") *S. chrysocarpa* (Desv.) H.S. Irwin & Barneby and having the baby drink some of the decoction [28, 33–35, 38].

A baby is at risk to get evil eye or ogri ai ("bad eye") by an envious or a malevolent glare that can inflict harm, suffering, or even death [28, 33–35, 38]. This condition is commonly treated by bathing the infant with Reckitt's Blue, which presumably has its origin in its whitening (i.e., cleansing) effect on laundry [28, 33–35, 38]. Ogri ai can presumably be prevented by rubbing asafetida or didibri kaka ("devil's feces")—the foul smelling dried latex from the rhizomes of the stinking gum *Ferula assafoetida* L. (Apiaceae)—in the baby's hair, and placing a gold bracelet with three black beads on its clothes [28, 33–35, 38].

4. Ethnopharmacological practices of Hindustani

4.1. The Hindustani community in Suriname

The first indentured laborers from (then British) India arrived on June 5, 1873, in Paramaribo with the sailing ship Lalla Rookh that had departed more than 3 months earlier from central depots in Calcutta [18, 19]. The 452 passengers—called "Hindustanis" by the Dutch—were mostly recruited from the modern-day states of Uttar Pradesh and Bihar in northern and eastern India, respectively [18, 19]. Important reasons to leave their homeland were the high unemployment and the substantial loss of traditional jobs due to the rapid industrialization of India [18, 19]. However, at least some of them might have been misled into believing that they were taken to a place of pilgrimage called Sri Ram which turned out to be Suriname [18, 19]. Sixty-three more shiploads with laborers arrived in Suriname, taking as many as 34,304 Hindustani to the Dutch colony until 1916, when this practice was discouraged by Mahatma Gandhi's movement for an independent India [18, 19].

Although formally considered laborers on a 5-year contract rather than slaves [18, 19], working conditions on the sugar and coffee plantations were more or less equal to slavery [18, 19]. Working hours were long, payment was low, housing was in former slave accommodations, and not completing assigned tasks was severely punished [18, 19]. This regularly led to bloody uprisings, the largest one of which occurred in 1902 at the Marienburg sugar factory in Commewijne, then the center of sugarcane processing in Suriname [18, 19]. Angry workers killed the Scottish supervisor James Mavor, and in retaliation the Dutch colonial forces killed 24 workers and wounded over 39 [18, 19]. The Hindustani fatalities were buried in a mass grave that has remained unidentified until today [18, 19].

Nevertheless, only one-third of the workers returned to India after the completion of their contract [18, 19]. The remaining two-thirds accepted the offer of free settlement rights on plantations plus a bonus of a 100 Dutch guilders for abandoning their right to a return passage [18, 19]. Several of them used their bonus money and their savings to grow rice on their small plots of land, particularly in the western district of Nickerie yielding them appreciable incomes [18, 19]. Even today, a number of Hindustanis own sizable rice farms in Suriname [51].

4.2. Ayurveda

All and all, the Hindustani community has economically and politically been very successful in the Surinamese society but has managed to keep their culture and traditions alive, strengthening the group identity [51]. This holds true for their religion, marriage rituals, customs in raising children, family and communal life, burial rites, as well as celebrations as Holi Phagwah, the festival of colors that celebrates the victory of good over evil and the arrival of spring, and Diwali, the festival of lights that rejoices the triumph of light over darkness [51]. Notably, Surinamese Hindi or Sarnami—a dialect based on Bhojpuri, the main language spoken in the parts of India, the Hindustani originated from—is the third-most spoken language in Suriname after Surinamese and Dutch [51].

The Hindustanis have also largely preserved their cultural and traditional medicinal practices which are strongly linked to Ayurvedic medicine or Ayurveda (Sanskrit for "knowledge of life") [52–54]. Ayurveda is probably one of the oldest forms of medicine [52–54]. It originates from India and dates back more than 3000 years ago, and is still one of the country's most important traditional health-care systems [52–54]. Up to 80% of Indians use Ayurvedic medications for a variety of conditions including complex ailments such as angina pectoris and diabetes mellitus [52–54]. Ayurvedic practitioners are educated in 180 training centers [52–54], and the huge intellectual property and economic interest are managed by the prominent Department of Ayurveda, Yoga and Naturopathy, Unani, Siddha, and Homeopathy [52–54]. India's government also supports laboratory and clinical research on Ayurvedic preparations [52–54].

Ayurvedic medicinal concepts are based on the belief that health and wellness depend on a delicate balance between mind, body, and spirit, and that imbalance results in disease [52–54]. This holistic approach is a fundamental aspect of Ayurveda [52–54]. Today, Ayurveda is widely practiced throughout the world and in many countries recognized as a form of complementary and alternative medicine [52–54]. The principal ingredients of Ayurvedic medications are preparations derived from leaves, fruits, seeds, bark, or roots from certain plants [52–54]. Hundreds of plant species are used for such preparations [52–54]. In addition, Ayurvedic medications may be prepared from animal products such as milk, bones, or fats, and/or minerals such as sulfur, lead, arsenic, copper sulfate, and gold [52–54].

4.3. Medicinal and ritual plants used by Hindustanis

The Hindustanis in Suriname also use a large variety of plants for their Ayurveda-based cultural and medicinal customs [55–57]. Several of these plants have been brought over from India but others have been discovered in Suriname or adopted from other cultures [55–57]. Examples of long known and very popular Ayurvedic medicinal plants are the neem *Azadirachta indica* A. Juss., 1830 (Meliaceae), the ashoka tree *Saraca asoca* (Roxb.) Willd. (Fabaceae), the Indian bael tree *Aegle marmelos* (L.) Corrêa (Rutaceae), the bitter melon *Momordica charantia* Linn (Cucurbitaceae), the jambolan *Syzygium cumini* (L.) Skeels (Myrtaceae), the turmeric *Curcuma longa* L. (1753) (Zingiberaceae), and the holy basil or tulsi *Ocimum tenuiflorum* L. (Lamiaceae) [55–57].

The bitter-tasting constituents of parts of *A. indica* are believed to boost the immune system and to treat many diseases, among others, colds, fevers, respiratory conditions, stomach ailments, high blood pressure, and/or diabetes mellitus [58]. Volatile substances emanating from *A. indica* leaves placed under the bed sheets would also treat chicken pox [59], and a tea from these parts of the plant is typically used as an internal cleanse [58]. These beneficial effects may be related to the anthelmintic, antifungal, antibacterial, and antiviral activities of nimbinin, one of the main bioactive compounds of *A. indica* [60].

The stem bark, flowers, and seeds from *S. asoca* are used against postmenopausal syndrome and gynecological disorders [61]. And preparations from various parts of *A. marmelos, M. charantia*, and *S. cumini* are extensively used for treating diabetes mellitus but so far without convincing scientific evidence [62–64]. However, a few studies suggest that the presumed blood glucose-lowering activity of *M. charantia* may depend on the way the medication is prepared: preparations from fresh leaves seem to elicit a better effect when compared to the widely available tablets or capsules [65].

C. longa and *O. tenuiflorum* are among the most popular Ayurvedic herbs. The powdered rhizomes from *C. longa* are an essential part of curry which is used as a spice in many Hindustani dishes [51]. *C. longa* preparations are furthermore used, among others, as a diuretic; to stimulate blood flow in the pelvic area; to treat fevers with jaundice, hepatitis, and malaria; to prevent excessive menstrual pain; to enhance mental functioning and well-being; and externally for herpes, bruises, wounds, and rheumatism [66]. The leaves from the aromatic plant *O. tenuiflorum*—either fresh, dried, powdered, or as a tea—would treat a similar variety of diseases including stress and a disturbed homeostasis [67].

Many of these plants are also considered sacred and are used in various Hindu rituals [51]. For instance, preparations from *A. indica* leaves, bark, and fruits are consumed during certain ceremonies, festivals, and commemorations; the fruits from *A. marmelos* are offered to Shiva, the god of yoga, meditation, and arts during religious rituals; a paste of turmeric in coconut oil is applied on the skin of the bride and the groom during pre-marriage rituals to make their skin bright and glowing; the flowers from *O. tenuiflorum* are used as a holy cleanser for food offerings during prayers; and *S. asoca* is worshipped during Chaitra, the first month of the Hindu calendar, marking the arrival of Spring.

5. Ethnopharmacological practices of Javanese

5.1. The Javanese community in Suriname

The first group of Javanese indentured laborers arrived in Paramaribo on August 9, 1890 [19, 20]. It consisted of 94 small farmers from villages in Central and East Java in the former Dutch East Indies [19, 20]. They had been recruited by the very influential Netherlands Trading Society established by the Dutch King Willem I, either by force, bribery, or manipulation [19, 20]. The approximately 40-day journey was hard, and many Javanese died on the ship, in-transit in The Netherlands, or upon arrival in Paramaribo [19, 20]. Those who survived were mainly set to work on sugarcane plantations in the district of Commewijne [19, 20].

This was deemed so successful that many more followed from 1894 on. In 1904, Javanese laborers were even specifically recruited to construct the Colonial Railways for the transport of sugarcane from surrounding plantations to the sugarcane factory in Marienburg [19, 20]. Contracts were signed for 5 years, but life in Suriname's countryside was brutal and wages were minimal [19, 20]. For this reason, thousands of Javanese returned to Indonesia or to The Netherlands, particularly after Indonesia's independence in 1954 [19, 20].

The influx of indentured workers from Java ceased in 1939 with the advent of the Second World War, and had brought a total of 32,956 Javanese in Suriname [19, 20]. Those who settled in Suriname received a plot of land and a reimbursement of 100 guilders repatriation money [19, 20]. They were initially kept isolated in the countryside, particularly after Governor Johannes C. Kielstra's (1933–1943) consent of Javanese farm villages with their own village head (the lurah) and chief committee [19, 20]. On the other hand, this secluded lifestyle strengthened the group identity, as they maintained the rich culture they had brought with them from Java [19, 20].

Nowadays, the Javanese community has been well integrated in the Surinamese society, but many of their traditions and rituals have been preserved [68–70]. This holds true not only for their language but also for their types of entertainment such as the wayang shadow puppet show accompanied by distinctive orchestral gamelan music, and Javanese ludruk theater that includes the centuries old tradition of storytelling through slow, graceful, and expressive dances [70]. An important ritual that has been preserved is the preparation of the sacrificial slamatan meal at seven specific time periods to commemorate the departed, including the day of passing and 1000 after his/her death [70].

5.2. Jamu

The Javanese have also maintained their traditional medicinal practices which are mainly based on medicinal plants and are referred to as Jamu [70]. Jamu is the widely practiced form of traditional medicine in Indonesia that probably has its origin in the Mataram Kingdom era in ancient Java, some 1300 years ago [71, 72]. Jamu is mostly based on plants, but materials from animals such as honey, royal jelly, bee larvae, milk, and chicken eggs are also used [71, 72].

Jamu products called jamus are in Indonesia traditionally available from (particularly female) peddlers and street-side vendors, but are nowadays also produced and retailed by large companies in dried form in sachet packaging or as tablets, capsules, and liquid drinks [71, 72]. The manufacturers of jamus are united in Gabungan Pengusaha Jamu, an Indonesian Herbal and Traditional Medicine Association [71, 72]. Together, they employ roughly 15 million workers, produce over 1200 different jamu products, and bring in annual revenues of more than US$ 73 million [71, 72].

Jamu is practiced in both Indonesia and Suriname by highly respected medicinal practitioners known as dukuns or tabibs [70, 71, 73]. The dukun is very influential and holds extensive knowledge about the preparation of the large variety of sometimes rather complicated jamus [70, 71]. An example is the very popular jamu galian consisting of different parts of eight plants that is widely used in Suriname as a general health-promoting tonic [70, 71, 73]. The dukun also plays an important role during, for instance, nyuwuk, a ritual to bring a person at ease by praying over and blowing three times over a glass of water that then must be drunk by the client [70, 71, 73]. Nyuwuk is often performed prior to examinations, circumcisions, or giving birth [70, 71].

5.3. Medicinal and ritual plants used by Javanese

Many plants incorporated in jamus belong to the family Zingiberaceae which have been brought from Java and are now cultivated in Suriname [74]. A few examples are the laos *Alpinia galanga* (L.) Willd., the pink and blue ginger *C. aeruginosa* Roxb., (1810), the temu giring *C. heyneana* Valeton & Zijp, the earlier mentioned *C. longa* that has its origin in Indian Ayurveda, the yellow ginger *C. xanthorrhiza* Roxb., the aromatic ginger *Kaempferia galanga* L., the bengle *Zingiber cassumunar* Roxb., and the bitter ginger *Z. zerumbet* (L.) Roscoe ex. Sm. [74]. For medicinal purposes, the macerated and/or decocted rhizomes are used, either from a certain species or from combinations of several species [74].

As the majority of Javanese is Muslim [2], jamus are usually prepared on Mondays and Thursdays which are assigned for fasting in Islam. They are used for treating a wide variety of conditions. For instance, the rhizomes from *A. galanga* would treat the fungal skin infection "lota" (pityriasis alba), stomach cramps, and dysentery [74]. And those from *C. xanthorriza* would help against liver ailments, eczema, constipation, and gallstones, and for cleansing the uterus after giving birth [74]. The mother is also advised to drink on a daily basis a decoction of *C. xanthorriza, C. aeruginosa,* and *Z. zerumbet* rhizomes together with leaves from *P. anisum* [73]. These apparent health benefits may be attributed, at least in part, to the anti-parasitic activity of *A. galanga* preparations and one of its bioactive constituents galangin [75, 76], and the anti-inflammatory and hepatoprotective effects of curcumin in *C. xanthorriza* products [77].

Jamus prepared from *C. longa* are used for treating, among others, inflamed gums, abscesses, menstrual pains, and skin rash, partially because of their antiseptic activity and refreshing effect [74]. The latter action may also help explain the application of a *C. longa*-based ointment called bobok for alleviating the discomfort of sprains, insect bites, and toothache [74]. Furthermore, the juice collected from *C. longa* rhizomes is, together with that from *Z. zerumbet* rhizomes, used for treating stomach ache, and together with the macerated rhizomes of *C. aeruginosa*, and *Z. zerumbet*, a grated onion, sugar, and a packet of cooked Glycine max soybeans, for treating pinworm infections in children [74]. The potential health benefits of *C. longa* may be ascribed to the antimicrobial and anti-inflammatory properties of curcuminoids in the plant [66].

Medicinal plants belonging to families other than the Zingiberaceae that are incorporated in popular jamus are the cat's whiskers *Orthosiphon grandiflorus* Bold. (Lamiaceae), the betel *Piper betle* L. (Piperaceae), the ketyi beling *Strobilanthes crispa* Blume (Acanthaceae), and the gambir *Uncaria gambir* (W. Hunter) Roxb., 1824 (Rubiaceae) [74]. An infusion of the leaves from *O. grandiflorus* and *S. crispa*, either separately or in combination, can be used against kidney stones and renal colics [74]. And rolled-up or macerated leaves from *P. betle* are placed in the nostrils to stop nose bleeding. *P. betle* leaves are also chewed together with those from *U. gambir* to heal inflamed gums [74]. There is at least some preclinical evidence to support these applications [78–81].

6. Closing remarks

As a result of its fascinating and tumultuous history, Suriname has become a treasure chest of traditional medicinal approaches and rituals based on plants. Traditions and rituals from every continent on Earth have found their way in the country and have largely been preserved. This is illustrated by the various examples given in this overview about Maroons and Creoles as well as Hindustanis and Javanese. However, the same applies to the rich Indigenous South American cultures, traditional Chinese medicine, and the cultures brought over by many other ethnicities in the country. Gradually, many of these traditions are finding their way to other ethnicities. This is likely to result in a unique and even richer traditional medical culture in the country.

For instance, the use of kowru dresis as well as many remedies and rituals against evil eye has its origin in Africa but is not anymore restricted to Maroons and Creoles and has become common practice in all ethnic groups in Suriname. The neem plant *A. indica*, the turmeric *C. longa*, and the bitter melon *M. charantia* have presumably been introduced in Suriname by Hindustanis but are now widely used throughout the country against a variety of conditions. And the broad use of the cat's whiskers *O. aristatus* for treating kidney stones and renal colics is attributable to the Javanese. This ethnic group is also responsible for the presence of many medicinal Zingiberaceae species in Suriname and the general use of the laos *A. galanga* against the skin disease lota.

Contributing to this pool are the traditional medicinal customs of the Indigenous which already had a profound influence on Maroon culture, and traditional Chinese medicine that has become, similarly to Indian Ayurveda, a form of complementary and alternative medicine that is worldwide respected. It is foreseeable that these cultural fusions—meetings of the mind—will lead to the development of a distinct form of herbalism in Suriname that will generate a unique array of medicines.

Author details

Dennis R.A. Mans*, Deeksha Ganga and Joëlle Kartopawiro

*Address all correspondence to: dennis_mans@yahoo.com

Department of Pharmacology, Anton de Kom University of Suriname, Paramaribo, Suriname

References

[1] Bakker E, Dalhuisen L, Donk R, Hassankhan M, Steegh F. Geschiedenis van Suriname: van stam tot staat (History of Suriname: from tribe to state). Zutphen: Walburg Pers; 1998.

[2] Algemeen Bureau voor de Statistiek/Conservation International Suriname. Suriname in cijfers 286-2012/04. (General Bureau of Statistics/Conservation International Suriname. Suriname in numbers 286-2012/04). Milieustatistieken (Environment Statistics). Paramaribo: Algemeen Bureau voor de Statistiek; 2012.

[3] Algemeen Bureau voor de Statistiek/Censuskantoor. Suriname in cijfers 2013/05. Resultaten achtste (8ste) volks- en woningtelling in Suriname (volume 1) (General Bureau of Statistics/ Census office. Suriname in numbers 2013/05. Results of the eight general census of Suriname). Demografische en sociale karakteristieken en migratie (Demographic and social characteristics and migration). Paramaribo: Algemeen Bureau voor de Statistiek; 2013.

[4] Hammond DS. Forest conservation and management in the Guiana Shield (Chapter 1). In: Hammond DS, editor. Tropical rainforests of the Guiana shield. Wallingford: CABI Publishing; 2005. p. 1–14.

[5] Algemeen Bureau voor de Statistiek. Suriname in cijfers 303-2014-04 (General Bureau of Statistics. Suriname in numbers 303-2014-04). Basis indicatoren (Basic indicators). Paramaribo: Algemeen Bureau voor de Statistiek; 2014.

[6] The World Bank. Suriname overview [Internet]. 2014. Available from: http://www.worldbank.org/en/country/suriname/overview [Accessed: 2016-09-12].

[7] Helman A. Cultureel mozaïek van Suriname. Bijdrage tot onderling begrip (Cultural mosaic of Suriname. A contribution to mutual understanding). Zutphen: De Walburg Pers; 1977.

[8] Versteeg AH. The history of prehistoric archeological research in Suriname. In: Wong TE, de Vletter DR, Krook L, Zonneveld JIS, van Loon AJ, editors. The history of earth sciences in Suriname. Amsterdam: Kon. Ned. Academie Wetenschappen & Toegepaste Geowetenschappen TNO; 1998. p. 203–234.

[9] Mann CC. 1491: New revelation of the Americas before Columbus. New York, NY: Knopf Publishing Group; 2005.

[10] Parry JH. The discovery of South America. New York, NY: Taplinger Publishing Co; 1979.

[11] British Empire: South America: Surinam—Brief history [Internet]. Available from: http://www.britishempire.co.uk/maproom/surinam.htm [Accessed: 2016-09-12].

[12] History of Jews in Suriname—Suriname Jewish community [Internet]. Available from: http://www.surinamejewishcommunity.com/history [Accessed: 2016-09-12].

[13] Goslinga CC. The Dutch in the Caribbean and on the Wild Coast 1580-1680. Gainesville: University Press of Florida; 1989.

[14] Oostindie G. Paradise overseas: the Dutch Caribbean: colonialism and its transatlantic legacies. Oxford: Macmillan Caribbean; 2005.

[15] Postma J. The Dutch in the Atlantic slave trade, 1600-1815. Cambridge: Cambridge University Press; 1990.

[16] Jagdew E. Vrede te midden van oorlog in Suriname. Inheemsen, Europeanen, Marrons en Vredesverdragen 1667–1863 (Peace amidst war in Suriname. Indigenous, Europeans, Maroons, and peace treaties 1667–1863) [thesis]. Paramaribo: Anton de Kom Universiteit van Suriname; 2014.

[17] Arends J. 2002. The history of the Surinamese Creoles I: a sociohistorical survey. In: Carlin E, Arends J, editors. Atlas of the languages of Suriname. Leiden: KITLV Press; 2002. p. 115–130.

[18] Tinker H. A new system of slavery: the export of Indian labour overseas 1830-1920. London: Oxford University Press; 1974.

[19] Hoefte R. In place of slavery: a social history of British Indian and Javanese laborers in Suriname. Gainesville: University Press of Florida; 1998.

[20] Djasmadi L, Hoefte R, Mingoen H, editors. Migratie en cultureel erfgoed: verhalen van Javanen in Suriname, Indonesië en Nederland (Migration and cultural heritage: stories of Javanese in Suriname, Indonesia and The Netherlands). Leiden: KITLV Press; 2010.

[21] Ankum-Houwink JC. Chinese kontraktarbeiders in in de 19e eeuw (Chinese contract workers in the 19th century). OSO. 1985;4:181–186.

[22] Hoefte R. Suriname in the long twentieth century. Domination, contestation, globalization. New York, NY: Palgrave Macmillan; 2014.

[23] Pakosie ARM. Maroon leadership and the Surinamese state (1760–1990). J Legal Plur. 1996;37–38:263–278.

[24] Fey T. Marrons van Suriname (Maroons from Suriname). Amsterdam: KIT Publishers; 2009.

[25] Parahoe M. Agro-biodiversity and relationship of people with the environment: a comparison of the Kwinti Maroons and Trio indigenous people, Suriname [thesis]. Mona: University of the West Indies; 2001.

[26] Herndon CN, Uiterloo M, Uremaru A, Plotkin MJ, Emanuels-Smith G, Jitan J. Disease concepts and treatment by tribal healers of an Amazonian forest culture. J Ethnobiol Ethnomed. 2009;5:27. DOI: 10.1186/1746-4269-5-27

[27] Hoogbergen WSM. The Boni-Maroon wars in Suriname. Leiden: Brill; 1990.

[28] Thoden Van Velzen HUE, van Wetering W. The great father and the danger: Religious cults, material forces, and collective fantasies in the world of the Surinamese Maroons. Dordrecht: Floris Publications; 1988.

[29] Stephen HJM. Geneeskruiden van Suriname: hun toepassing in de volksgeneeskunde en in de magie (Herbal medicines from Suriname: their applications in folk medicine and wizardry). Amsterdam: De Driehoek; 1979.

[30] Onwuanibe RC. The philosophy of African medicinal practice. J Opin. 1979;9:25–28.

[31] World Health Organization. WHO traditional medicine strategy 2002–2005. Geneva: World Health Organization; 2002.

[32] Chitindingu E, George G, Gow J. A review of the integration of traditional, complementary and alternative medicine into the curriculum of South African medical schools. BMC Med Educ. 2014;14:40. DOI: 10.1186/1472-6920-14-40

[33] Wooding CJ. Winti: een Afro-Amerikaanse godsdienst in Suriname. Een cultuurhistorische analyse van de religieuze verschijnselen in de Para (Winti: an African-American religion in Suriname. A cultural-historical analysis of religious phenomena in Para). Meppel: Krips Repro BV; 1972.

[34] Wooding CJ. Traditional healing and medicine in Winti: a sociological interpretation. J Opin. 1979;9:35–40.

[35] Vossen T, Towns A, Ruysschaert S, Quiroz D, van Andel T. Consequences of the trans-Atlantic slave trade on medicinal plant selection: plant use for cultural bound syndromes affecting children in Suriname and Western Africa. PLoS One. 2016;9(11):e112345. DOI:10.1371/journal.pone.0112345

[36] Veth, B. Gebruiks- en medicinale planten van de Wayana Indianen in Frans Guyana en Suriname (Useful and medicinal plants of the Wayana Indians in French Guiana and Suriname). Utrecht: Nationaal Herbarium Nederland, Universiteit Utrecht; 1990.

[37] Dragtenstein F. Trouw aan de blanken. Quassie van Nieuw Timotibo, twist en strijd in de 18e eeuw in Suriname (Loyalty to Whites. Quassie van Nieuw Timotibo, strife and struggle in the 18th century in Suriname). Amsterdam: NiNsee/KIT Publishers; 2004.

[38] Van Andel TR, Ruysschaert S. Medicinale en rituele planten van Suriname (Medicinal and ritual plants of Suriname). Amsterdam: KIT Publishers; 2011.

[39] Carney JA, Rosomoff RN. In the shadow of slavery: Africa's botanical legacy in the Atlantic World. 6th ed. Berkeley: University of California Press; 2009.

[40] May AF. Sranan oso dresi. Surinaams kruidenboek (Surinamese folk medicine. A collection of Surinamese medicinal herbs). Paramaribo: De Walburg Pers; 1982.

[41] Titjari. Famiri-encyclopedia foe da natoera dresi-fasi. Gezinskruidenboek van de natuurgeneeswijzen. Natuurgeneeswijzen uit het zonnige Suriname (Encyclopedia of plant-based forms of treatment. Folk medicines from sunny Suriname). Amsterdam: Sangrafoe; 1985.

[42] Heyde H. Surinaamse medicijnplanten (Surinamese medicinal plants). 2nd ed. Paramaribo: Westfort; 1987.

[43] Slagveer JL. Surinaams groot kruidenboek: Sranan oso dresie (Surinamese herbal medicines). Paramaribo: De West; 1990.

[44] Sedoc NO. Afrosurinaamse natuurgeneeswijzen: bevattende meer dan tweehonderd meest gebruikelijke geneeskrachtige kruiden (Afro-Surinamese natural remedies: over two hundred commonly used medicinal herbs). Paramaribo: Vaco Press; 1992.

[45] Lemli J. The mechanism of action of sennosides. Ann Gastroenterol Hepatol (Paris). 1996;32:109–112.

[46] Chevalier A. Natural health: encyclopedia of herbal medicine. New York, NY: Dorling Kindersley; 2000.

[47] Shojaii A, Abdollahi Fard M. Review of pharmacological properties and chemical constituents of *Pimpinella anisum*. ISRN Pharmaceutics. 2012, 510795. DOI: 10.5402/2012/510795

[48] Patel JR, Tripathi P, Sharma V, Chauhan NS, Dixit VK. Phyllanthus amarus: ethnomedicinal uses, phytochemistry and pharmacology: a review. J Ethnopharmacol. 2011;138:286–313.

[49] Sati H, Sati B, Saklani S, Bhatt PC, Mishra AP. Phytochemical and pharmacological potential of *Aristolochia indica*: a review. Res J Pharmaceut Biol Chem Sci. 2011;2:647–654.

[50] Shibata S. A drug over the millennia: pharmacognosy, chemistry, and pharmacology of licorice. Yakugaku Zasshi. 2000;120:849–862.

[51] Hira S. 125 jaar sociaal-economische ontwikkeling in Suriname (125 years of social-economic development in Suriname). In: Hassankhan M, Hira S, editors. Van Gya en Boodheea tot Lachmon en Djwalapersad. Grepen uit 125 jaar maatschappelijke ontwikkeling van Hindostanen (From Gya and Boodheea to Lachmon and Djwalapersad. Impressions from 125 years social development of Hindustanis). Paramaribo/Den Haag: IMWO/Nauyuga/Amrit; 1998. p. 10–26.

[52] Chopra A, Doiphode VV. Ayurvedic medicine. Core concept, therapeutic principles, and current relevance. Med Clin North Am. 2002;86:75–89.

[53] Ravishankar B, Shukla VJ. Indian systems of medicine: a brief profile. Afr J Tradit Complement Altern Med. 2007;4:319–337.

[54] Kessler C, Wischnewsky M, Michalsen A, Eisenmann C, Melzer J. Ayurveda: between religion, spirituality, and medicine. Evid Based Complement Alternat Med. 2013. DOI: 10.1155/2013/952432

[55] Raghoenandan UPD. Etnobotanisch onderzoek bij de Hindoestaanse bevolkingsgroep in Suriname (An ethnobotanical investigation among Hindustanis in Suriname). [thesis]. Paramaribo: Anton de Kom Universiteit van Suriname; 1994.

[56] Ramharakh S. Planten gebruik door Surinaamse Hindoestanen in Nederland (The use of medicinal plants by Surinamese Hindustanis in The Netherlands). Utrecht: Nationaal Herbarium Nederland, Universiteit Utrecht, Utrecht; 2005.

[57] Haripersaud PP. Collecting biodiversity [thesis]. Utrecht: Universiteit Utrecht; 2009.

[58] Alzohairy MA. Therapeutics role of *Azadirachta indica* (neem) and their active constituents in diseases prevention and treatment. Evid Based Complement Alternat Med. 2016. DOI: 10.1155/2016/7382506

[59] Kumar VS, Navaratnam V. Neem (*Azadirachta indica*): prehistory to contemporary medicinal uses to humankind. Asian Pac J Trop Biomed. 2013;3:505–514.

[60] Hossaina MA, Al-Toubia WAS, Welia AM, Al-Riyamia QA, Al-Sabahiba JN. Identification and characterization of chemical compounds indifferent crude extracts from leaves of Omani neem. J Taibah Univ Sci. 2013;7:181–188.

[61] Singh S, Krishna THA, Kamalraj S, Kuriakose GC, Valayil JM, Jayabaskaran C. Phytomedicinal importance of *Saraca asoca* (Ashoka): an exciting past, an emerging present and a promising future. Curr Sci. 2015;109:1790–1801.

[62] Muralidharan L. Beneficial effects of *Aegle marmelos* leaves on blood glucose levels and body weight changes in alloxan-induced diabetic rats. J Med Plants Stud. 2014;2:46–49.

[63] Grover JK, Yadav SP. Pharmacological actions and potential uses of *Momordica charantia*: a review. J Ethnopharmacol. 2004;93:123–132.

[64] Kumar A, Ilavarasan R, Jayachandran T, Deecaraman M, Aravindan P, Padmanabhan N, Krishan MRV. Anti-diabetic activity of *Syzigium cumini* and its isolated compound against streptozotocin-induced diabetic rats. J Med Plants Res. 2008;2:246–249.

[65] Chen Q, Chan LL, Li ET. Bitter melon (*Momordica charantia*) reduces adiposity, lowers serum insulin and normalizes glucose tolerance in rats fed a high fat diet. J Nutr. 2003;133:1088–1093.

[66] Kunnumakkara B, Bordoloi D, Padmavathi G, Monisha J, Roy NK, Prasad S, Aggarwal BB. Curcumin, the golden nutraceutical: multitargeting for multiple chronic diseases. Br J Pharmacol. 2016. DOI: 2016. DOI: 10.1111/bph.13621

[67] Ravi P, Elumalai A, Eswaraiah MC, Kasarla R. A review on krishna tulsi, *Ocimum tenuiflorum*. Linn. Int J Res Ayurveda Pharmacy 2012;3:291–293.

[68] Superlan P. The Javanese in Surinam: ethnicity in a plural society [thesis]. Urban and Champaign: University of Illinois; 1976.

[69] Derveld FER. Politieke mobilisatie en integratie van de Javanen in Suriname (Political mobilization and integration of Javanese in Suriname). Bouma's Boekhandel. Groningen: Bouma's Boekhandel; 1982.

[70] De Waal Malefijt A. The Javanese of Surinam. Assen: van Gorcum; 1963.

[71] Beers S-J. Jamu: the ancient Indonesian art of herbal healing. North Clarendon: Tuttle Publishing; 2013.

[72] Elfahmi KR, Woerdenbag HJ, Kayser O. Jamu: Indonesian traditional herbal medicine towards rational phytopharmacological use. J Herbal Med. 2014;4:51–73.

[73] Al Makmun MT, Widodob SE. Construing traditional Javanese herbal medicine of headache: transliterating, translating, and interpreting Serat Primbon Jampi Jawi. Procedia - Soc Behav Sci. 2014;134:238–245.

[74] Tjong Ayong G. Het gebruik van medicinale planten door de Javaanse bevolkingsgroep in Suriname (The use of medicinal plants by the Javanese in Suriname). Paramaribo: Instituut voor de Opleiding van Leraren; 1989.

[75] Al-Adhroey AH, Nor ZM, Al-Mekhlafi HM, Mahmud R. Median lethal dose, antimalarial activity, phytochemical screening and radical scavenging of methanolic *Languas galanga* rhizome extract. Molecules. 2010;15:8366–8376. DOI:10.3390/molecules15118366

[76] Kaur A, Singh R, Dey CS, Sharma SS, Bhutani KK, Singh IP. Antileishmanial phenylpropanoids from Alpinia galanga (Linn.) Willd. Indian J Exp Biol. 2010:48:314–331.

[77] Priyadarsini KI. The chemistry of curcumin: from extraction to therapeutic agent. Molecules. 2014;19:20091–20112. DOI:10.3390/molecules191220091

[78] Premgamone A, Sriboonlue P, Disatapornjaroen W, Maskasem S, Sinsupan N, Apinives C. A long-term study on the efficacy of a herbal plant, *Orthosiphon grandiflorus*, and sodium potassium citrate in renal calculi treatment. Southeast Asian J Trop Med Public Health. 2001;32:654–660.

[79] Dwivedi V, Tripathi S. Review study on potential activity of *Piper betle*. J Pharmacogn Phytochem. 2014;4:93–98.

[80] Nurraihana H, Norfariza-Hanoon NA. Phytochemistry, pharmacology and toxicology properties of *Strobilanthes crispus*. Int Food Res J. 2013;20:2045–2056.

[81] Mesfin Yimam M, Lee Y-C, Kim T-W, Moore B, Jiao P, Hong M, Kim H-J, Nam J-B, Kim M-R, Oh J-S, Cleveland S, Hyun E-J, Chu M, Jia Q. Analgesic and anti-inflammatory effect of UP3005, a botanical composition containing two standardized extracts of *Uncaria gambir* and *Morus alba*. Pharmacogn Res. 2015;7(Suppl 1):S39–S46.

10

Romanian Aromatic and Medicinal Plants: From Tradition to Science

Radu Claudiu Fierascu, Irina Fierascu, Alina Ortan, Sorin Marius Avramescu, Cristina Elena Dinu-Pirvu and Daniela Ionescu

Abstract

From ancient times, plants have been used by humans for food, fodder, fibre and medicinal purposes. Several plants were empirically considered as treatments for a large array of illness and medical conditions. Each community had specific natural remedies, based on the geographical area, environmental conditions and other factors. Thus, the use of plants can be considered as part of the intangible cultural heritage of each community. In the geographical area of today's Romania, the ancient inhabitants, Dacians, had very good knowledge regarding the use of plants for medicinal purposes, as presented by several historical sources. The present work describes protocols for the extraction and purification of natural extracts, analytical characterisation, *in vitro* and *in vivo* evaluation of their potential applications as well as some practical examples of their application on selected Romanian native medicinal and aromatic plants. The presented results offer scientific support to their traditional use, suggesting in the same time some modern applications, for example in the nanotechnology field.

Keywords: aromatic and medicinal plants, Romanian, traditional remedy, scientific evidence

1. Introduction

1.1. Traditional use of medicinal and aromatic plants

The first human's tries to treat diseases were aiming for the environmental plants, so natural products could be considered the main mean of diseases treatment across the globe until the advent of scientific medicine. During their evolution on Earth, plants have developed the ability to synthesize certain chemical compounds for protection in the fight against world's predators, such as insects, fungi, herbivorous mammals, etc.

Although some of these compounds are toxic to predators, they proved to have beneficial effects in the treatment of human diseases. In the past centuries, the practice of empirical use of plants for therapeutic purposes was passed either in writing or orally, from generation to generation. Thus, the oldest way of treatment, phytotherapy, whose beginnings lie in Palaeolithic and whose traces are preserved in folk medicine up to our days, was developed on an empirical base, but also in the context of a magic vision of the world, where the symbol, the analogy and the correspondences principle have played and are playing an important role in the choice of useful plants [1–3].

People always appealed to nature, mainly to plants, for treating and curing various diseases; harvesting plants with everything they prove useful and their complete exploitation gave humans the opportunity to familiarize with their curative properties [4]. The first more precise data about the use of plants for healing in what is today Romania were given by the Greek doctor Discorides (doctor in Nero's army) in the five-volume treatise on plants "De Materia Medica", the precursor of all modern Pharmacopoeia and one of the most important botanical atlases in history. He pointed out that in Dacia numerous plant species were used on a large scale, making a vague and incomplete description of them. Published in 77, the book was describing 600 species of medicinal plants, of which 40 species were specific to Dacia's territory. Among these species, 27 plants have Daco-Thracian names, 8-Latin and 5-Greek, which is a confirmation of the age of phytotherapy in Romania [2, 3, 5, 6].

Over the time, the inhabitants of Romania's lands kept the continuity of rich traditions in the use of plants from spontaneous flora, which proved to be effective in curing physical or psychological suffering (injuries, fractures, bleeding, poisoning, animal bites, sunstroke, frostbite, infectious diseases, etc.).

Due to its geographic position, with a varied landscape and a climate favourable for rich vegetation, Romania is the meeting place of the Eurasian and Mediterranean flora. Here, grow more than 3600 species of higher plants, of which over 700 have become medicines, thanks to the long experience of the Romanian people in their use to cure diseases. In the Romanian plant heritage, there are numerous wild and cultivated plants that have different uses [1–9].

1.2. Short presentation of plants selected for the study

Among the Romanian traditional plants, *Heracleum sphondylium* L. (hogweed) occupies a special role due to its extremely intense vitalizing effects, therefore being called "Romanian Ginseng". The plant is known since antiquity, from the time of Plinius the Elder, under the name of *Heracleum*, derived from Heros, Heracles, Hercules, who had discovered its medical effect. It is an herbaceous plant, perennial or biannual that belongs to the family of *Apiaceae*, frequently found in meadows, scrublands, rarely in forests, from the plain region up to the mountains. The flowers are grouped in rich clusters, white or pink pal. The Romanian name of the plant comes from the leaves' shape which resembles a bear's paw. The herbal medicine uses the whole plant (especially leaves, buds, roots and seeds). The leaves and the buds are harvested from April to October; the whole plant is harvested during flowering, while the roots are harvested in spring and autumn. It is dryed in the shadow, in a thin layer. Heracleum's root and seeds quickly refresh and rejuvenate the body, increase exercise capacity and psychological tone, eliminate sterility, impotence and frigidity. It is a remedy indicated to the third age, relieving the discomforts of the premature physical decline, restoring tone and appetite for life [2, 3, 5, 6].

Anethum graveolens L. (dill) is an herbaceous, annual, terofite, vegetable, spicy, aromatic, cultivated and sub-spontaneous plant, which belongs to the *Apiaceae* family. It is known and cultivated since antiquity by Egyptians, Greeks, Romans and Gauls. In Romania, it is grown throughout the country, especially in assorted cultures. The stem, leaves and fruits have therapeutic uses in the traditional human medicine and in cult or traditional veterinary medicine. The harvesting of the stems and leaves is made when inflorescence is formed, while the harvesting of fruits is made when they are mature. From ancient times, culinary and medicinal uses were attributed to the dill. Decoction of the dill's seeds is used to treat stomach aches; the tea obtained by boiling the floriferous stems and dried inflorescences of dill is used to treat kidney diseases, hearts diseases and atherosclerosis and to increase lactation at women. Also, crushed dill's seed are used to treat intestinal worms at children. The dill is recommended in anorexia, indigestions, difficult digestion, heart diseases, urinary diseases, haemorrhoids, flatulence, various internal and external inflammations and menstrual pains [2, 5].

Taraxacum officinalis (L.) Weber ex F.H. Wigg (dandelion) is an herbaceous and perennial plant, which belongs to the *Asteraceae* family, common throughout Romania, in sunny places or in semidarkness, forests, meadows, pastures, on the roadside, from plains until subalpine area. The whole plant is harvested in spring, before and after the flowering, aerial parts or just the leaves are harvested in spring and the root is harvested in autumn or in early spring. Drying is made in the shadow, in a thin layer, in very airy places. The root and aerial parts of the plant have therapeutic uses in human and veterinary medicine, cult and traditional. Since Dacian times, the flowers and the juice resulting from squeezing dandelion's leaves were used in various skin disorders, the root was used in rheumatic diseases, the decoction of the leaves was used to treat liver diseases, while the decoction from the root was used to treat kidney diseases and against bleeding. The dandelion is recommended in liver diseases, urinary disorders, circulatory disorders, obesity, constipation, haemorrhoids, anaemia, cataracts, acne and endocrine diseases. In addition, the traditional medicine uses the plant to stimulate the pancreatic secretion, in the treatment of cancer and as an easy purgative in preventing constipations [2, 6].

Arctium lappa L. (burdock) is an herbaceous and biannual plant, which belongs to the *Asteraceae* family, common throughout Romania, from plain to mountain areas, wild lands, roadsides, along fences and flood groves. Known since antiquity by Geto-Dacians, the burdock was one of the most important and the oldest medicine practiced by our human folk medicine. The uses of the plant passed under the name of empirically remedies. Raw leaves were put on wounds and swellings; they were used to relieve the fever, to treat corns and to remove back pains. Tackling the lost hair and the stimulation of their growth was made by washing the head with broth resulting from boiling the burdock's leaves and stems. The harvesting of burdock's roots is made in spring for the 2 years plants and in autumn for the 1 year plants. After washing, the aerial plants are cleaned and dried at the sun, in thin layer. The leaves are harvested without petiole, in May–June, before flowering and dry in the shadow in one place. The roots show the therapeutically importance for the human and veterinary medicine. They have stronger and laster detoxifying effects, with an impressive range of uses, from food poisoning, skin diseases or rheumatism to glandular or metabolism disorders. In the long term, they have beneficial effects on the activity of the liver and gallbladder and they prevent diabetes and tumour diseases. In case of respiratory diseases and flu, the burdock is a valuable remedy, helping to stop the growth of the microorganisms, reducing fever and preventing complications. It is used the decoction, infusion, hot steeping, tincture and powder of burdock's root [6].

Anthriscus sylvestris (L.) Hoffm. (wild chervil) and *Anthriscus cerefolium* (L.) Hoffm. (the garden species) are herbaceous, biannual (respectively annual), terofite plant, belonging to the *Apiaceae* family, with pleasant smelling, white flowers arranged in small umbrellas, related with parsley and carrot. It is common in temperate regions, on the roadsides and forests, in pastures and hay fields. In the Romanian folk medicine, the aerial flowered parts of the plant are used, harvested in May-June, dried in a thin layer in well ventilated spaces. It has been used traditionally as a stimulant, diuretic, anti-haemorrhoidal, antipyretic, anti-inflammatory and analgesic. In the human folk medicine, it is also used in digestive disorders, having slightly laxative action, in bronchitis and chronic lung diseases, as an antitussive. Externally, it is used in inflammations of the eyelid, dermatitis and eczemas [4].

2. Obtaining and characterisation of natural extracts with biomedical applications

2.1. Extraction and separation of active compounds

The concentration of biologically active compounds of natural extracts directly depends on a series of factors, such as genomic composition, biological value of the cultivar, maturity stage of the plant, climatic zone, environmental conditions, post-harvest and storage conditions, as well as *the extraction methods applied* [10]. Processing of medicinal plants can be divided into two stages: *primary processing*, which consists of plants drying, conditioning and packaging, and *advanced processing* that consists of transforming raw materials obtained from primary processing into the desired final product. Extracts may be categorized according to several parameters, as follows [10]: considering the *nature of the solvent* extracts may be: aqueous extracts (infusion or maceration-type), hydroalcoholic extracts (tincture-type), oily extracts, medicinal vinegars (macerated in vinegar) or medicinal wines (macerated in wine); considering the *obtaining method*: selective extract (targeting the compounds of interest), non-selective extracts (tincture, macerated type, etc.), extracts obtained by pressing (fruit and vegetables juice); considering the *parts of the plant* subject to extraction: partial extract (only certain anatomical parts of the plant) or total extract (whole plant); considering the *water content* of the plant (humidity): extract obtained from dried plant or fresh plant extract; considering the *method of preparation*: simple, successive or multiple extracts.

Specific biologically active compounds are obtained from the vegetal products (different parts of plants or various mixtures of aromatic and medicinal plants) using appropriate solvents. To obtain water-soluble active substance at a pH close to neutral one (such as acids, bases, salts, sugars, phenols and polyphenols, amino acids, glycosides, gums, tannins, enzymes) water is used as solvent. Given that water is not a good solvent for resins, alkaloid, and oils - type compounds, etc., for obtaining them, alkaline or acidified water can be used. By-products as volatile oils, pigments, lecithin, resins, etc., are obtained using alcohol as a solvent (alcoholic or hydroalcoholic extracts). To prepare extractive solutions, different concentrations are used, ensuring the best yield, but also different solvents, depending on the nature of the substance to be extracted or the nature of raw material. When preparing extracts, it must be taken into account the influence of the following factors: *nature of the solvent* (water for salts of alkaloids, glycosides, sugars, proteins, enzymes, tannins, etc.; alcohol 50 or 70% for volatile oils, hydrocarbons, tannins, alkaloids bases and their salts, glycosides, resins, chlorophyll, etc.; ethyl ether for alkaloid bases, resins, volatile oils, etc.; ethanol for polyphenols, reducing compounds, alkaloids, salts, amino acids, polyphenolic glycosides, sterol glycosides), *the shredding degree of plant, the ratio between the amount of plant and solvent, time and temperature*. The extraction techniques can be *batch processes* (maceration, percolation, infusion, decoction, accelerated solvent extraction, microwave-assisted extraction, supercritical fluid extraction) or *continuous processes* (organic solvents continuous extraction, continuous percolation, Soxhlet extraction) [10].

Maceration is the extraction process for slightly soluble and thermosensitive principles, which consists of treating the vegetal product with a solvent, for well-established time periods, followed by separation by filtration or decantation; maceration time depends on the type of used solvent. *Percolation* is the cold extraction process using solvents in counterflow. *Infusion* is used for the extraction of compounds that are not affected by high temperature and consists of wetting the shredded vegetal material with water, followed by the addition of boiling water and leaving them in contact for a specific period of time (usually 30 min). This process is not used for plants containing volatile oils; in this case, the shredded vegetal product is wetted with a diluted alcohol solution, followed by the method described above. *Decoction* is a technique commonly used for roots, rhizomes and bark, and it is similar with infusion process: the plant is soaked in cold water, macerated, heated water is added and then brought near boiling temperature (this method is also not suitable for plants containing high content of volatile oils). *Microwave extraction* is the technique that uses microwave energy to heat the solvent and sample, in order to increase the rate of mass transfer between the substances dissolved in sample matrix and solvent, contributing to their easier passage into the solvent [11]. *Ultrasonic extraction* involves the use of ultrasounds with varying frequencies, increasing the permeability of cell walls, thus favouring the extraction of biologically active compounds with considerably yields [12, 13]. *Supercritical fluid extraction* (alternative to classical solvent extraction) is performed with supercritical fluids (CO_2), at critical pressure (74 bar) and low temperature [14, 15]. *Continuous extraction* in special equipments (Soxhlet type) is based on a large difference between the boiling points of the solvent and the targeted compounds, representing a highly efficient method [16]. *Extraction via alcoholic fermentation* is the extraction technology based on fermentation processes and *in situ* generation of alcohol. *Continuous extraction with organic solvents* is based on the continuous solvent recycling in the mass of vegetal material. *Accelerated solvent extraction* is a method based on the use of high temperature and pressure in order to accelerate the kinetics of dissolution and to break the bonds of analyte/matrix interaction. It has the advantage of using smaller amounts of raw materials, resulting in high extraction yields [17]. *Cold extraction* methods is used for plants with thermosensitive biologically active compounds (maceration, percolation and counterflow extraction); for thermostable active principles, other methods (Soxhlet extraction, decoction, microwave or accelerated solvent extraction, etc.) are selected.

At the basis of extraction of *volatile oils* from vegetal products are their physico-chemical properties, especially high vapour pressure and solubility in non-aqueous volatile solvents and fatty substances. Vegetal materials subjected to extraction can be both fresh and dried, as a whole or fragmented (leaves, grass), crushed (groundwater bodies) or as sawdust (wood). Choosing appropriate extraction method is based on the amount of oil in vegetal product, disposing and physico-chemical properties. For example, by pressing may be processed vegetal materials with high content of volatile oil, for the ones with medium content is preferably to use steam distillation and for the ones with low content—volatile solvents or lipophilic substances extraction [18, 19]. The main methods for *obtaining* volatile oils are as follows: *hydrodistillation* has several disadvantages: esters hydrolysis caused by the high temperature, obtaining other compounds (such as coumarins), oxidation of alcohols, aldehydes and ketones; the main advantage is the direct obtaining of volatile oil; *steam distillation*—oils having superior quality are obtained, compared with the hydrodistillation; *organic solvents extraction*—especially used for obtaining thermosensitive natural compounds that cannot be obtained by steam distillation; the active principles are isolated and then the solvent is removed by distillation; *animal fat extraction* is a technique exclusively used in cosmetics, and it is applied for fresh flowers. This process enables the extraction of natural fragrances without altering the composition, and it is suitable even for small amounts of plant material [20]; *extraction with liquefied gases*—applies especially for flowers, in the cosmetics industry, using high pressure and supercritical fluids. Using this method are obtained better quality and less colourful extracts than those obtained with organic solvents, rich in waxes and fatty components [21–23]. *Pressing extraction* is applied to aromatic and medicinal plants with high content of volatile oils. It is a suitable method to obtain essential oils from citrus fruits and consists of mechanical pressing, obtaining volatile oils but also mucilage, pectin, proteins, liposoluble colorants, etc. *Adsorption on an adsorbent material* is applied for the extraction of odorants from flowers by their adsorption on a substrate such as activated charcoal, alumina, etc. *Purification and separation* of biologically active compounds can be achieved by chromatographic techniques, membrane techniques, as well as liquid-liquid extraction. *Chromatographic techniques* are effective methods of separation and purification of organic compounds, based on the components distribution of a mixture between two phases: one fixed and one mobile; *liquid-liquid extraction* is applied for the separation of compounds of interest from impurities and is based on solubility difference of the extracted component in one or more solvents immiscible or partially miscible between them. *Membrane techniques* are categorized according to the size of particles to be filtered as follows: microfiltration—the process used for the separation of particles ranging in size from 0.1 to 10 μm; ultrafiltration—used for the separation at low pressure of colloidal substances and compounds with molecular weight between 500 and 500,000 Da, such as viruses, bacteria, colloidal substances biomolecules; nanofiltration—process at low pressure through which the molecules with the size of approximately 0.001 μm are removed; reverse osmosis (hyperfiltration)—process where an important factor is the osmotic pressure [24].

2.2. Analytical characterisation of extracts/active compounds

The plants are considered in our days as established sources of pharmaceutical, aromatic and industrial compounds. Various biocompounds gives the colour, odour or therapeutic actions. Used as pure compounds [25], impregnated in different supports [26–28] or used as intermediaries (for example for nanoparticle phytosynthesis) [29], bioactive compounds offers a natural health source. The potential applications of medicinal plants are determined by their compositional profile and possible synergies between those compounds. Nevertheless, as previous stated, the composition of the natural extracts varies with a series of factors. So, a variation in the phytochemical profiles of extract of the same plant, harvested from different areas, in different seasons or using different techniques is inherent [30]. In the following paragraphs, we will present the main methods used for the analytical characterisation of natural extracts.

2.2.1. Phytochemical assays

The phytochemical assays are currently used for the preliminary assessment of the extracts composition, following some major type of compounds, such as sesqui- and monoterpenoids, phenolics, anthocyanins, flavonoids, saponins, oligomeric proanthocyanidins, flavan-3-ols, tannins, o-quinone or other parameters, such as the polyphenol index or the potential browning. *The terpenoids* (especially simpler mono- and sesquiterpenoids) represents the main constituents of the essential oils. The non-volatile di- and tri-terpenoids are usually obtained from plants, tree gums and resins [31]. *Sesquiterpene alcohols* represent substances consisting of 15 carbon atoms and contain an alcohol group. They usually accompany other compounds that are in excess in some oils, having specific antidepressant and sedative action [32]. *Sesquiterpene hydrocarbons* are compounds containing 15 carbon atoms, usually accompanying monoterpenes compounds in the volatile fraction. They possess anti-inflammatory, anti-allergic and emmenagogue action [32]. *Polyphenolic carboxylic acids* belong to the heteroside group, having an acetal structure. To this group belong a series of well-known phenolic heterosides such as rosmarinic, caffeic, gentisic, vanillic, siringic acid [32]. *Triterpenic compounds* are actually triterpenic saponozides with a pentacyclic chemical structure, with immunostimulatory, pharmacodynamic, antimicrobial, anti-inflammatory and hypoglycaemic action [32]. *Saponins* are natural occurring substances with sterol or triterpenic structure that, in colloidal solution with water, foams under stirring [32]. *Flavonoids* are natural occurring phenolic substances containing plant pigments. Their anti-inflammatory, anti-allergic and antioxidant properties are well-established [32]. *Phenolics* represent the naturally occurring compounds with one or more aromatic rings and one or more hydroxyl groups. They are the most abundant secondary metabolites of plants. Their widespread in the plant kingdom makes them also one of the most studied classes of natural occurring compounds. They are of special interest not only due to their antioxidant activity, but also due to their presence in plant foods and beverages [33]. The *anthocyanins* are pigments found in flowers, fruits, leaves, roots that change colour depending on the cell pH. The most known anthocyanins are: peonin, malvin, cyanin, rutin, etc. [32]. *Tannins* are naturally occurring plant compounds with a very complex chemical structure (comprising of several phenolic hydroxyl and carboxyl groups). They possess antidiarrheal, antifungal, antiviral and antiseptic properties [32].

The phytochemical assays usually involve a specific reaction, standard substances and spectrophotometric measurements at specific wavelengths [34]. In the following paragraphs will be presented the most common photochemical assays; it must be mentioned that other particular recipes and standards are also used in the literature. The presented recipes could also be applied for the study of essential oils, with proper dilution in alcohols.

The total sesquiterpenoids are determined through the reaction between 98% acetyl chloride, 70% perchloric acid and the extract. The determinations are performed by scanning the 350–800 nm region and measuring at 608 nm. The standard used for calibration is α-santalol, and the results are presented as μg/mg of extract [34, 35]. *The total monoterpenoids* determination involves the reaction of the extract with 2% vanillin-H_2SO_4 reagent, the heating and cooling of the mixture and reading the absorbance at 608 nm. The most common standard is linalool [34, 36]. The results are presented as μg linalool equivalents. One of the earliest phytochemical assays, the *total phenolics content*, is also the most encountered in the literature. The determination involves the reaction between extract, Folin-Ciocalteu reagent and sodium carbonate. The absorbance is measured at 765 nm with a gallic acid calibration curve [34, 37–39]. The results are presented as gallic acid equivalents (GAE) or as percent [38]. *The total anthocyanins* are determined through the reaction of the extract, n-butanol:HCl (95:5) and 2% $NH_4Fe(SO_4)_2$ solution in 2 M HCl, with the absorbance reading at 550 nm. The standard used is cyanidin chloride [34, 40]. *The total flavonoids* content is determined by the reaction of the extract with ethanol, aluminium chloride (10%), 1 M potassium acetate in bidistilled water [39, 41]. The absorbance is recorded at 415 nm and rutin is used as standard. The results are presented as rutin equivalent. *The total saponins* are determined by the reaction between the extract, 8% vanillin in ethanol and 72% H_2SO_4; the absorbance is recorded at 544 nm, using as standard sapogenin [34]. The results are presented as mg saponins/g dry weight. The determination of *oligomeric proanthocyanidins* involves the reaction of the extract 0.5% vanillin reagent and 4% HCl in methanol. The absorbance is recorded at 500 nm, and catechin is used as standard [34]. The results are presented as catechin equivalents. *Determination of total polyphenols and casein/BSA(bovine serum albumin)/PVPP (polyvinylpolypyrrolidone)-bound tannins*—the extract diluted with water reacts with BSA or casein or PVPP; polyphenols are determined as above for total phenolics; absorbance is recorded at 720 nm on a catechin calibration curve and the *bound tannins* = (total polyphenols) – (unbound polyphenols); the result are presented as mg catechin/g dry plant extract [34]. *Total flavan-3-ols* are determined from the reaction between the extract and p-dimethylaminocinnamaldehyde (DMACA) (0.1% in 1N HCl in methanol); the absorbance is measured at 640 nm; catechin is used as standard and the results are presented as mg catechin/g dry plant extract [34, 42]. *The polyphenol index, potential browning and soluble o-quinone content* is determined following the same recipe as presented for the total polyphenols and casein/BSA/PVPP-bound tannins, reading the absorbance at 280 nm (for polyphenol index), 320 nm (for potential browning) and 437 nm (soluble *o*-quinone) [34].

2.2.2. Chromatographic methods

The main objective of the analytical methods is to determine both quantitatively and qualitatively the target compounds from plant extract. It is a difficult task since generally an extract contain numerous compounds (some of them being highly labile) with a broad range of polarities, volatility, molecular weight and quantities. Therefore, it is unrealistic to believe that a complete evaluation of an extract can be performed using a single method. Several aspects must be taken into consideration for appropriate selection of analytical methods: what type of information we need from the sample, amount of sample available for analysis, relative quantities of different components present in the sample. Due to the extract complexity, the analytical tools fitted for this task fall mainly in the chromatographic methods area: thin-layer chromatography (TLC) [43], gas chromatography (GC) [44], high-performance liquid chromatography and capillary electrophoresis (CE) [45]. These techniques show a good performance in plant extract analysis due to simple treatment required for samples and diversity of detectors corresponding to different molecules properties (**Table 1**).

Chromatographic methods represent a suitable choice for nearly all biomolecules that come across in plant extracts. These methods have the advantages of high specificity and also allow us to determine a large number of compounds in a single analysis and to benefit from a high dynamic range. Impact of gas chromatography in biomolecules analysis is somewhat hindered by low thermostability of some of these species which involve the necessity of time consuming and expensive pretreatment of samples, like derivatisation [46, 47].

TLC has been improved in the last years and has a large potential to determine some group of compounds using different detection methods and colouring reagents. Although high-performance thin-layer chromatography (HPTLC) has a good efficiency, the limiting factors in its use remain the low resolution and reproducibility [48, 49]. In contrast, *HPLC* use increase tremendously in the last years due to high efficiency and flexibility. Some certain advantages over other methods are as follows: different separation techniques, large range of HPLC columns suitable for all type of extracts, optimization of measurement using various mobile phases, gradient and isocratic approach extend the options during analysis, reverse phase techniques allow simultaneous analysis of compounds with large differences in properties. In addition, HPLC can be used as preparative or purification method, most analysis require ambient temperature, in most cases analysis are performed in short time interval, large number of detectors and the possibility to be connected in series are available.

Counter-current chromatography (CCC) is a special form of chromatography using only liquid-liquid partition without solid support [50]. This approach give the possibility to overcome some of the classic techniques drawbacks such us: column deactivation, samples contamination, etc. CCC was constantly improved during the years in terms of efficient separation in a short period of time hence the recent development in this field are focused on high-speed

Methods	Target biomolecules	Sample preparation	Detector
GC	Non-polar, thermostable	Difficult, derivatisation	FID, TCD, NPD, MS, HePD
TLC	Large range	Simple	Colour reagents
HPLC	Polar	Simple	UV-VIS, RI, MS, ELSD, NMR, fluorescence
CE	Ionic	Simple	UV, MS

Table 1. Characteristics of the main chromatographic techniques used for the study of natural extracts.

CCC (HSCCC) with two main technology high performance centrifugal partition chromatography (HPCPC), and fast centrifugal partition chromatography (FCPC). The performance of these methods allows the separation of plant extracts with complex matrix such us: separation of non-polar compounds, isolation of vitamin B12, chiral resolution of carboxylic acids, complete resolution of isoleucine, DCCC of anthocyanins, etc.

A further improvement of analytical methods in the biological samples is represented by hyphenation techniques, which are a combination or coupling of two or more analytical techniques using an appropriate interface. Most common link between techniques is represented by separation methods (chromatography) with an online spectroscopic detection technology (mass spectrometry or NMR). Also hyphenation techniques can be extended in both ways: in the separation parts (two separation methods) or in the spectrometry zone (two or more spectrometry methods) such us: SPE-LC-MS, LC-PDA-MS, LC-MS-MS, LC-NMR-MS. Albeit these techniques are more expensive than former methods the advantages overcome the capital costs: fast analysis, better automation, large number of sample processed in a period of time, higher reproducibility, less contamination, etc.

Most common and established hyphenation technique is *GC-MS* with a large number of improvements comparing with the components techniques used separately: direct transfer of components from GC to MS, accurate chemical identification of target compounds, possibility to expand analytical capability using the same equipment (GC-MS-MS) or even GC-MS^n). However, the same restrictions apply for biomolecules as in the case of using GC combined with classic detectors: cannot detect non-volatile, polar and thermally labile compounds, requires time consuming sample preparation (hydrolysis/derivatisation).

LC-MS is another relatively frequently used method that became more and more used in biological samples analysis. LC-MS advantages compared to GC-MS are evident: higher sensitivity and specificity, easy sample preparation (aqueous matrix is frequent but forbidden in GC or GC-MS), co-eluting compounds can be more easily separated, can be applied to detect non-volatile, polar and thermally labile compounds, several mass analysers can be used: quadrupole ion traps, time of flight (TOF), time of flight reflection (TOFR) and ion cyclotron resonance (ICR). Among major disadvantages there are lack of mass spectral libraries, hindering of the analyses by matrix effect, high capital costs and the need for qualified operators [51].

A novel hyphenation technique is represented by *LC-HMRS* (liquid chromatography-high resolution mass spectrometry) with sensitivity sub pictogram level that distinguishes compounds with the same nominal mass but different exact mass, avoids development of time-consuming protocols like in LC-MS/MS and requires operators with less experience. The main advantage of *continuous-flow HPLC-NMR* [52] is its simplicity, although the technique is less sensitive than other hyphenated methods previously described. This is mostly due to the limited residence time of the analytes in the flow cell, but also because the volume of most HPLC peaks exceeds the volume of the NMR flow-cell, thereby placing much of the analyte outside the cell during data acquisition. But still these methods remain an important direction in the development of methods for biological samples characterization.

2.2.3. *Other methods*

Besides the above presented analytical methods, other techniques are currently applied for the characterisation of natural extracts.

The *UV-Vis absorption spectroscopy* is one of the oldest methods of molecular spectroscopy very adequate in characterizing chemical extracts. This technique can be used both to obtain a general spectra of the extracts, but also for other types of measurements such phytochemicals assays. In the UV-Vis spectrophotometric measurements, the biologically active compounds present specific wavelengths (for phenolic acids adsorption shows between 220 and 280 nm, flavonoids, quinones and furanocoumarins between 290 and 420 nm, chlorophylls 600–660 nm, carotenoids between 400 and 500 nm, sesquiterpenoids at 608 nm and so on) [39, 41, 53]. *Fourier transform infrared spectroscopy* (*FTIR*) is based on the detection of molecular vibrations and is a technique particularly suitable for samples that may contain many pigments, being able to detect both organic functional groups and inorganics [54]. With a spectra library, FTIR can provide considerable information useful to the analysis, due to the presence of peaks in specific regions [29, 39, 55–57]. Very often used complementary with FTIR, *Raman spectroscopy* offers information on the molecular vibrations of a system and can be used for qualitative and quantitative determinations [58, 59]. *Nuclear magnetic resonance spectroscopy* (*NMR*) is used to determine the properties of atoms or molecules by exploiting the magnetic properties of the atomic nuclei. It is currently used for qualitative and quantitative determination on natural extracts, either by itself or combined with other techniques [60, 61]. *Matrix-assisted laser desorption/ionisation* (*MALDI*) represents a technique used in mass spectrometry that allows the analysis of thermally labile and high molecular weight compounds (synthetic polymers, biopolymers, macromolecules, etc.). Most often, for biochemistry applications, MALDI is associated with TOF (time-of-flight mass spectrometer) [62]. Less encountered, the *X-ray diffraction (XRD)* can be used for the identification and quantification of natural crystalline compounds, either from dried extracts or in liquid matrixes [63, 64].

By determining the concentrations of carbon, hydrogen, nitrogen, sulphur or oxygen, the *elemental analysis* technique can be an important step in characterizing chemical extracts, given that it can provide information that can be corroborated with other analyse results to get a complex image of the sample [65]. Very often, the elemental composition of an extract is needed, as the mineral components can enhance the therapeutic applications of plants, while other elements can be hazardous for human health [66]; also, the trace element profile can very well be used to characterize a specific soil-plant system [67]. The mineral composition of the extracts is most often quantified using *inductively coupled plasma* (*ICP*) techniques [68] (with variants *atomic/optic emission spectrometry—ICP-AES/OES* and *mass spectrometry—ICP-MS*) or *atomic absorption spectroscopy* (*AAS*) (also with several variants). Lately, with the development of the technique, *X-ray fluorescence* is also used for the elemental characterisation of extracts, having the advantages of rapid and multi-element analysis, lower analysis costs and the possibility of portable instruments [29].

2.3. *In vitro* protocols for the evaluation of natural extracts

The *in vitro* characterisation methods cover a very large area of applications. The most common application is the evaluation of the *antioxidant activity*. Among the methods for evaluating the antioxidant potential, the most encountered in the literature data are as follows: *DPPH assay*—a method based on the reduction of DPPH-free radical, quantified by absorbance reading at 517 nm [39]. The *Trolox equivalent antioxidant capacity* (*TEAC*) measures the antioxidant capacity of a given substance compared with the standard Trolox. Commonly, the antioxidant capacity is determined using the ABTS decolourisation assay [69]. *The ferric-reducing ability of plasma* (FRAP) assay measures reduction of the ferric iron induced by antioxidants. The method measures the absorption changes at 593 nm generated by the reduction of it is based on the reduction of the complex of ferric iron and TPTZ to the ferrous form at low pH [70]. *The ferrous oxide-xylenol orange* (FOX) assay directly measures the peroxide-dependent oxidation of Fe(II) to Fe(III) in acidic environment. The absorbance is measured at 560 nm [71]. The *ORAC assay* (oxygen radical absorbance capacity) measures the oxidative degradation of a fluorescent molecule (β-phycoerythrin or fluorescein) by a radical source (AAPH). The antioxidants protect the fluorescent molecule by quenching, thus inhibiting the fluorescence decay [72]. The *HORAC assay* (hydroxyl radical antioxidant capacity) is based on the oxidation of fluorescein by hydroxyl radicals, free radicals being generated by hydrogen peroxide. The hydroxyl radical mediated oxidation of fluorescein is blocked by the antioxidants present in the samples [70]. *TRAP method* (total radical antioxidant potential) is based on the influence of antioxidants on the fluorescence decay of R-phycoerythrin (R-PE) during a controlled peroxidation reaction, using as radical generator ABAP [70]. The total oxyradical scavenging capacity (TOSC) assay measures the decrease in ethylene production caused by antioxidants. In the presence of antioxidants, KMBA inhibits the thermal hydrolysis of ABAP. The determinations are carried out through gas-chromatography. In the last decades, new electrochemical methods emerged having several advantages when compared with the classical methods: sensitivity, fastness, simple and inexpensive instrumentation, small volumes of samples. The electrochemical methods cover a large area of electrochemical techniques [73].

Another very important group of *in vitro* methods is represented by the *antimicrobial assays*. All the antimicrobial techniques involve the determination of the effect of the sample against relevant strains, compared with a negative control (the solvent used for extraction) and a positive control (an appropriate antibiotic). *The agar diffusion test* (or the Kirby-Bauer antibiotic testing) represents a highly standardized assay [74]. The media used is Mueller-Hinton, at a pH between 7.2 and 7.4. The inoculation is made with a 0.5 McFarland broth culture. *The plate-hole diffusion assay* is commonly used to evaluate the antibacterial potential of natural products. The test material diffuses from pre-cut wells through agar seeded with bacteria. The antibacterial effect is evaluated by the clear zone surrounding the well [75]. *The well diffusion assay* is performed in order to establish the antimicrobial potential of extracts both on bacteria and fungi. Few drops of extract are placed in the appropriate wells and, after incubation, the zones of inhibition in millimetres are measured [75]. *The agar dilution method* involves the incorporation of extracts with varying concentrations into an agar medium (using serial two-fold dilutions), followed by inoculation with the test microbial onto the surface of the plate. The minimum inhibitory concentration is determined as the lowest at which the sample completely inhibits the microbial growth [75]. *The broth micro- or macro-dilution* represents one of the basic techniques for establishing the antimicrobial potential of natural extracts. The procedure uses two-fold dilutions of the sample in a liquid growth medium dispensed in tubes of minimum 2 mL (macrodilution) or in 96-well microtitration plate (microdilution).

After inoculation, the tubes or plates are incubated under suitable conditions. The MIC determinations for this method are more difficult, so often viewing devices are used for reading microdilution tests. *The liquid-dilution method* can determine whether a sample has a cidal or static action at a certain concentration. The minimal bactericidal or fungicidal concentration (MBC or MFC) can be determined using completely inhibited dilution cultures and assessing growth (static) or no-growth (cidal) after incubation [76]. *The disc diffusion technique* represents a modified version of the Kirby-Bauer assay. It involves the use of discs impregnated with the test substance for the determination of inhibition area, by comparison with a standard substance [75]. *The agar slant scheme* is particularly useful for the storage of bacteria over extended periods. Agar slants also aids at the identification of bacteria by characteristic patterns of movement [77]. In *the cup plate method*, the test samples diffuse from a cup through an agar layer in a Petri dish; after incubation, around the cup appears zones of inhibition. Similarly, *the agar well procedure* involves the formation of wells in the agar media and the addition of samples and standard in the respective wells [77].

The *antiviral potential* of extracts can be evaluated using some cell-based assays. The most encountered techniques are plaque inhibition assay, plaque reduction assay, inhibition of virus-induced cytopathic effect (CPE), virus yield reduction assay and endpoint titration technique (EPTT). *The plaque inhibition assay* is based on the infection of a monolayer of host cells (pre-incubated with a solution containing the sample) with the targeted virus at various concentrations (expressed as plaque forming units—*pfu*); the surface of the layer is also covered with a sample-containing solution. After incubation, the plaques are stained (for example, with neutral red) and counted; the percent of inhibition is calculated by reference to negative control (without sample) [76]. *The plaque reduction assay* implies the mixing of the sample (or controls) with the viral suspension, incubation and subsequently addition of the mixture to host cells. The overlay used in this case is composed of agar or carboxymethyl cellulose. After specific periods of time, the *pfu* are measured by microscopy, fluorescent antibodies or specific dyes [78]. *The virus-induced cytopathic effect* (*CPE*) *assay* is particularly useful for the evaluation of the effect on viruses that induce CPE, but not form plaques. It is based on the detection of structural changes in host cells that are caused by viral invasion, with and without treatment with a non-toxic dose of tested substance [76]. *The virus yield reduction assay* is a two-step procedure. The cells (incubated with the tested materials) are infected with specific viruses. After incubation, the supernatants are collected and the virus titers are determined. *The endpoint titration technique* involves the determination of virus titer reduction, using 2-fold dilutions of the tested substance [76]. For the quantification of viruses, modern methods developed can complete the presented assays: tuneable resistive pulse sensing, flow cytometry, quantitative polymerase chain reaction (*qPCR*), enzyme-linked immunosorbent assay (ELISA), etc. [76].

Unlike the previous presented assays, the *antiparasitic assays* are highly species-specific. Several studies were published, especially covering the tropical infectious diseases, such as leishmaniasis, malaria, African sleeping sickness or Chagas disease [76]. In order to perform the *in vitro* assays, the models used for each illness (*Leishmania donovani, Plasmodium falciparum, Trypanosoma brucei*, respectively, *Trypanosoma cruzi*) are incubated in specific growth medium (with or without host cells) with the tested materials. By evaluating the parasite multiplication and total parasite burdens (using methods specific for each spe-

cies), the results can be expressed as % reduction (compared to control), IC_{50} and IC_{90} (50% and 90% inhibitory concentration).
The *cytotoxicity assays* are commonly used in *in vitro* studies. The assays study the effect of tested substances on specific cellular lines. The cytotoxic effect can be manifested in a series of cell fates: the cells may undergo *necrosis* (premature death of cells by lysis) can stop growing and dividing (decrease in cell viability) or they can undergo *apoptosis* (controlled cell death). As the cytotoxic compounds often compromise the cell membrane integrity, *the cellular membrane integrity assays* are the most common ways to determine the cytotoxicity of specific compounds. The cellular integrity can be determined either by determining the effect produced inside the cells of specific vital dyes (for example, *trypan blue* or *propidium iodide*, dyes that are excluded from the healthy cells) [79] or by monitoring the passing to the outside of substances normally sequestered inside the cells (such as *lactate dehydrogenase—LDH*). Other methods of monitoring the cytotoxicity are the colorimetric methods (MTT assay, XTT assay, MTS assay, sulforhodamine B (SRB) assay, other water-soluble tetrazolium salts—WSTs assay, etc.) [80]. *The neutral red assay* can be also used to measure cell viability, as living cells take it up and concentrate it in the lysosomes. *The protein assay* represented an indirect measurement of cell viability, measuring the protein content of viable cells after washing of the treated plates [80].

The genotoxicity assays represents a very important parameter when proposing new drugs (either of natural origin or synthetic ones), determining aberrations in the affected cells (chromatid and chromosome gaps, chromosome breaks, chromatid deletions, fragmentation, translocation, complex rearrangements, etc.). The most used assays are the *Ames test, in vitro chromosome aberration assay, in vitro micronucleus test* and *comet assay*. The *Ames test* represents an *in vitro* assay for bacterial gene mutations using strains of *Salmonella typhimurium* developed by Ames et al. [81]. The general procedure involves the spreading of bacteria on agar plate containing small histidine amounts, allowing it to develop for a short time and have the opportunity to mutate. The surviving bacteria after histidine depletion are those that gain the histidine-producing ability trough mutation. The mutagenicity potential of the tested substance will be proportional to the number of colonies observed. In the *in vitro chromosome aberration assay*, cell cultures are exposed to the test substance, with and without an exogenous source of metabolic activation. At specific intervals, the cells are treated with a metaphase-arresting substance, harvested, stained and analysed in order to determine the presence of chromosome aberrations [82]. For the *in vitro micronucleus test*, cell cultures are exposed to the test substance, with and without an exogenous source of metabolic activation. The cells are grown to allow the formation of micronuclei in interphase cells, harvested and analysed for the presence of micronuclei. For the *comet assay* or single cell gel electrophoresis, cells are embedded in agarose on a microscope slide and are lysed, followed by electrophoresis staining and observation by fluorescence microscopy. A particularly interesting application of the cytotoxicity assays is the evaluation of *anticancer potential* of natural products. In order to establish the anticancer effect, the previously presented assays for cell viability are applied on a series of specific cancerous cells, like bladder cancer (i.e. UM-UC-3), breast cancer (MCF-7), colon cancer (HCT116), cervical cancer (HeLa), gastric cancer (BGC823), kidney cancer (M-1), leukaemia (Jurkat), lung cancer (SHP-77), melanoma (A375), pancreatic adenocarcinoma (SW-1990), ovarian cancer (A2780) and others. Many studies present the anti-cancer effects of various natural extracts [83].

2.4. *In vivo* protocols for the evaluation of natural extracts

When exploring crude natural extracts, the use of *in vivo* assays can prove to be problematic, as many of those bioassays can be expensive, time-consuming (turnaround time approximately 2 months) and require high-level expertise. Also, the screening of crude extracts, consisting of multiple components, can be questionable. Thus, many scientists uses the *in vitro* assays for screening the natural extracts and reserve the *in vivo* assays for purified compounds [84]. The *in vivo* methods currently used can be divided by the biological entities subjected to test into assays using plant systems and assays using animals. Several types of *plant-using assays* are available, i.e. specific-locus tests (using maize, corn, etc.) [85] or *Arabidopsis* multilocus assay [86], appropriate for genetic risk assessment. Cytogenetic and chromosomal aberration tests were developed using *Tradescantia* [87] and, respectively, onions or beans [29]. Also, DNA adducts analysis is applicable to somatic and germinal plant cell systems [88] and cucumber seeds can be used for the study of the germination inhibitory effect [39]. What all those tests have in common is the recognized quality of plants to be very goof indicators of genotoxic and cytotoxic effects.

The *animal-using assays*, in contrast, are much more regulated by the national and international legislation. In Europe, studies involving animals for experimental and other scientific purposes have to be carried out in compliance with EU legislation (Directive 2010/63/EU) [89]. For all *in vivo* methods, the tested samples are administered to the test animals (fishes, mice, rats, etc.) at a definite dosage, described by the specific method. After a period of time, the animals are usually sacrificed and blood or tissues are used for the assay [70]. Practically, for most of the already presented *in vitro* assays, there is an *in vivo* correspondent. However, due to the legislation and moral issues raised by the use of animal *in vivo* models, the current focus is on the development of viable *in vitro* alternatives. Before any *in vivo* study can be performed, *the acute toxicity* of any tested material should be established. This is expressed as the concentration that is lethal to 50% of the test organisms in a specific time interval. The test organism could be vertebrate organisms, but for obvious reasons, very often testing on invertebrate is preferred (for example, the *Daphnia magna assay*) [41]. The animal models can be used for the evaluation of the *antioxidant potential*, in assays such as ferric reducing ability of plasma, reduced glutathione (*GSH*) estimation, glutathione peroxidase (*GSHPx*) estimation, glutathione S-transferase (*GSt*), superoxide dismutase (*SOD*) method, γ-glutamyl transpeptidase activity (*GGT*) assay, glutathione reductase (*GR*) assay, lipid peroxidation (*LPO*) assay, *LDL* assay or catalase assay [70]. For the evaluation of *anti-diabetic potential* of natural extracts, the test animals (usually rodents) are induced diabetes (i.e. with *streptozotocin*) and the variation of peak blood glucose is recorded [90]. The *anti-inflammatory potential* can be evaluated using paw-oedema assay (induced by carrageenin, dextran, kaolin, etc.) and observation of the effect of the tested material on the evolution of the oedema [91]. The *gastroprotective effect* can be determined using animals to which gastric ulcer is induced (usually using absolute ethanol). After treatment, the animals are sacrificed, and gastric tissues are collected to evaluate the ulcers and to measure enzymatic activity [92]. For the evaluation of *anti-microbial* and *anti-viral potential,* the microbial strain or virus is induced to the test animals and the effectiveness of the natural extract is subsequently evaluated [93, 94]. The *antitumor activity* can be determined on tumour bearing animals (i.e. Ehrlich ascites carcinoma-induced or Dalton's ascites lymphoma induced animals). The effect is determined using survival time, haematological studies, lipid peroxidation, solid tumour mass, etc. [95]. The *antipyretic activity* can be evaluated using animals with induced pyrexia (i.e. by Brewer's yeast). The animals' temperatures are measured at specific time intervals after treatment [96]. The *analgesic effect* can be determined using either the hot plate test (pain reflex in response to an external thermal stimulus is observed after treatment) or the acetic acid induced writhing test (after treatment, 0.7% acetic acid is administered and the constriction of abdomen, turning of trunk and extension of hind legs are observed) [96]. Other several assays can be performed using *in vivo* models, such as *subacute/subchronic oral/dermal toxicity, eye/dermal irritation, reproduction toxicity, chromosome aberration, micronucleus assay, carcinogenicity, aquatic toxicology, bioaccumulation*, very often provided by specific companies [97].

3. Evaluation of some traditionally used plants

The following paragraphs will shortly present selected results published by the authors, regarding the obtaining, characterisation and application of natural extracts from selected medicinal and aromatic plants, presented in Section 1.2.

Recently, our group presented the preliminary evaluation of the crude hydroalcoholic extract (50% ethanol) obtained from the upper aerial part of *Heracleum sphondylium* L. subsp. *Sphondylium* [39]. The evaluation consisted of chemical evaluation, as well as antifungal, antioxidant and germination inhibitory properties. The chemical evaluation consisted of UV-Vis, FTIR and GC-MS analyses, as well as phytochemical assays—total phenolics, total terpenoids and total flavonoids. The tested extract revealed good antioxidant potential (determined by the DPPH assay) and good antifungal properties (evaluated by *in vitro* disc diffusion testing, against *Aspergillus niger* and *Penicillium hirsutum*, using miconazole nitrate as positive control). These findings support the traditional use of hogweed as a natural antifungal and antioxidant. The *germination inhibitory effect*, determined on seeds of *Cucumis sativus* Cornichon Wisconsin, recommends its use for the development of environmentally friendly and safe bio-herbicide. The described antifungal and germination inhibitory effects are most probably due to the content in furanocoumarins and total phenolics, as found by analytic determinations.

The essential oils extracted from various parts of *Anethum graveolens* L. (fruits, flowers and leaves), characterised by gas chromatography [98], TLC or phytochemical assays [99], were the subject of several pharamacognostic and applications studies previously published, revealing not only their composition [98, 99], consisting of flavonoids (aglycones and glycosides), hydroxycinnamic acid derivatives, coumarins, sterols, terpenoids (e.g. carvone) and mucilages, but also the antifungal activity (against *Candida albicans* [98]) determined by disk diffusion method, using as positive standard miconazole impregnated disc) and the possibilities of incorporating the essential oils in liposomal delivery vehicles [100–102]. The entrapment of *A. graveolens* essential oils in such delivery vehicles represents a very important step in developing topical pharmaceuticals capitalizing their good antimicrobial properties.

The hydroalcoholic extracts (40% alcohol) obtained from the leaves of *Taraxacum officinalis* (L.) Weber ex F.H. Wigg and roots of *Arctium lappa* L. were characterised using HPLC, phytochemical assays and absorption emission atomic spectrometry (to determine the mineral content) [7]. The content in total polyphenols and total flavone derivatives was found to be higher in the burdock extract compared with the dandelion extract. Several polyphenol carboxylic acids (caffeic, chlorogenic, ferulic, cichoric, cinaric) and flavone derivatives (rutin, quercetrin, quercetin, luteolin, apigenin) were identified in the two extracts by means of HPLC. Also, several minerals (Ca, Mg, Na, K, Mn, Fe, Zn, Cu) were quantified, minerals that could offer the extracts antioxidant properties [7]. The extracts exhibited bactericidal effects against *Escherichia coli* and *Salmonella abony enterica* [8].

Anthriscus with two variations (wild chervil—*A. sylvestris* (L.) Hoffm. and garden chervil—*A. cerefolium* (L.) Hoffm.) represented the subject of an ethnomedicinal and a phytochemical and pharmacological study [4] and of a paper dealing with the obtaining, characterisation and applications of hydroalcoholic extracts (50% ethanol) [41]. The previously mentioned review paper [4] contained the botanical and ethnomedicinal presentation of *A. sylvestris*, the phytochemical profile of its roots, aerial parts and fruits, and its possible applications, such as antitumor, anti-microbial, anti-inflammatory, antioxidant and biotechnology applications. *A. cerefolium* extracts were obtained from the aerial parts, via classical hydroalcoholic method and microwave extraction [41]. The extracts were characterised using UV-Vis, GC-MS and phytochemical assays. The sample obtained by microwave extraction was not only richer in terpenoids, flavonoids and phenolic compounds, but also had a better antifungal (against *A. niger* and *P. hirsutum* fungal lines) and antioxidant activity (as determined by the DPPH assay and a chemiluminescence method). Finally, the paper described the applications of the extracts in nanotechnology, for the phytosynthesis of silver nanoparticles. The nanoparticles obtained using the microwaves-extract had smaller dimensions (evaluated by UV-Vis, SEM and TEM) and enhanced antifungal and antioxidant properties. The phytosynthesised nanoparticles presented a relatively good stability in time; also, no evidence of toxicity exhibited by the silver nanoparticles was shown by an *in vivo* toxicity assay (*Daphnia magna* bioassay) [41].

The present work aims not to exhaustively present the obtaining and characterisation methods of natural extracts, but to bring its contribution to the field of phytochemistry, by addressing the most common methods for obtaining/characterisation of natural products, supported by some examples from our previously published works.

Acknowledgements

This work was partially supported by the Romanian UEFISCDI—"Partnerships in priority areas" program, project number 176/01/07/2014 (PN-IIPT-PCCA-2013-4-0953). All the authors had an equal contribution to the present work.

Author details

Radu Claudiu Fierascu[1], Irina Fierascu[1], Alina Ortan[2*], Sorin Marius Avramescu[3], Cristina Elena Dinu-Pirvu[4] and Daniela Ionescu[5]

*Address all correspondence to: alina_ortan@hotmail.com

1 The National Institute for Chemistry and Petrochemistry—ICECHIM, Bucharest, Romania

2 University of Agronomic Sciences and Veterinary Medicine, Bucharest, Romania

3 University of Bucharest, Research Centre for Environmental Protection and Waste Management, Bucharest, Romania

4 "Carol Davila" University of Medicine and Pharmacy, Bucharest, Romania

5 S.C. HOFIGAL EXPORT IMPORT S.A., Bucharest, Romania

References

[1] Parvu C., Enciclopedia plantelor, Plante din flora Romanie (*Plants encyclopedia, Plants from Romanian flora*). Bucharest: Ed. Tehnica; 2002.

[2] Scarlat M.A., Tohanescu M. Mic tratat de fitomedicina (*Small treaty of phytomedicine*). Ploiesti: World Galaxy; 2003.

[3] Tudor I., Minoiu M. Plantele medicinale miraculoase din flora Romaniei (*Miraculous medicinal plants from Romanian flora*). Bucharest: Artmed; 2004.

[4] Olaru O.T., Nitulescu G.M., Ortan A., Dinu-Parvu C.E. Ethnomedicinal, phytochemical and pharmacological profile of *Anthriscus sylvestris* as an alternative source for anticancer lignans. Molecules. 2005;**20**:15003–15022.

[5] Bojor O., Popescu O. Fitoterapie traditionala si moderna (*Traditional and modern phytotherapy*). Bucharest: Fiat lux; 2001.

[6] Milica C. Medicina naturista. Tainele tineretii, sanatatii si frumusetii (*Naturist medicine. Secrets of youth, health and beauty*) v.1 and 2. Iasi: Doxologia; 2013.

[7] Ionescu D., Popescu M., Rizea G.D., Mihele D., Bulearca G., Ivopol M., et al. Polyphenols and minerals, antioxidants in the plants used in the natural treatment of hepatobilliary disorders. Rev. Chim. 2014;**65**(5):507–511.

[8] Ionescu D., Predan G., Rizea G.D., Mihele D., Ivopol G., Ionita C. Antimicrobial activity of some hydroalcoholic extracts of artichoke (*Cynara scolymus*), burdock (*Actium lappa*) and dandelion (*Taraxacum officinale*). Bull. Transilvania Univ. Basov. 2013;**6**(55):113–120.

[9] Ionescu D. Studii privind influenta unor noi preparate de natura vegetala cu actiune hepato-colecistica asupra parametrilor biochimici la animale (*Studies on the influence of new preparations of plant acting on the liver and gallbladder biochemical parameters in animals*) [PhD thesis]. Bucharest:2014.

[10] Handa S.S., An overview of extraction techniques for medicinal and aromatic plants. In: Handa S.S., Khanuja S.P.S., Longo G., Rakesh D.D., editors. Extraction technologies for medicinal and aromatic plants. Trieste: Int. Centre Sci. High Technol; 2008.

[11] Deng C.H., Xu X.Q., Yao N., Li N., Zhang X.M. Rapid determination of essential oil compounds in *Artemisia selengensis* Turcz by gas chromatography–mass spectrometry with microwave distillation and simultaneous solid-phase microextraction. Anal. Chim. Acta. 2006;**556**:289–294.

[12] Chen L., Jin H., Ding L., Zhang H., Li J., Qu C., et al. Dynamic microwave assisted extraction of flavonoids from *Herba epimedii*. Sep. Purif. Technol. 2007;**59**(1):50–57.

[13] Schinor E.C., Salvador M.J., Turatti I.C.C., Zucchi O.L.A.D., Dias D.A. Comparison of classical and ultrasound-assisted extractions of steroids and triterpenoids from three *Chresta* spp. Ultrason. Sonochem. 2004;**11**(6):415–421.

[14] McHugh M., Krukonis V., Brenner H. Supercritical Fluid Extraction, Principles and Practice. 2nd ed. Amsterdam: Elsevier B.V.; 1994.

[15] Paun-Roman G., Radu G.L. Obtinerea unor principii biologic active din plante in forma purificata si concentrate prin tehnologii avansate (*Obtaining biologic active principles from plants in a concentrated and purified form, using advanced technologies*). In: Cascaval D., Galaction A.I., editors. Biotehnologia, intre stiinta si arta. Iasi: Ed. Venus; 2007. p. 61–94.

[16] Butler M.S. The role of natural product chemistry in drug discovery. J. Nat. Prod. 2004;**67**(12):2141–2153.

[17] Fines-Neuschild S., Boucher E., de Vernal A., Gelinas Y., Leclerc P. Accelerated solvent extraction—An efficient tool to remove extractives from tree-rings. Dendrochronol. 2015;**36**:45–48.

[18] Lawrence B.M. Commercial essential oils: Truths and consequences. In: Swift K.A.D., editor. Advances in flavours and fragrances: From the sensation to the synthesis. Cambridge: Royal Society of Chemistry; 2002. pp. 57–83.

[19] Ortan A. Nanostructuri lipidice – vectori de distributie pentru principii active volatile (*Lipid nanostructures - distribution vectors for active volatile principles*). Bucharest, Romania: Ed. Printech; 2013.

[20] Hui Y. H., editor. Handbook of food products manufacturing, Vol.1, Hoboken, New Jersey: Wiley; 2007.

[21] Bhat S.V., Nagasampagi B.A., Sivakumar M. Chemistry of natural products. India: Springer Science & Business Media; 2005. 840 p.

[22] Keville K., Green M. Aromatherapy: a complete guide to the healing art. 2nd ed. USA: Crossing Press; 2008. 256 p.

[23] Garland S. The complete book of herb and spices. UK: Frances Lincoln; 2004. 288 p.

[24] Paun G., Gheorghe O., Diaconu M. Curs procesare avansata a plantelor medicinale (*Course Advanced processing of medicinal plants*). 2011. Available from: http://medplanet.dbioro.eu/doc/Curs%20procesare%20avansata%20RO.pdf

[25] Bucar F., Wube A., Schmid M. Natural product isolation – how to get from biological material to pure compounds. Nat. Prod. Rep. 2013;**30**:525–545.

[26] Mustapa A.N., Martin A., Sanz-Moral L.M., Rueda M., Cocero M.J. Impregnation of medicinal plant phytochemical compounds into silica and alginate aerogels. J. Supercrit. Fluids. 2016;**116**:251–263.

[27] Stoica R., Pop S.F., Ion R.M. Evaluation of natural polyphenols entrapped in calcium alginate beads prepared by the ionotropic gelation method. J. Optoel. Adv. Mat. 2013;**15**(7–8):893–898.

[28] Lima S.S.P., Lucchese A.M., Araujo-Filho H.G., Menezes P.P., Araujo A.A.S., Quintans-Junior L.J., et al. Inclusion of terpenes in cyclodextrins: preparation, characterization and pharmacological approaches. Carbohydr. Polym. 2016;**151**:965–987.

[29] Sutan N.A., Fierascu I., Fierascu R.C., Manolescu D.S., Soare L.C. Comparative analytical characterization and in vitro citogenotoxic activity evaluation of *Asplenium scolopendrium* L. leaves and rhizome extracts prior to and after Ag nanoparticles phytosynthesis. Ind. Crops Prod. 2016;**83C**:379–386.

[30] Dhami N., Mishra A.D. Phytochemical variation: How to resolve the quality controversies of herbal medicinal products? J. Herb. Med. 2015;**5**(2):118–127.

[31] Gutensohn M., Dudareva N. Tomato Fruits-A Platform for Metabolic Engineering of Terpenes. In: O'Connor S.E., editor. Methods in Enzymology. Synthetic Biology and Metabolic Engineering in Plants and Microbes Part B: Metabolism in Plants. 576th ed. Amsterdam: Elsevier B.V.; 2016. pp. 333–359. doi:10.1016/bs.mie.2016.03.012

[32] Istudor V. Farmacognozie, Fitochimie, Fitoterapie (*Pharmacognosy, Phytochemistry, Phytotherapy*). vol. 2 ed. Bucharest: Editura Medicala; 2001.

[33] Dai J., Mumper R.J. Plant phenolics: extraction, analysis and their antioxidant and anticancer properties. Molecules. 2010;**15**:7313–7352. doi:10.3390/molecules15107313

[34] Misra B.B., Dey D. Phytochemical analyses and evaluation of antioxidant efficacy of *in vitro* Callus extract of East Indian sandalwood tree (*Santalum album* L.). J. Pharmacog. Phytochem. 2012;**1**:7–16.

[35] Jones C.G., Ghisalberti E.L., Plummer J.A., Barbour E.L. Quantitative co-occurrence of sesquiterpenes; a tool for elucidating their biosynthesis in Indian sandalwood, *Santalum album*. Phytochemistry. 2006;**67**(22):2463–2468. doi:10.1016/j.phytochem.2006.09.013

[36] Doneva-Sapceska D., Dimitrovski A., Bojadziev T., Milanov G., Vojnovski B. Free and potentially volatile monoterpenes in grape varieties from the Republic of Macedonia. Bull. Chem. Technol. Macedonia. 2006;**25**(1):51–56 .

[37] Singleton V., Rossi J. Colorimetry of total phenolics with phosphomolybdic phosphotungstic acid reagents. Am. J. Enol. Viticult. 1965;**16**:144–158.

[38] ISO 14502–1:2005, Determination of substances characteristic of green and black tea-1: Content of total polyphenols in tea-Colorimetric method using Folin-Ciocalteu reagent.

[39] Fierascu R.C., Padure I.M., Avramescu S.M., Ungureanu C., Bunghez R.I., Ortan A., et al. Preliminary assessment of the antioxidant, antifungal and germination inhibitory potential of *Heracleum sphondylium* L. (*Apiaceae*). Farmacia. 2016;**64**(3):403–408.

[40] Porter L.J., Hrstich L.N., Chan B.G. The conversion of procyanidins and prodelphinidins to cyanidin and delphinidin. Phytochemistry. 1986;**25**:223–230.

[41] Ortan A., Fierascu I., Ungureanu C., Fierascu R.C., Avramescu S.M., Dumitrescu O., et al. Innovative phytosynthesized silver nanoarchitectures with enhanced antifungal and antioxidant properties. Appl. Surf. Sci. 2015;**358**:540–548

[42] Arnous A., Makris D.P., Kefalas P. Effect of principal polyphenolic components in relation to antioxidant characteristics of aged red wines. J. Agricult. Food Chem. 2001; **49**(12):5736–5742.

[43] Jesionek W., Majer-Dziedzic B., Choma I.M. Separation, identification and investigation of antioxidant ability of plant extract components using TLC, LC-MS and TLC-DPPH. J. Liq. Chromatogr. Relat. Technol. 2015;**38**(11):1147–1153.

[44] Seenivasagan T., Paul A.V.N. Gas-chromatography and electroantennogram analysis of saturated hydrocarbons of cruciferous host plants and host larval body extracts of *plutella xylostella* for behavioural manipulation of cotesia plutellae. Ind. J. Exp. Biol. 2011;**49**(5):375–386.

[45] Rivasseau C., Boisson A.M., Mongelard G., Couram G., Bastien O., Bligny R. Rapid analysis of organic acids in plant extracts by capillary electrophoresis with indirect UV detection: directed metabolic analyses during metal stress. J. Chromatogr. A. 2006;**1129**(2):283–290.

[46] Akhgari A., Laakso I., Seppanen-Laakso T., Yrjonen T., Vuorela H., Oksman-Caldentey K.M., et al. Determination of terpenoid indole alkaloids in hairy roots of *Rhazya stricta* (*Apocynaceae*) by GC-MS. Phytochem. Anal. 2015;**29**(5):331–338.

[47] Qureshi M.N., Stecher G., Sultana T., Abel G., Popp M., Bonn G.K. Determination of carbohydrates in medicinal plants-comparison between TLC, mf-MELDI-MS and GC-MS. Phytochem. Anal. 2011;**22**(4):296–302.

[48] Sripathi S.K., Poongothai G., Lalitha P. Identification of pinitol in plants extracts by HPTLC. J. Chem. Pharmaceut. Res. 2011;**3**(5):544–549.

[49] Turkmen Z., Mercan S., Cengiz S. An HPTLC method for the determination of oleandrin in Nerium plant extracts and its application to forensic toxicology. J. Planar. Chromatogr. - Modern TLC. 2013;**26**(3):279–283.

[50] Wang J., Yu J., Li L., Liu C.M., Zhang Y., Wang Q. Isolation of high purity ginsenosides from plant extract of panax ginseng by high performance centrifugal partition chromatography coupled with evaporative light scattering detection. J. Liq. Chromatogr. Relat. Technol. 2013;**36**(5):583–590.

[51] Fong S.Y., Wong Y.C., Zuo Z. Development of a SPE-LC/MS/MS method for simultaneous quantification of baicalein, wogonin, oroxylin A and their glucuronides baicalin, wogonoside and oroxyloside in rats and its application to brain uptake and plasma pharmacokinetic studies. J. Pharm. Biomed. Anal. 2014;**97**:9–23.

[52] Staerk D., Lambert M., Jaroszewski W.J. HPLC-NMR techniques for plant extract analysis. In: Kayser O., Quax W.J., editors. Medicinal plant biotechnology: from basic research to industrial applications. Weinheim: Wiley Verlag GmbH; 2006. pp. 29–48.

[53] Bunghez F., Socaciu C., Zagrean F., Pop R.M., Ranga F., Romanciuc F. Characterisation of an aromatic plant-based formula using UV–Vis spectroscopy, LC–ESI(+)QTOF-MS and HPLC-DAD analysis. Bull. UASVM Food Sci. Technol. 2013;**70**(1):16–24.

[54] Scoog D.A., Holler F.J., Hrouch S.R. Principles of instrumental analysis. 6th ed. USA: Cengage Learning; 2006. 1056 p.

[55] Gonzales G.F., Miranda S., Nieto J., Fernandez G., Yucra S., Rubio J., et al. Red maca (*Lepidium meyenii*) reduced prostate size in rats. Reprod. Biol. Endocrinol. 2005;**3**(6):1–9.

[56] Ragavendran P., Sophia D., Raj C.A., Gopalakrishnan V.K. Functional group analysis of various extracts of *Aerva lanata* (L) by FTIR spectrum. Pharmacol. onLine 2011;**1**:358–364.

[57] Chaudhuri C., Pathak A.K., Sevanan M. Phytochemical screening and antimicrobial activity of extracts from leaves and stem of *Ecbolium linneanum*. Bangladesh J. Pharmacol. 2011;**6**:84–91.

[58] Edwards H.G.M., Farwell D.W., de Oliveira L.F.C., Alia J.M., Le Hyaric M., de Ameida M.V. FT-Raman spectroscopic studies of guarana and some extracts. Anal. Chim. Acta. 2005;**532**(2):177–186.

[59] Chylinska M., Szymanska-Chargot M., Zdunek A. FT-IR and FT-Raman characterization of non-cellulosic polysaccharides fractions isolated from plant cell wall. Carbohydr. Polym. 2016;**154**:45–54.

[60] Yan K.J., Chu Y., Huang J.H., Jiang M.M., Li W., Wang Y.F., et al. Qualitative and quantitative analyses of compound danshen extract based on 1H NMR method and its application for quality control. J. Pharm. Biomed. Anal. 2016;**131**:183-187.

[61] Karioti A., Giocaliere E., Guccione C., Pieraccini G., Gallo E., Vannacci A., et al. Combined HPLC-DAD–MS, HPLC–MS^n and NMR spectroscopy for quality control of plant extracts: The case of a commercial blend sold as dietary supplement. J. Pharm. Biomed. Anal. 2014;**88**:7–15.

[62] Lopez-Garcia M., Garcia M.S.D., Vilarino J.M.L., Rodriguez M.V.G. MALDI-TOF to compare polysaccharide profiles from commercial health supplements of different mushroom species. Food Chem. 2016;**199**:597–604.

[63] Martins F.T., dos Santos M.H., Coelho C.P., Barbosa L.C., Dias G.C., Fracca M.P., et al. A powder X-ray diffraction method for detection of polyprenylated benzophenones in

plant extracts associated with HPLC for quantitative analysis. J. Pharm. Biomed. Anal. 2011;**54**(3):451–457.

[64] Leonell F., Mostarda A., De Angelis L., Lamba D., Demitri N., La Bella A., et al. Proof of the structure of the *Stemodia chilensis* tetracyclic diterpenoid (+)-19-acetoxystemodan-12-ol by synthesis from (+)-podocarpic acid: X-ray structure determination of a key intermediate. J. Nat. Prod. 2016;**79**(4):1155–1159.

[65] Rodrigues D., Freitas A.C., Sousa S., Amorim M., Vasconcelos M.W., da Costa J.P., et al. Chemical and structural characterization of *Pholiota nameko* extracts with biological properties. Food Chem. 2017;**216**:176–185.

[66] Kostic D., Mitic S., Zarubica A., Mitic M., Velickovic J., Randjelovic S. Content of trace metals in medicinal plants and their extracts. Hem. Ind. 2011;**65**(2):165–170.

[67] Kabata-Pendias A. Trace Elements in Soils and Plants. 4th ed. London: CRC Press; 2010.

[68] Soare L.C., Visoiu E., Bejan C., Dobrescu C.M., Fierascu I., Iosub I., et al. Research on the in vitro bioaccumulation capacity of lead in some *Pteridophyte* species of the Romanian flora. Rev. Chim. 2015;**12**:2017–2020.

[69] Rice-Evans C.A., Miller N.M. Total antioxidant status in plasma and body fluids. Meth. Enzimol. 1994;**234**:279–293.

[70] Alam M.N., Bristi N.J., M. Rafiquzzaman. Review on *in vivo* and *in vitro* methods evaluation of antioxidant activity. Saudi Pharm. J. 2013;**21**:143–152.

[71] Sochor J., Ruttkay-Nedecky B., Babula P., Adam V., Hubalek J., Kizek R. Automation of methods for determination of lipid peroxidation. In: Catala A., editor. Lipid peroxidation. Rijeka: InTech; 2012. doi:10.5772/45945

[72] Tomer D.P., McLeman L.D., Ohmine S., Scherer P.M., Murray B.K., O'Neill K.L. Comparison of the total oxyradical scavenging capacity and oxygen radical absorbance capacity antioxidant assays. J. Med. Food. 2007;**10**:337–344.

[73] Pisoschi A.M., Cimpeanu C., Predoi G. Electrochemical methods for total antioxidant capacity and its main contributors determination: a review. Open Chem. 2015;**13**:824–56.

[74] Bauer A.W., Kirby W.M.M., Sherris J.C., Turck M. Antibiotic susceptibility testing by a standardized single disk method. Am. J. Clin. Pathol. 1966;**36**:493–496.

[75] Balouiri M., Sadiki M., Ibnsouda S.K. Methods for *in vitro* evaluating antimicrobial activity: a review. J. Pharm. Anal. 2016;**6**(2):71–79.

[76] Cos P., Vlietinck A.J., Berghe D.V., Maes L. Anti-infective potential of natural products: how to develop a stronger *in vitro* proof-of-concept. J Ethnopharmacol. 2006;**106**:290–302

[77] Ullah N., Parveen A., Bano R., Zulfiqar I., Maryam M., Jabeen S., et al. *In vitro* and *in vivo* protocols of antimicrobial bioassay of medicinal herbal extracts: a review. Asian Pac. J. Trop. Dis. 2016;**6**(8):660–667.

[78] Schmidt N.J., Dennis J., Lennette E.H. Plaque reduction neutralization test for human cytomegalovirus based upon enhanced uptake of neutral red by virus-infected cells. J. Clin. Microbiol. 1976;**4**(1):61–66.

[79] Riss T.L., Moravec R.A. Use of multiple assay endpoints to investigate the effects of incubation time, dose of toxin, and plating density in cell-based cytotoxicity assays. Assay Drug Dev. Technol. **2**(1):51–62.

[80] Fan F., Wood K.V. Bioluminescent assays for high-throughput screening. Assay Drug Dev. Technol. 2007;**5**(1):127–136.

[81] Ames B.N., Durston W.E., Yamasaki E., Lee F.D. Carcinogens are mutagens: a simple test system combining liver homogenates for activation and bacteria for detection. Proc. Natl. Acad. Sci. 1973;**70**(8):2281–2285.

[82] Stammberger I., Czich A., Braun K. Drug discovery and evaluation. In: Vogel H.G., Hock F.J., Maas J., Mayer D., editors. Genotoxicity. Heidelberg: Springer; pp. 829–840.

[83] Kittakoop P. Anticancer drugs and potential anticancer leads inspired by natural products. Stud. Nat. Prod. Chem. 2015;**44**:251–307.

[84] Attaway D.H., Zaborsky O.R., editors. Marine biotechnology, Vol. 1, Pharmaceutical and bioactive natural products. New York: Springer Science+Business Media; 1993.

[85] Griffiths A.J.F., Miller J.H., Suzuki D.T., Lewontin R.C., Gelbart W.M. An introduction to genetic analysis. 7th ed. New York: W.H. Freeman; 2000.

[86] Redei G., Acedo G., Andhu S. Sensitivity, specificity and accuracy of the *Arabidopsis* assay in the identification of carcinogens. U.S. Environ. Prot. Ag., Washington, D.C. 2002:EPA/600/D-84/105.

[87] Misik M., Ma T.H., Nersesyan A., Monarca S., Kim J.K., Knasmueller S. Micronucleus assays with *Tradescantia pollen* tetrads: an update. Mutagenes. 2011;**26**(1):215–221.

[88] Teaf C.M., Middendorf P.J. Mutagenesis and genetic toxicology. In: Williams P.L., James R.C., Roberts S.M., editors. Principles of toxicology: environmental and industrial applications. 2nd ed. Hoboken: John Wiley & Sons; 2000. pp. 293–264.

[89] Directive 2010/63/EU of the European parliament and of the Council on the protection of animals used for scientific purposes. 2010.

[90] Ali R.B., Atangwho I.J., Kuar N., Ahmad M., Mahmud R., Asmawi M.Z. *In vitro* and *in vivo* effects of standardized extract and fractions of *Phaleria macrocarpa* fruits pericarp on lead carbohydrate digesting enzymes. BMC Complement. Alt. Med. 2013:201313:39.

[91] Lattanzio F., Greco E., Carretta D., Cervellati R., Govonic P., Speroni E. *In vivo* anti-inflammatory effect of *Rosa canina* L. extract. J. Ethnopharmacol. 2011;**137**(1):880–885.

[92] Al Batran R., Al-Bayaty F., Abdulla M.A., Al-Obaidi M.M., Hajrezaei M., Hassandarvish P., et al. Gastroprotective effects of *Corchorus olitorius* leaf extract against ethanol-induced gastric mucosal haemorrhagic lesions in rats. J. Gastroenterol. Hepatol. 2013; **28**(8):1321–1329.

[93] Itelima J.U., Agina S.E. *In vivo* antimicrobial activity of plant species on *Escherichia coli* O157:H7 inoculated into albino rats. World J. Microbiol. 2014;**1**(1):002–009.

[94] Betz U.A., Fischer R., Kleymann G., Hendrix M., Rubsamen-Waigmann H. Potent *in vivo* antiviral activity of the herpes simplex virus primase-helicase inhibitor BAY 57–1293. Antimicrob Agents Chemother. 2002;**46**(6):1766–1772.

[95] Robertson S., Narayanan N., Kapoor B.R. Antitumour activity of *Prosopis cineraria* (L.) Druce against Ehrlich ascites carcinoma-induced mice. Nat Prod Res. 2011;**25**(8):857–862.

[96] Bhowmick R., Sarwar S., Dewan S.M.R., Das A., Das B., Uddin M.M.N., et al. *In vivo* analgesic, antipyretic, and anti-inflammatory potential in Swiss albino mice and *in vitro* thrombolytic activity of hydroalcoholic extract from *Litsea glutinosa* leaves. Biol. Res. 2014;**47**(1):56.

[97] http://www.genpharmtox.de/downloads/Toxicology.pdf

[98] Ortan A., Ferdes M., Dinu Pirvu C. Comparative microbiological activity of volatile oils from *Anethum graveolens* species. Stud. Univ. V. Goldis, Life Sci. Ser. 2012;**22**(4):531–535.

[99] Ortan A., Popescu M.L., Gaita A.L., Dinu-Pirvu C., Campeanu G. Contributions to the pharmacognostical study on *Anethum graveolens*, dill (*Apiaceae*). Rom. Biotechnol. Lett. 2009;**14**(2):4342–4348.

[100] Ortan A., Ferdes M., Rodino S., Pirvu C., Draganescu D. Topical delivery system of liposomally encapsulated volatile oil of *Anethum graveolens*. Farmacia. 2013;**61**(2):361–370.

[101] Ortan A., Dinu Parvu C., Ghica M.V., Popescu L.M., Ionita L. Rheological study of a liposomal hydrogel based on Carbopol. Rom. Biotechnol. Lett. 2011;**16**(S1):47–54.

[102] Ortan A., Campeanu G., Dinu Pirvu C., Popescu L. Studies concerning the entrapment of *Anethum graveolens* essential oil in liposomes. Rom. Biotechnol. Lett. 2009;**14**(3):4411–4417.

11

Medicinal Plants in the Northwestern China and their Medicinal Uses

Liu Dongling, Wang Yinquan and Tian Ling

Abstract

The Northwestern China is a typical arid and semi-arid region of inner Asia, where some important medicinal species such as *Angelica sinensis, Radix astragali, Radix codonopsis, Radix et rhizoma rhei, Radix glycyrrhizae, Lycium barbarum* L are found and grew in the mountains areas, or desert areas. Among them, *A. sinensis, R. astragali* and *R. glycyrrhizae* are frequently used in traditional Chinese medicines and herbal prescriptions, thus encouraged many researchers to investigate and develop them. Our purpose is to provide a review of recent advances about three typical medicinal plants of *A. sinensis, Astragalus membranaceus* and *R. glycyrrhizae* in Northwestern China, mainly referring to botanical identity, chemical constituents, pharmacological studies, application in formulation, safety and cultivation practices. That will provide some valuable information for the further study and development of medicinal plants in Northwestern China.

Keywords: medicinal plants, Northwestern China, *Angelica sinensis, Radix astragali, Radix glycyrrhizae*

1. Introduction

Approximately 8300 wild plant species of known medicinal species in the Northwestern China, some 400 species are used in traditional Chinese medicines (TCM) or by drug manufacturing units in China. Most of these medicinal plants grow in the arid and semi-arid marginal mountains areas, or desert areas of Northwestern China.

This chapter aims to provide a review of recent advances in the fields of botanical identity, chemical constituents, pharmacological studies, application in formulation, safety and cultivation practices about three typical medicinal plants of *Angelica sinensis, Astragalus membranaceus* and *Radix glycyrrhizae* in Northwestern China.

2. *Angelica sinensis*

当归 (Danggui, *A. sinensis*)

2.1. Botanical identity

A. sinensis is the root of *A. sinensis* (*Oliv.*) *Diels* (Umbelliferae family). The genus Angelica is comprised of over 90 species, a total of 45 angelica species are currently distributed in China, of which 32 are endemic [1]. It is mainly cultivated in the southeastern parts of Gansu Province, occurring in Yunnan, Sichuan, Shaanxi and Hubei and showing strong ecological adaptability at altitudes of 1500–2000 m above sea level in China. Photographs of *A. sinensis* are shown in **Figure 1**. As a perennial herb, *A. sinensis* grows to heights of approximately 0.4–1 m (Flora of China). The whole root is yellowish-brown to brown, about 25 cm long, and irregularly cylindrical with some branch roots stemming from the lower end. The leaves have alternating ovate blades that can range in size between 8 and 18 cm long and 15–20 cm wide. The fruit is elliptical to ovate, and the flowers have 4–7 cm long stems and compound umbels [2].

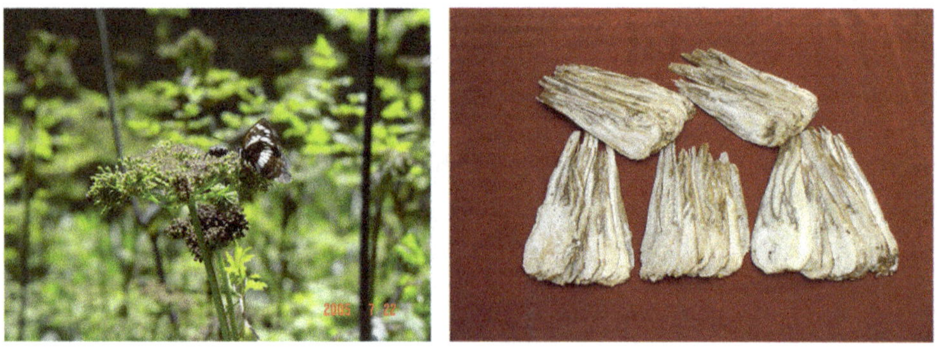

Figure 1. Photographs of *A. sinensis*.

2.2. Chemical constituents

Studies have shown that *A. sinensis* contains polysaccharides, flavonoids, volatile oils, trace elements, amino acids and vitamins, which account for approximately 0.4–0.7% of the total content. Phthalides, polysaccharides and organic acids are the main chemical components concerned to the bioactivities and pharmacological properties of *A. sinensis* [3]. Phthalides, as one of the characteristic components, have used for the quality control of *A. sinensis*. Ligustilide is also used as an important component for assessing the quality of *A. sinensis*, which can account for 0.5–5.0%, and the concentration of Z-ligustilide in *A. sinensis* varies within the range of 1.26–37.7 mg/g [4]. *A. sinensis* is rich in all types of amino acids, containing as many as 17 types and accounting for approximately 6.5% of the total chemical composition of *A. sinensis*. The seven types of non-synthesized amino acids are essential, and content variations can cause great differences among the amino acids extracted [5]. Flavonoids have also been isolated from *A. sinensis,* and total flavonoids have been shown to provide with antibacterial and antioxidant activities [6]. Moreover, phospholipids, adenine, uracil and choline were recently found in *A. sinensis,* a total reported nucleosides content with the range of 1.507–3.119 mg/g [7]. The plant also contains vitamin B12, vitamin A and xanthotoxin, as well as several microelements, including sodium, potassium, calcium, iron, copper, zinc and manganese, among others [8]. In addition, 8,11-dyhydroxyl-ligustilide, 2,7-hydrox-ligustilide and magnolol have been found in *A. sinensis* [9]. The major organic acids in *A. sinensis* are shown in **Figure 2**.

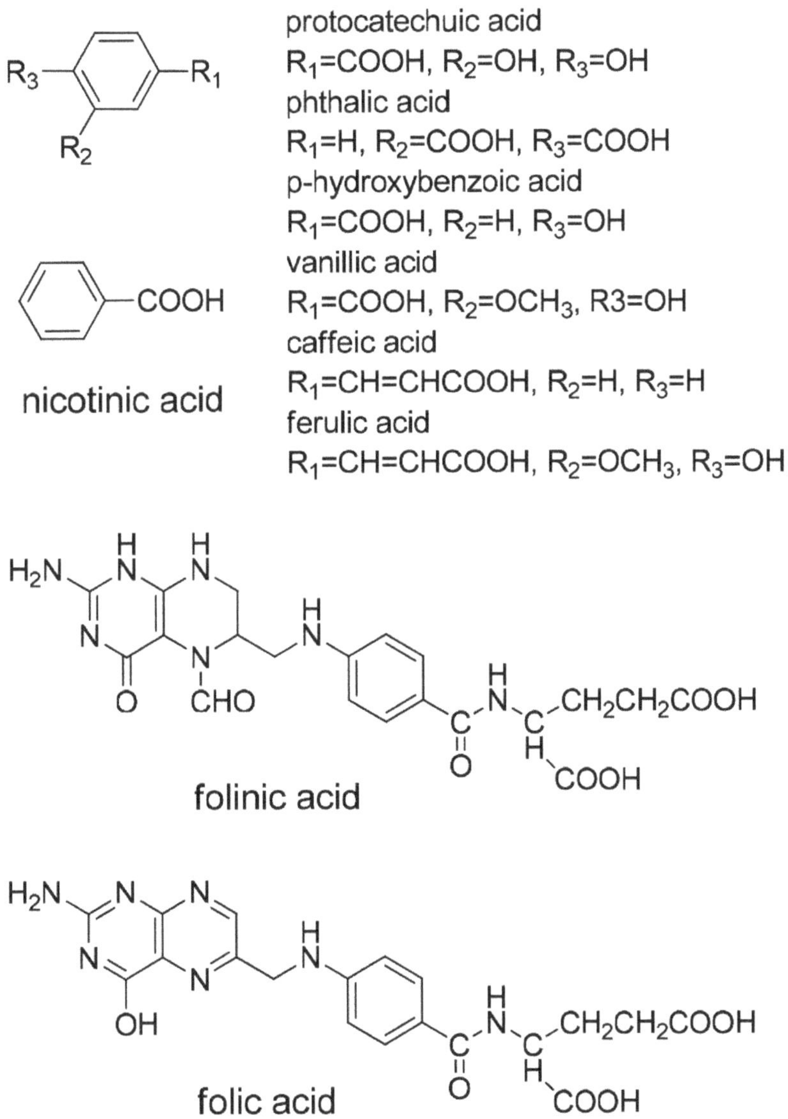

Figure 2. Chemical structures of the major organic acids in *A. sinensis* [10].

2.3. Pharmacological studies

A. sinensis has been used for thousands of years as a health food and drug in Asian countries and also as a dietary supplement in women's care in Europe. In China, the roots of *A. sinensis* have been extensively used in traditional medicine and have been primarily used for treatment of gynecological disease such as dysmenorrhea and amenorrhea and blood disease such as blood deficiency [10]. Modern pharmacological research indicated that *A. sinensis* also exerted pharmacological activities of anticancer, neuroprotective effect [11], antioxidant [12], hepatoprotective effect [13], radioprotection [14], immunoregulation [15], anti-inflammatory [16], antifungal effects and mosquito deterrence [17].

2.4. Application in formulation

These are ready-made combinations of herbs available to the general public to treat certain conditions without reference to a complete system of medicine. One company alone manufactures 280 of these formulations, designed for specific indications. Of these, 71 contain danggui [10]. Some of the herbs are traditionally put together ("Classic Pairs"), such Danggui and Chuanxiong Rhizoma (Ligusticum chuanxiong) or Danggui and *Radix astragali* or in "Standard Combinations". Danggui Buxue Tang is available in various formulations ranging from the TCM "Drug Pair" *A. sinensis* and *R. astragali* in a ratio of 5:1. Its suggested use for gynecological disorders such as anemia, infertility, has proved to be of potential for the perimenopause and menopause [18]. Moreover, there are also some popular formulations for Women's Health: Si Wu Tang (four substance decoction) formulated with varying ratios of *A. sinensis* (dang gui), *Radix rehmanniae* (shu di huang), *Radix paeoniae alba* (bai shao yao) and *Rhizoma ligustici* (chuan xiong). It is traditionally used as a decoction. Its function is to tonify and activate blood, smooth the liver and regulate menstruation [19].

2.5. Safety

It was reported that no obvious acute toxicity appeared through oral *A. sinensis* polysaccharide iron complexes (APIC) in mice and the maximum tolerated dose (MTD) of APIC in mice was 4800 mg/kg, 1920 times the adult daily dose. Thus, APIC was considered safe for oral use [20]. The toxicity of *A. sinensis* injection in the chick embryo chorioallantoic membrane model was explored. Results indicated that survival of chick embryos was not inhibited by *A. sinensis* injection. Furthermore, there were no differences between the treatment groups and the negative control, indicating that the resulting toxicity was very limited. Acute toxicity studies indicate that administration of *A. sinensis* produces no effects at doses up to 5000 mg/kg; similar results were observed in sub-chronic studies [21]. Therefore, *A. sinensis* is "generally recognized as safe (GRAS)" by the FDA but a number of side effects have been reported.

2.6. Cultivation practices

At present, the market supply of angelica is cultivated varieties. The proper field production altitude is from 2000 to 2500 m above sea level, while the proper seedling field is from

2500 to 2700 m above sea level. The annual average temperature of 4.5–5.7°C and average rainfall of 570–650 mm are suited for cultivating *A. sinensis*. It is also advisable to choose soil with a rich organic matter content, gray cinnamon soil and a neutral to weak alkaline of pH. The seedling fields should be chosen in uncultivated land, shifting land and especially in fertile uncultivated land with thick soil layer from 2500 to 2700 m above sea level. The most appropriate seedling field is a cool and humid place, short sunshine duration, and north-facing slope at an incline from 5 to 25°. The sowing time begins during the early to mid-June. After sowing, the seedling fields need to be kept humid and covered by grass cover in order to make it grow early, even and strong. The seedlings should be stored with a cellaring or piled storage before the ground freezing. There are two methods for seedlings storage. Crop rotation is a key measure of controlling soil-borne disease in cultivation practices of *A. sinensis*. The crop rotation in previous crop had better grains with a rotation cycle of 3 years. The optimal transplanting period is the middle of April. The reserve density is 9–12 plats/m^2. Combined with tillage, weeding should be carried out timely during growing period. Early bolting stage usually occurs in the middle of June, so it should be timely to remove of the plants of early bolting in case of water and fertilizers waste and affecting normal plants growing. Organic manure (4500–7500 kg/ha) as base fertilizer with timely topdressing the nitrogen, phosphorus and potassium (NPK) fertilizer should be combined. Ditylenchus destructor and root rot disease are the main diseases during the growth period of *A. sinensis*. The strategy of integrated pest management (IPM) is relied mainly on agricultural control while making insecticide chemical control subsidiary for controlling the diseases. The optimal harvest period of *A. sinensis* is during the mid-to-end of October. Fumigating by burning broad bean stalks and branches of poplars and/or willows is a traditional drying method. Introducing a modern drying technology for improving quality and increasing processing efficiency is the direction of future efforts. Dried angelica should be stored in clean, cool, dry, ventilates, moisture-resistant and smelling free storehouse, and a regularly checking store process is very necessary.

3. *Radix astragali*

黄芪 (Huangqi, *R. astragali*)

3.1. Botanical identity

R. astragali has a long history of medicinal use in Chinese herbal medicine and is one of the most popular herbal medicines worldwide. It is the dried root of *A. membranaceus* (Fisch.) Bge. (*A. membranaceus*) or *A. membranaceus* (Fisch.) Bge. var. mongholicus (Bge.) Hsiao. *A. membranaceus* and *A. membranaceus* var. mongholicus are mainly grown in Northwest China as well as in Mongolia and Korea, and they have some different botanical characteristics.

A. membranaceus var. mongholicus is a perennial herb, 50–150 cm high, with a straight, long and cylindrical root, measuring 20–50 cm, diameter 1–3.5 cm. Its stems are erect, with branches in the upper part, and are quilted with pubescence. It has an odd-pinnate, alternate, petiole base with lanceolate stipules, 25–37 leaflets, elliptical small leaves 4–9 mm long, and apex with long white pubescence. It has 10–25 flowers, racemes axillary, bracts linear-lanceolate, calyx tubular, calyx teeth—5, corolla yellow, butterfly, upper petal obovate triangular, glabrous, stamens—10, ovary stalked, ovate pods oblong, apex beaked, and significantly textured. The flowering period is from June to July, whereas fruiting is from August to September. It generally grows on hillsides, beside ditches, or in woodland and is found in Heilongjiang, Jilin, Liaoning, Inner Mongolia, Tibet and other places.

A. membranaceus has lobular 13–31 pieces, elliptic or ovate-lanceolate small leaves, length 7–30 mm, width 4–10 mm, corolla light yellow, ovary puberulous, ovate pod oblong 2–2.5 cm and apex beaked with a black undercoat (**Figure 3**). It grows on sunny hill-slopes, sandy riverbanks or shrub edges. This species is found in Heilongjiang, Jilin, Liaoning, Inner Mongolia, Tianjin, Beijing, Shanxi, Gansu and other places [22]. Moreover, both species are cultivated in the Northeast China, and they are gathered in the spring and autumn.

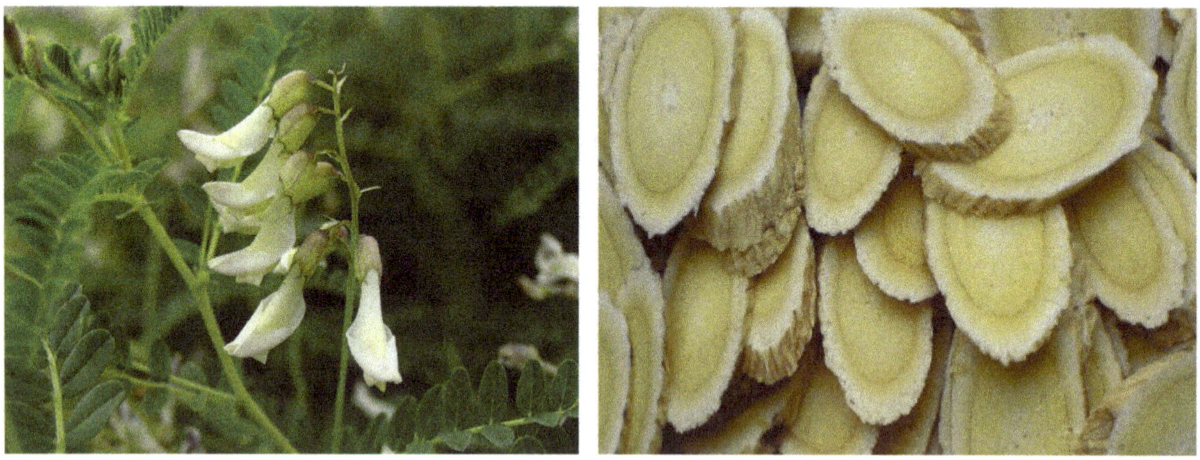

Figure 3. Photographs of *A. membranaceus*.

3.2. Chemical constituents

To date, *A. membranaceus* have been isolated and identified more than 100 compounds. Some of the compounds are shown in **Figure 4** [23]. Its major active constituents include triterpene saponins, flavonoids and polysaccharides. Other components found in the herb include γ-aminobutyric acid, L-canavanine, phytosterols (and other volatile oils) [24], fatty acids, choline, betaine, sterols, 3-hydroxy-2-methylpyridine, (−)-syringaresinol, (+)-lariciresinol, lupenone [25], bifendatatum, coumarin and amino acids [26]. Trace elements including zinc, iron, copper, magnesium, manganese, calcium, sodium, potassium, rubidium, silver, chromium, tin, vanadium and cobalt may also be present in varying quantities [27].

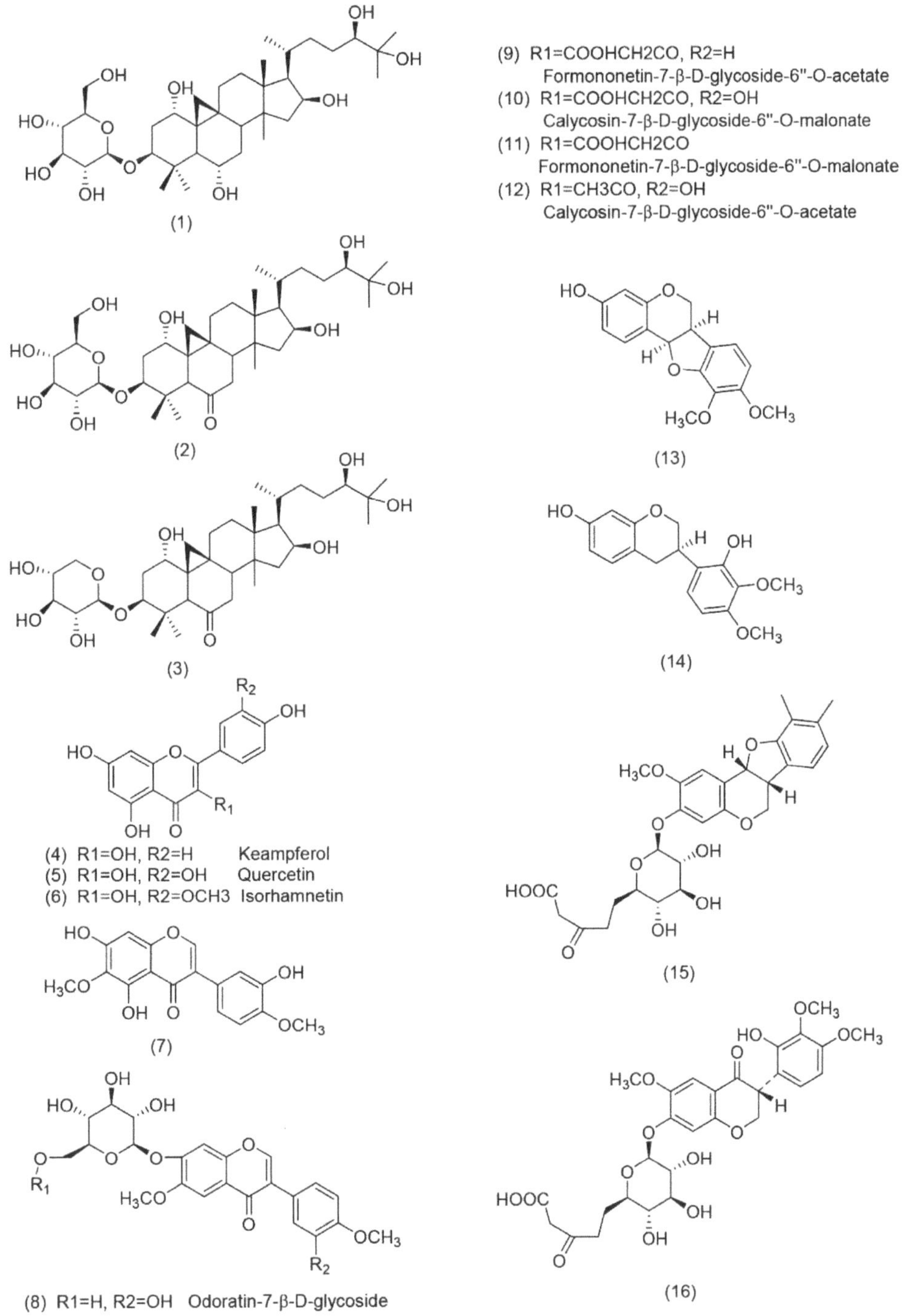

Figure 4. Chemical structures of the major compounds from Astragalus [23].

3.3. Pharmacological studies

The Chinese name Huangqi is the symbol of the "yellow leader" in china, linking to the yellow root and its status as one of the most important tonic herbs in traditional Chinese medicine (TCM). It was recorded in "Shen Nong Ben Cao Jing", the first book of Chinese herbal medicine, and was classified under the group of "qi"-tonifying drugs [28]. Huangqi is one of the 50 fundamental herbs used in TCM and was included in many TCM preparations with a wide range of biological functions [23]. In traditional Chinese medicine, *A. membranaceus* has been used for the treatment of general weakness and chronic illness and to increase overall vitality. Modern pharmacological studies indicated that *A. membranaceus* showed different peripheral effects such as immune modulation [29], anti-diabetic activity [30], anti-oxidative and anti-inflammatory actions [31], antitumor activity [32], antiviral actions [33] and enhancement of cardiovascular functions, the protection of cardiovascular function might be explained in terms of protection against membrane lipid peroxidation [34].

3.4. Application in formulation

A. membranaceus has been formulated as the main ingredients TCM formulations to treat patients with "qi"-deficiency symptoms, which present as a lack of strength, anorexia, edema, abscesses and spontaneous sweating. Other indications include shortness of breath, spontaneous sweating and frequent cold, night sweating and edema [35]. Some TCM herbal formulations included *A. membranaceus* have been evaluated and screened. A TCM formulation called "Shi-quan-da-bu-tang", comprising Astragalus and Ligusticum, has shown to improve the therapeutic efficacy of chemotherapy and radiation in various animal and clinical studies [36]. The prescription is capable of prolonging survival, preventing the recurrence of malignancies and increasing resistance to immunosuppression that resulted from antineoplastic and radiotherapy drugs through stimulation of the macrophages to produce IL-6 and tumor necrosis factor (TNF), and is most effective in stimulating hematopoietic factors and interleukin (IL) production [29]. Bu-Zhong-Yi-Qi-Tang was determined to be the most commonly prescribed formula for treating elderly patients with weakness and fatigue, especially for female AD patients. Bu-Zhong-Yi-Qi-Tang led to elevated levels of dopamine and noradrenaline in the cortical tissues of mice, as well as improved attention, learning function and memory [37]. Bu-Zhong-Yi-Qi-Tang was also used to treat elderly patients with weakness and fatigue [38].

3.5. Safety

Generally, *R. astragali* was regarded as a safe drug, no incidence of poisoning related with the use of *R. astragali* or its main active ingredients, has been reported *in vivo* or *in vitro* so far. It is determined that the LD50 of a crude extract of *R. astragali* is 40 g/kg using intraperitoneal injection (i.p.) in rats [39], and that did not show any adverse effects when raw herb was given to rats by lavage at the high dose 100 g/kg [40]. Moreover, the herbal extract (0.5 g/kg, i.p.) was injected to rats for 1 month, which caused no abnormal changes in food intake, urine/fecal production or behavior [41] Recently, the sub-chronic toxicity of the Astragalus extract, consisting of its active polysaccharides and saponins, has been evaluated the safety dosage range in clinical application. The application ranges 5.70–39.90 g/kg in rats, which are equivalent to 70 and 35 times in humans (0.57 g/kg, say, average body weight 70 kg), respectively [23, 42].

3.6. Cultivation practices

R. astragali is fond of coolness and drought tolerance but could not endure high temperature. An appropriate altitude of cultivating sites is from 1000 to 1500 m above sea level. The annual average temperature of 2–5°C and average rainfall of 250–350 mm are suited for cultivating. Sandy loam with rich organic matter content, good drainage and deeper is preferred. Seed coat of *R. astragali* is hard and difficult to germinate after sowing, so seed treatment should be done before sowing seeds. Seed was soaked with 70–80% sulfuric acid for 3–5 min, then quickly rinse, wash with running water. The sowing time of nurturing seedlings begins the early April. In cultivation practices, combined with soil preparation before planting, applying 45,000 to 60,000 kg/ha of manure and 25 to 30 kg/ha of phosphate fertilizer were recommended. Adopting

Seedling transplanting is usually used in the spring, by 20 cm apart in the row, 40 cm spacing between rows and 225,000 plants/ha. Combined with tillage, weeding should be carried out timely during growing period. The main disease in growing periods of *R. astragali* is powdery mildew; it can be used by 1000 time liquid mildothane 1000 time liquid spraying 2–3 time. The harvest period of *R. astragali* is during October to November and is dried using technology of freeze drying or solar drying.

4. *Radix glycyrrhizae*

甘草 (Gan cao, *R. glycyrrhizae*)

4.1. Botanical identity

R. glycyrrhizae is an ancient Greek word for the "sweet root," which was later called liquiritia and finally liquorice in Latin. As perennial shrub, it belongs to the leguminous Fabaceae (Leguminosae) family and exists about 20 species and grows mainly in Central Asia, Southwestern Asia and the Mediterranean region. The Chinese liquorice, *Glycyrrhiza uralensis Fish.* (*G. uralensis*), and the European liquorice, *Glycyrrhiza glabra L.* (*G. glabra*), are the most common ones among cultivated species. *G. glabra* is a more western species, found in Spain, Italy, Turkey, the Caucasus, Central Asia and the western China, whereas *G. uralensis* is distributed in Central Asia, Mongolia and China [43]. Photographs of *G. uralensis* are shown in **Figure 5**.

In the Northwest of China, *G. uralensis* mainly contains botanical characteristic as follows: calyx 5-lobed, two teeth than under three short; anther size (five big, five small), anther cell united at the top, different length of filaments. The ground part of different level is glands, glandular hairs and bristles, cilia, viscose or shen raised. A variety of underground part of the root and rhizome sweet taste needs to supplement the characteristics of some legumes as moniliform, ovule 1–11. The root and rhizome sweet including glycyrrhizin, glycyrrhizic acid, not sweet taste is some kind of glycyrrhetinic acid or glycyrrhetinic acid compounds (glycyrrhizic acid two yuan), some kinds of the above substances are not contained [44].

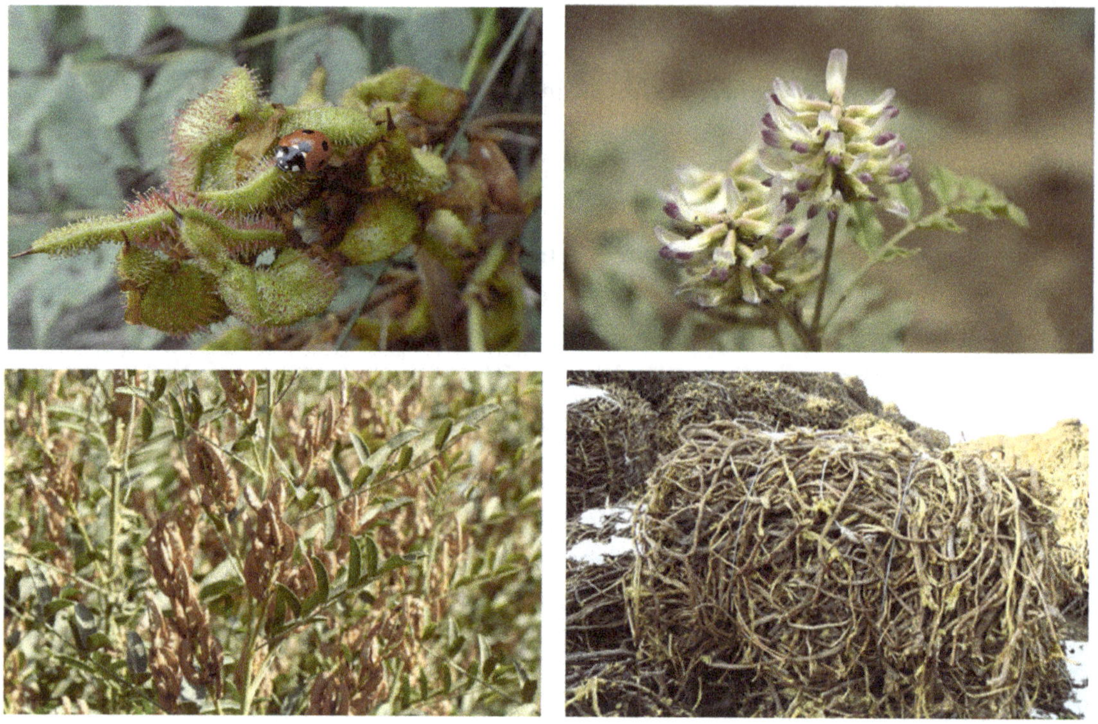

Figure 5. Photographs of *G. uralensis* are shown.

4.2. Chemical constituents

G. uralensis, commonly known as Chinese licorice, is an ancient herb of the legume family that is native to Asia. Its root is known to produce a variety of phytochemicals, plant secondary metabolites, including many terpenoids saponins (glycyrrhizic acid and glycyrrhetinic acid) and flavonoids flavonoids (liquiritin, isoliquiritin, liquiritigenin, isoliquiritigenin and glabridin). Among them, glycyrrhizin (I), liquiritin (II), isoliquiritin (III), liquiritigenin (IV) and isoliquiritigenin (V) (**Figure 6**) are believed to be bioactive contents [45].

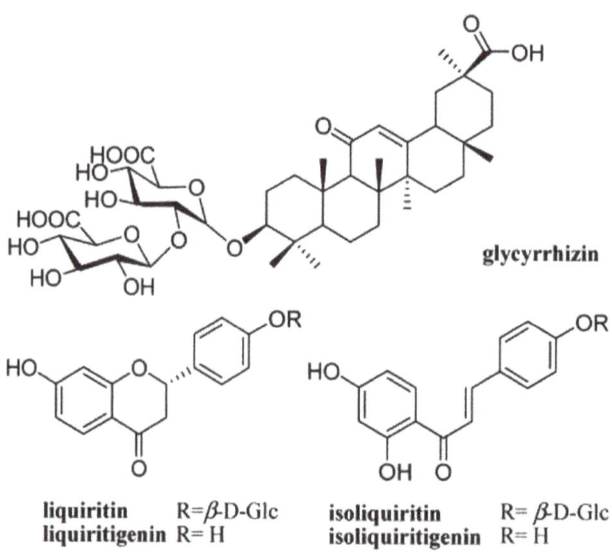

Figure 6. Structure of glycyrrhizin (I), liquiritin (II), isoliquiritin (III), liquiritigenin (IV) and isoliquiritigenin (V) [45].

4.3. Pharmacological studies

R. glycyrrhizae is one of the most famous herbal drugs used in TCM and has been used for several centuries. It has been frequently used in different formulations for the purposes of nourishing Qi (vital energy and functional activity of life), reducing spasms and pain, moistening the lungs and relieving coughs, detoxification, anti-inflammation and treating gastric ulcers [46]. According to modern pharmacological studies, its major constituents revealed various activities, providing concrete evidence for its extensive therapeutic use. The main saponin, glycyrrhizin, and its aglycone, glycyrrhetinic acid, has shown anti-inflammatory, anti-ulcer, hepatoprotective, immunomodulatory [47] and anti-virus activities; flavonoids, including flavanones such as liquiritin apioside, liquiritin and liquiritigenin, and chalcones, such as isoliquiritin apioside, isoliquiritin, isoliquiritigenin, etc., have shown antitussive, anti-inflammatory, anti-allergic and anti-tumor effects [48]. In addition, glycycoumarin, a species-specific compound to *G. uralensis*, has antispasmodic and antibacterial activities.

4.4. Application in formulation

A systematic database was constructed to investigate the frequency of reporting formulations and crude drugs described in Shang-Han-Lun (known as the Treatise on Cold Damage Disorders), a famous prescription in TCM. It consists of 112 kinds of genuine formulations from a total of 430 formulations but due to overlapping or repetition. The best three frequently mentioned prescription were Da-cheng-qi-tang (DCQT), Guizhi-tang (GZT) and Shaoyao-gancao-tang (SYGCT) [46]. Da-cheng-qi-tang, also known as Dai-joki-to in Japanese, is a formulation composed mainly of Rhizoma Rhei and Cortex Magnoliae used for the treatment of interior heat- and excess-syndrome. Clinically, DCQT was widely prescribed to promote the recovery of gastrointestinal motility after abdominal surgery and to treat acute abdominal diseases, such as acute pancreatitis, adhesive bowel obstructions and acute appendicitis [49]. Guizhi-tang contains *R. glycyrrhizae*, Ramulus Cinnamoni and Radix Paeoniae as major crude drugs and is used for the treatment of exterior cold- and deficiency-syndrome [46]. Shaoyao-gancao-tang (SYGCT) in Chinese or Shakuyaku-kanzo-to in Japanese is a traditional herbal formula used for analgesic purposes and consists of two herbs, the Radix of Paeonia lactiflora Pall.; PL and the Radix et Rhizome of *G. uralensis*; GU, in a ratio of 1:1. SYGCT has been clinically and pharmacologically applied to prevent muscle cramps and inhibit the contraction of skeletal muscle [50], reduce uric acid, regulate autonomic functions [51], relax intestinal smooth muscle [52] and relieve painful peripheral neuropathy [53].

4.5. Safety

The acute toxicities of licorice extract containing approximately 53% glycyrrhizin have similar acute toxicity doses and are low in mice and rats. Glycyrrhizin administered 70 mg/kg intravenously has shown acute toxic effects of convulsions and slight hemolysis in mice, whereas toxic effects did not see at lower doses of glycyrrhizin. The majority of short-term toxicity effects on the pituitary-adrenal axis have indicated that glycyrrhizin induced the pseudoaldosteronism at dose and time dependent manner, but the establishment of a clear no observed effect levels (NOEL) is difficult due to the differences in agents tested, animals used and end-points studied. The 90-day NOEL for licorice extract (53% glycyrrhizin) in rats is at the range of 0.31–0.63 g/kg, which delivers approximately glycyrrhizin 165–334 mg/kg [54]. However, for glycyrrhizin, the 30-day NOEL in rats is below 15 mg/kg [55]. In contrast, a two-year disodium glycyrrhizinate administered as high as 229 mg/kg/day or females administered as high as 407 mg/kg/day in mice showed no significant effects on average body weights or mortality, nor any signs of tumorgenicity among male animals. Other studies *in vivo* showed no teratogenic effects when glycyrrhizin salts were given maternally to mice, rats, hamsters or rabbits during gestation at doses up to 1000 mg/kg/day. However, dominant lethal testing in male rats suggests that an intake of glycyrrhizin 4000–5000 mg/kg/day could result in mutagenic effects in offspring [56]. Microbial experiments indicated that licorice extract and glycyrrhizinates were non-genotoxic and had some anti-genotoxic effects.

4.6. Cultivation practices

A climate condition with an average height of 1000–1500 m above sea level, annual average temperature of 6–8°C and average rainfall of 150–300 mm is suited for cultivating glycyrrhiza. Soil types of chestnut soil, brown soil, sierozem, dark loessial soils, salinized desert meadow soil and a weak alkaline (pH of 8–9) are the most suited for the cultivation of glycyrrhiza. The seedling fields should be chosen in the land of flat terrain, layers deep and fertile soil. Sow the seeds in drills 3–4 cm deep and 20 cm apart. The proper seed sowing time is in the end of April to early of May. Lifting seedling is in the day before transplanting. Transplanting is same as sowing time. Each plot at planting time, spacing of 10–15 cm and 25–30 cm row spacing planting are generally adopt. An under-mulch-drip irrigation or drip irrigation is usually a much better irrigation mode. Combined with tillage, weeding should be carried out timely during growing period. About 45,000 kg/ha of organic manure as base fertilizer with irrigation topdressing PK should be combined depending on soils and plant nutrition. Adopting measure of agricultural and biological prevention and cure control the diseases of rust disease, powdery mildew and brown spot, as well as insects of leaf beetle and *Porphyrophora sophorae* (Arch.). Seed breeding for 3–4 years, rhizomes multiply for 2–3 years can be harvested. When the stems and leaves withered in late September and early October, licorice roots could be excavated. Owing to deep roots, licorice should dig deep and not be broken or hurt the root bark. After sorting taproot and lateral root and removing reed head and bristles dried in the sun to a half dry state, tied into small, and then the sun to totally dry.

Acknowledgements

This work was supported by the National Natural Science Foundation (81260616, 81660625 and 81603407) and the Natural Science Foundation of Gansu Province (148RJZA061).

Author details

Liu Dongling[1, 2], Wang Yinquan[1, 3*] and Tian Ling[1]

*Address all correspondence to: kjkfpp@163.com

1 Gansu University of Chinese Medicine, Lanzhou, PR China

2 Key Laboratory of Traditional Chinese Medicine Quality and Standard, Lanzhou, PR China

3 Northwest Collaborative Innovation Center for Chinese Medicine, Lanzhou, PR China

References

[1] She, M.L., Pu, F.T., Pan, Z.H. Apiaceae. Flora of China Editorial Committee (ED), Flora of China Vol. 14. Missouri Botanical Garden Press, St. Louis, Missouri, 2005. pp. 1–205. (In Chinese)

[2] Zhao, R.M., Chen, H., Guo, F.X., Wang, Y., Zhang, S.Z., Wang, Q.R. Comparative study on distributed feature of wild *Angelica sinensis* resources and the different in growth characteristics with its cultivars to Min County of Gansu. Acta Prataculturae Sin.; 2014. 23: 29–37.

[3] Fang, L., Xiao, X.F., Liu, C.X., He, X. Recent advance in studies on *Angelica sinensis*. Chin. Herb. Med.; 2012. 4: 12–25. DOI: 10.3969/j.issn.1674-6384.2012.01.004

[4] Chen, X.P., Li, W., Xiao, X.F., Zhang, L.L., Liu, C.X. Phytochemical and pharmacological studies on *Radix Angelica sinensis*. Chin. J. Nat. Med.; 2013. 11: 577–587. DOI: 10.1016/S1875-5364(13)60067-9

[5] Jia, Z.S., Guan, T.Y., Cao, G.J. Study on the content of amino acid and micro-element. Amino Acids Biot. Resour.; 1992. 2: 49. (In Chinese)

[6] Li, G.C., Wei, W.T., Gao, T.J., Li, L.J. Study on the extraction for total flavonoids from *Angelica sinensis* (Oliv.). Diels and its antibacterial effect. Lishizhen Med. Mater. Med. Res.; 2010. 22: 310–311. (In Chinese)

[7] Cao, Y., Yan, H., Duan, J.A., Qian, D.W., Song, B.S., Guo, S., Hem, Z.Q. Analysis of nucleosides in the dried roots of *Angelica sinensis* from different regions. Chin. J. Pharm. Anal.; 2010. 30: 2026–2030. (In Chinese)

[8] Cao, Z.Y., Fang, J.H., Lu, W., Shen, X. Determination of trace elements for *Angelica sinensis* by ICP-OES with microwave digestion. Stud. Trace Elem. Health; 2011. 28: 18–20. (In Chinese)

[9] Zhao, X.J., Wang, H.F., Zhao, D.Q., Ji, H.X., Pei, Y.H., Bai, J. Isolation and identification of the chemical constituents from roots of *Angelica sinensis (Oliv.) Diels*. J. Shenyang Pharm. Univ.; 2013. 30: 182–185. (In Chinese)

[10] Wei, W.L., Zeng, R., Gu, C.M., Qu, Y., Huang, L.F. *Angelica sinensis* in China—A review of botanical profile, ethnopharmacology, phytochemistry and chemical analysis. J. Ethnopharmacol.; 2016. 190: 116–141. DOI: 10.1016/j.jep.2016.05.023

[11] Bunel, V., Antoine, M.H., Nortier, J., Duez, P., Stévigny, C. Nephroprotective effects of ferulic acid, Z-ligustilide and E-ligustilideisolated from *Angelica sinensis* againstcisplatin toxicity *in vitro*. Toxicol. In Vitro; 2015. 3: 458–467. DOI: 10.1016/j.tiv.2014.12.017

[12] Wang, L.Y., Tang, Y.P., Liu, X., Zhu, M., Tao, W.W., Li, W.X., Duan, J.A. Effects of ferulic acid on antioxidant activity in *Angelicae Sinensis Radix, chuanxiong Rhizoma,* and their combination. Chin. J. Nat. Med.; 2015. 13: 401–408. DOI: 10.1016/S1875-5364(15)30032-7

[13] Hua, Y., Xue, W., Zhang, M., Wei, Y., Ji, P. Metabonomics study on the hepatoprotective effect of polysaccharides from different preparations of *Angelica sinensis*. J. Ethnopharmacol.; 2014. 151: 1090–1099. DOI: 10.1016/j.jep.2013.12.011

[14] Zhao, L., Wang, Y., Shen, H.L., Shen, X.D., Nie, Y., Wang, Y., Han, T., Yin, M., Zhang, Q.Y. Structural characterization and radioprotection of bone marrow hematopoiesis of two novel polysaccharides from the root of *Angelica sinensis* (*Oliv.*) *Diels*. Fitoterapia; 2012. 83: 1712–1720. DOI: 10.1016/j.fitote.2012.09.029

[15] Wang, J.M., Ge, B.L., Li, Z.H., Guan, F.X., Li, F.F. Structural analysis and immunoregulation activity comparison of five polysaccharides from *Angelica sinensis*. Carbohydr. Polym.; 2016. 140: 6–12. DOI: 10.1016/j.carbpol.2015.12.050

[16] Saw, C.L., Wu, Q., Su, Z.Y., Wang, H., Yang, Y., Xu, X., Huang, Y., Khor, T.O., Kong, A.N. Effects of natural phytochemicals in *Angelica sinensis* (Danggui) on Nrf2-mediated gene expression of phase II drug metabolizing enzymes and anti-inflammation. Biopharm. Drug Dispos.; 2013. 34: 303–311. DOI: 10.1002/bdd.1846

[17] Wedge, D.E., Klun, J.A., Tabanca, N., Demirci, B.D., Ozek, T., Baser, K.H., Liu, Z., Zhang, S., Cantrell, C.L., Zhang, J. Bioactivity-guided fractionation and GC/MS fingerprinting of *Angelica sinensis* and *Angelica archangelica* root components for antifungal and mosquito deterrent activity. J. Agric. Food Chem.; 2009. 57: 464–470. DOI: 10.1021/jf802820d

[18] Xie, Q.F., Xie, J.H., Dong, T., Su, J.Y., Cai, D.K., Chen, J.P., Liu, L.F., Li, Y.C., Lai, X.P., Tsim, K.W., Su, Z.R. Effect of a derived herbal recipe from an ancient Chinese formula, Danggui Buxue Tang, on ovariectomized rats. J. Ethnopharmacol.; 2012. 144: 567–575. DOI: 10.1016/j.jep.2012.09.041

[19] Upton R. American Herbal Pharmacopoeia and Therapeutic Compendium-Dang Gui Root Scotts Valley. CA, USA. 2003.

[20] Wang, Y.D., Wang, H.Y., Li, L., Zhang, C.G., Zhang, G.X., Zhang, Y., Liu, C.E. Anti-fatigue activity of *acanthopanax gracilistylus* wine. Chin. J. Health Lab. Technol.; 2009. 19: 1404–1405. (In Chinese)

[21] Yang, L.X., Dou, W.Y., Yan, C.L., Liu, T.H., Wei, D.W. Study on toxicity of *Angelica sinensis* injection and *Astragalus membranaceus* injection in chorioallantoic membrane model. Chin. J. Exp. Trad. Med. Form.; 2009. 15: 46–48. (In Chinese)

[22] Yan, L., Wan, T., Zhang, Z., Wang, R.X., Sun, B.W.. Analysis on botanical characters of *Astragalus membranaceus Bunge.* and *A. membranaceus var. mongholicus* (*Bunge.*) *Hsiao.* J. Inner Mongolia Agric. Univ.; 2001. 22: 71–77. (In Chinese)

[23] Fu, J., Wang, Z., Huang, L., Zheng, S., Wang, D., Chen, S., Zhang, H., Yang, S. Review of the botanical characteristics, phytochemistry, and pharmacology of *Astragalus membranaceus* (Huangqi). Phytother. Res.; 2014. 28: 1275–1283. DOI: 10.1002/ptr.5188

[24] Tang, W. Eisenbrand, G. Chinese Drugs of Plant Origin. Springer-Verlag, Beijing, 1992. pp. 191–197. (In Chinese)

[25] Subarnas, A., Oshima, Y., Hikino, H. Isoflavans and a pterocarpan from Astragalus mongholicus. Phytochemistry; 1991. 30: 2777–2780. DOI: 10.1016/0031-9422(91)85143-N

[26] Huang, K.C. The Pharmacology of Chinese Herbs. CRC Press, Boca Raton, 1999. (In Chinese)

[27] Mills, S., Bone, K. Principles and Practice of Phytotherapy. Churchill Livingstone, Edinburgh, 2000.

[28] Auyeung, K.K., Han, Q.B., Ko, J.K. *Astragalus membranaceus*: A review of its protection against in flammation and gastrointestinal cancers. Am. J. Chin. Med.; 2016. 44: 1–22. DOI: 10.1142/S0192415X16500014

[29] Yoshida, Y., Wang, M.Q., Liu, J.N., Shan, B.E., Yamashita, U. Immunomodulating activity of Chinese medicinal herbs and *Oldenlandia diffusa* in particular. Int. J. Immunopharmacol.; 1997. 19: 359–370. DOI: 10.1016/S0192-0561(97)00076-3

[30] Agyemang, K., Han, L., Liu, E., Zhang, Y., Wang, T., Gao, X. Recent advances in *Astragalus membranaceus* anti-diabetic research: Pharmacological effects of its phytochemical constituents. Evid. Based Complement. Alternat. Med.; 2013: 654643. DOI: 10.1155/2013/654643

[31] Ryu, M., Kim, H.E., Chun, M., Kang, S., Shim, B., Yu, Y.B., Jeong, G., Lee, J.S. *Astragali Radix* elicits anti-inflammation via activation of MKP-1, concomitant with attenuation of p38 and Erk. J. Ethnopharmacol.; 2008. 115: 184–193. DOI: 10.1016/j.jep.2007.09.027

[32] Shen, H.H., Wang, K., Li, W., Ying, Y.H., Gao, G.X., Li, X.B., Huang, H.Q. Astragalus membranaceus prevents airway hyperreactivity in mice related to Th2 response inhibition. J. Ethnopharmacol.; 2008. 116: 363–369. DOI: 10.1016/j.jep.2007.12.002

[33] Liu, Y.H., Sun, S., Zhang, H.Q., Zhang, Y.T., Xia, B. 2D NMR study on cycloartane triterpenoids from *Astragalus membranaceus var. mongholicus*. J. China Pharm. Univ.; 2008. 39: 15–19. (In Chinese)

[34] Toda, S., Shirataki, Y. Inhibitory effects of *Astragali Radix*, a crude drug in Oriental medicines, on lipid peroxidation and protein oxidative modification by copper. J. Ethnopharmacol.; 1999. 68: 331–333. DOI: 10.1002/ptr.5188

[35] Hong, Y. Oriental Materica: A Concise Guide. Oriental Healing Arts Institute, Long Beach, 1986.

[36] McCulloch, M., See, C., Shu, X.J., Broffman, M., Kramer, A., Fan, W.Y., Gao, J., Lieb, W., Shieh, K., Colford, J.M. Jr. Astragalus-based Chinese herbs and platinum-based chemotherapy for advanced non-small-cell lung cancer: Meta-analysis of randomized trials. J. Clin. Oncol.; 2006. 24: 419–430. DOI: 10.1200/JCO.2005.03.6392

[37] Shih, H.C., Chang, K.H., Chen, F.L., Chen, C.M., Chen, S.C., Lin, Y.T., Shibuya, A. Anti-aging effects of the traditional Chinese medicine Bu-zhong-yi-qi-tang in mice. Am. J. Chin. Med.; 2000. 28: 77–86. DOI: 10.1142/S0192415X00000106

[38] Toshiaki, K., Nobuhiko, S., Eiichi, T., Shinya, S., Yutaka, S., Hiroshi, O., Hideki, O., Katsutoshi, T. Assessment of effects of traditional herbal medicines on elderly patients with weakness using a self-controlled trial. Geriatr. Gerontol. Int.; 2004. 4: 169–174. DOI: 10.1111/j.1447-0594.2004.00246.x

[39] Wagner, H.B., Xiao, P.G., Chen, J., Michler, M.G. *Radix Astragali* (Huangqi): Chinese Drug Monographs and Analysis Germany. Verlag, Wald, 1997. pp. 1–17.

[40] Bensky, D., Gamble, A. Chinese Herbal Medicine: Materia Medica, Revised Edition. Eastland Press, Seattle, 1993.

[41] Chang, H., But, P. Pharmacology and Applications of Chinese Materia Medica, Vol. 2. World Scientific, Singapore, 1987. pp. 1041–1046.

[42] Yu, S.Y., Ouyang, H.T., Yang, J.Y., Huang, X.L., Yang, T., Duan, J.P., Cheng, J.P., Chen, Y.X., Yang, Y.J., Qiong, P. Subchronic toxicity studies of *radix astragali* extract in rats and dogs. J. Ethnopharmacol.; 2007. 110: 352–355. DOI: 10.1016/j.jep.2006.09.024

[43] Hayashi, H., Sudo, H. Economic importance of licorice. Plant Biotechnol.; 2009. 26: 101–104. DOI: 10.5511/plantbiotechnology.26.101

[44] Li, X.Y. A study of the system and new taxa of Genus Glycyrrhiza L. Bull Bot. Research.; 1993. 13: 4–43. (In Chinese)

[45] Guo, Z., Wu, Y., Wang, R., Wang, W., Liu, Y., Zhang, X.Q., Gao, S., Zhang, Y., Wei, S. Distribution patterns of the contents of five active components in taproot and stolon of *Glycyrrhiza uralensis*. Biol. Pharm. Bull.; 2014. 37: 1253–1258. DOI: 10.1248/bpb.b14-00173

[46] Katakai, M., Akamaru, T., Tani, T. An analysis of the frequency of formulations and crude drugs described in (Shan-Han-Lun). Yakushigaku Zasshi; 2002. 37: 28–35.

[47] Isbrucker, R.A., Burdock, G.A. Risk and safety assessment on the consumption of Licorice root (Glycyrrhiza sp.), its extract and powder as a food ingredient, with emphasis on the pharmacology and toxicology of glycyrrhizin. Regul. Toxicol. Pharmacol.; 2006. 46: 167–192. DOI: 10.1016/j.yrtph.2006.06.002

[48] Asl, M.N., Hosseinzadeh, H. Review of pharmacological effects of Glycyrrhiza sp. and its bioactive compounds. Phytother. Res.; 2008. 22: 709–724. DOI: 10.1002/ptr.2362

[49] Wan, J.B., Bai, X., Cai, X.J., Rao, Y., Wang, Y.S., Wang, Y.T. Chemical differentiation of da-cheng-qi-tang, a chinese medicine formula, prepared by traditional and modern decoction methods using uplc/q-tofms-based metabolomics approach. J. Pharm. Biomed. Anal.; 2013. 83: 34–42. DOI: 10.1016/j.jpba.2013.04.019

[50] Hinoshita, F., Ogura, Y., Suzuki, Y., Hara, S., Yamada, A., Tanaka, N., Yamashita, A., Marumo, F. Effect of orally administered shao-yao-gan-cao-tang (shakuyaku-kanzo-to) on muscle cramps in maintenance hemodialysis patients: A preliminary study. Am. J. Chin. Med.; 2003. 31: 445–453. DOI: 10.1142/S0192415X03001144

[51] Wu, T.H., Chen, L.C., Yang, L.L. Hypouricemic effect and regulatory effects on autonomic function of Shao-Yao Gan-Cao Tang, a Chinese herbal prescription, in asymptomatic hyperuricemic vegetarians. Rheumatol. Int.; 2007. 28: 27–31. DOI: 10.1007/s00296-007-0385-7

[52] Satoh, H., Tsuro, K. Pharmacological modulation by Shakuyakukanzoto (Shao-Yao-Gan-Cao-Tang) and the ingredients in rat intestinal smooth muscle. Chin. Med.; 2011. 2: 62–70. DOI: 10.4236/cm.2011.22012

[53] Hidaka, T., Shima, T., Nagira, K., Ieki, M., Nakamura, T., Aono, Y., Kuraishi, Y., Arai, T., Saito, S. Herbal medicine Shakuyaku-kanzo-to reduces paclitaxel-induced painful peripheral neuropathy in mice. Eur. J. Pain; 2009. 13: 22–27. DOI: 10.1016/j.ejpain.2008.03.003

[54] Komiyama, K., Kawakubo, Y., Fukushima, T., Sugimoto, K., Takeshima, H., Ko, Y., Sato, T., Okamoto, M., Umezawa, I., Nishiyama, Y. Acute and subacute toxicity test on the extract from Glycyrrhiza. Oyo Yakuri; 1977. 14: 535–548.

[55] Rossi, T., Fano, R.A., Castelli, M., Malagoli, M., Ruberto, A.I., Baggio, G., Zennaro, R., Migaldi, M., Barbolini, G. Correlation between high intake of glycyrrhizin and myolysis of the papillary muscles: an experimental in vivo study. Pharmacol. Toxicol.; 1999. 85: 221–229. DOI: 10.1111/j.1600-0773.1999.tb02012.x

[56] Sheu, C.W., Cain, K.T., Rushbrook, C.J., Jorgenson, T.A., Generoso, W.M. Tests for mutagenic effects of ammoniated glycyrrhizin, butylated hydroxytoluene, and gum Arabic in rodent germ cells. Environ. Mutagen.; 1986. 8: 357–367. DOI: 10.1002/em.2860080305

12

Cardiac Glycosides in Medicinal Plants

Nagy Morsy

Abstract

Plant active metabolites are under intensive examinations around the world to supplement the drugs with minimal side effects. Thus, there is vast potential to explore the possible medicine from the plant sources. Cardiac glycosides are a unique group of secondary metabolites that they are considered one of the most useful drugs in therapeutics. In this review, cardiac glycosides and their analogues are presented. The structure and distribution in plants, as well as structure elucidations, synthetic routes, and chemical analysis, are shown. In addition, the pharmacological activities, mode of action studies, and structureactivity relationships are discussed.

Keywords: cardiac glycosides, distribution in nature, structure features, structure elucidation, chemical analysis, pharmacological activities, structure-activity relationships

1. Introduction

Many research efforts have been done toward the proofs of the use of plant species in medicinal treatments in recent years. The effect of plants used has been examined traditionally to support treatment of various diseases. Cardiac glycosides are a group that comprises the most drug-like molecules subjected to several investigations and they were proved to be fruitful in developing potential drugs [1–5]. They are chemical compounds responsible for the poisoning of livestock and the treatment of congestive heart failure. Extracts or latexes of cardiac glycosides plants have been applied to poison arrows in Africa, Asia, and South America for use in hunting and fighting. It is expected to be evolved as a defense way in plants. Cardiac glycosides are steroids having the ability to exert specific powerful action on the cardiac muscle. A very small amount can exert a beneficial simulation on diseased heart. These compounds are primarily valuable in the treatment of congestive heart failure. They increase the force of heart contraction without a concomitant increase on oxygen consumption. Consequently, the myocardium becomes more efficient pump and is able to meet the demands of circulatory system [6–8].

2. Structure diversity of cardiac glycosides

Cardiac glycosides are a group comprising two main classes of compounds that differ in the structure of their aglycone as shown in **Figure 1**. Cardiac glycosides are either C23 or C24 steroids with a basic nucleus of cyclopentanoperhydro phenanthrene substituted at C17. Cardenolides have a five-membered lactone group in the C17 with α, β-unsaturated γ-lactone ring (butenolide), whereas the other group, the bufadienolides, was first discovered as skin poisons in toads. The C17 substituent with a doubly unsaturated six-membered lactone ring (α-pyrone). Plants can produce both cardenolides and bufadienolides. Another group, isocardenolides, has the double bond of butenolid ring at position 21 or 22 instead of position 20 as shown in **Figure 1**. Most clinical attention was directed to the cardenolides owing to their therapeutic use. Digoxin and digitoxin are the two most widely used digitalis inotropes. There are two million patients receiving these cardenolides in the US. In general, some isocardenolides appeared to be devoid from any cardiac activity [9].

Cardiac glycosides, cardenolides, and bufadienolides, bear a structure resemblance to the steroid saponins and have the same solubility and foaming characteristics. They are also distinguished from other steroid glycosides by a 14-hydroxy group and some peculiar sugar incorporated in their skeleton. Other substituent groups may be present, for example, additional hydroxyl groups at C-1, 11, 12, 16, and 19. The sugars are always linked at C-3. Some members have an aldehyde group rather than methyl group at C-19 [10].

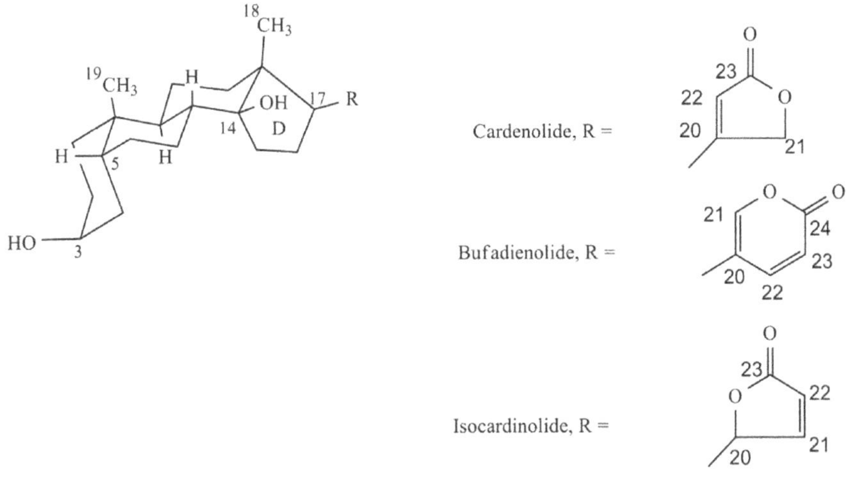

Figure 1. Structures of cardiac glycosides.

These compounds are also characterized by its unusual "U shape." This "U shape" has an A/B and C/D *cis* and B/C trans ring junctions. On the other hand, the adrenocortical steroids typically possess an A/B, B/C, and C/D all having trans conformation, while the bile salts characteristically have an A/B *cis* and B/C, trans orientation [10]. Although cardiac glycosides are more abundant than aglycones, some aglycones of cardiac glycosides are used for congestive heart failure and commercially available like digoxigenin, gitoxigenin, strophanthidin, and ouabagenin as shown in **Figure 2**. The most commercially important plant sources of cardiac glycosides are *digitalis purpurea, D. lanata, Strophanthus gratus,* and *Strophanthus kombé* [6]. **Figure 2** shows the structure of some common cardiac aglycones.

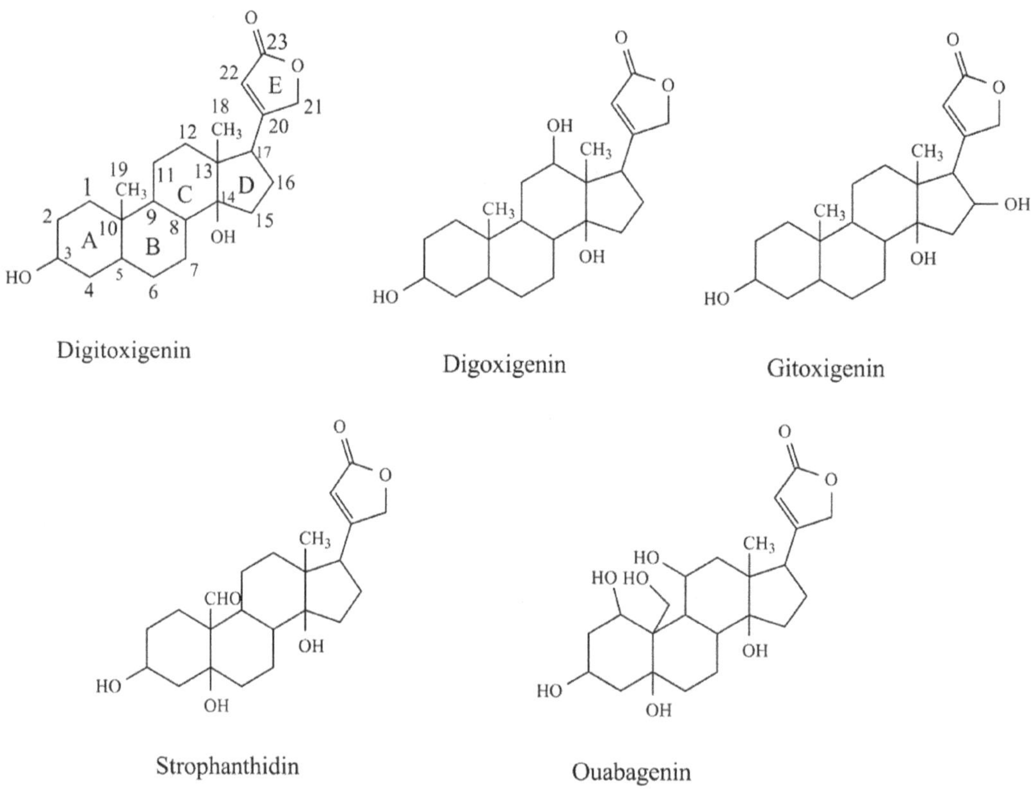

Figure 2. Structures of some common cardiac aglycones.

The sugar moieties are mostly attached to the aglycone at C-3 by β-linkage and are composed of up to four sugar units. It may include glucose or rhamnose together with other deoxy sugars whose natural occurrence is, so far, known only in association with cardiac glycosides [11–15]. **Figure 3** shows the structures of some examples of sugar residues attached to cardenolides,

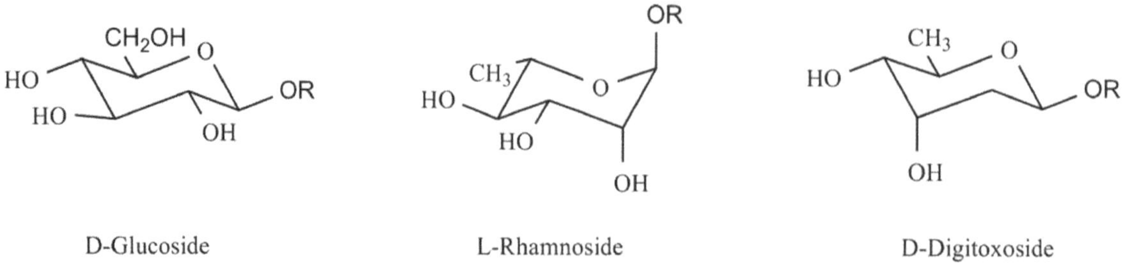

Figure 3. Examples of sugar residues attached to cardenolides.

which occur in the pyranoid form [11]. To differentiate between sugars with a hydroxyl group at C–2 and 2-deoxy-sugar chemically, hydrolysis is the first choice [16]. The latter are almost completely hydrolyzed by boiling in 0.05 N mineral acid in 50% aqueous methanol for 30 min, whereas the former sugars are not completely affected by this procedure.

3. Distribution in plant kingdom

Cardiac glycosides occur in small amounts in the seeds, leaves, stems, roots, and bark of plants of wide geographical distribution. Many species grow in tropical regions and have been employed, in the past, by natives of Africa, Asia, and South America for preparation of arrow poisons [17]. In plants, cardenolides appear to be confined to the angiosperms. They are more abundant in families Apocynaceae and Asclepiadaceae (now subsumed in Apocynaceae). However, it could be also found in some plants belonging to Liliaceae, Ranunculaceae, Moraceae, Leguminosae, Scrophulariaceae, Cruciferae, Sterculiaceae, Euphorbiaceae, Tiliaceae, and Celastraceae [18]. Some of the plants' genera containing natural cardenolides are illustrated in **Table 1**.

Family	Genera
Apocynaceae	*Adenium, Acokanthera, Strophanthus, Apocynum, Cerbera, Thevetia, Nerium, Carissa, Urechites*
Asclepiadaceae (subsumed in Apocynaceae)	*Gomphocarpus, Calotropis, Pachycarpus, Asclepias, Xysmalobium, Cryptostegia, Menabea, Periploca*
Moraceae	*Antiaris, Antiaropsis, Naucleopsis, Maquira, Castilla*
Leguminosae	*Coronilla*
Scrophulariaceae	*Digitalis, Isoplexis*
Cruciferae	*Erysimum, Cheiranthus*
Sterculiaceae	*Mansonia*
Tiliaceae	*Corchorus*
Celastraceae	*Euonymus, Lophopetalum*

Table 1. Some common plants containing natural cardenolides.

The bufadienolides occur in plants of families: Hyacinthaceae (Syn. Liliaceae), Crassulaceae, Iridaceae, Melianthaceae, Ranunculaceae, and Santalaceae. Two genera of Hyacinthaceae are known to produce them (Urginea and Bowiea). Several compounds of bufadienolides had been isolated from *Urginea maritima*, which is commonly known as Squill. It is worthy to mention that the genus *Urginea* is an aggregate of six species and it has been used in medicine since ancient times because of its powerful digitalis-like effect. There are various animal sources for bufadienolides, e.g., Buffo (toad), Photinus (fireflies), and Rhabdophis (snakes) [19].

4. Extraction and purification of cardiac glycosides

The isolation and identification of pure cardiac glycosides from their crude mixture faced some difficulties in the past due to its low quantity or its presence as a complex mixture. Reichstein's group [16] suggested the defatting of dried and powdered seeds, and/or leaves with petroleum ether followed by digestion with water at 0°C to extract polysaccharides and hydrolytic enzymes. One of the most common methods of extraction of cardiac glycosides is the prior protection of plant material by its maceration in toluene and allowing it to stand for many days at 25–37°C to avoid the enzymatic hydrolysis. Then, it is followed by exhaustive extraction with water-alcohol mixture. The aqueous extract could be evaporated to a small volume under vacuum at 50°C. Fats could then be removed by extraction with petroleum ether and the aqueous syrup of glycosides is diluted with an equal volume of water. Tannic acid and other polyphenolic and acidic products are precipitated with freshly prepared lead hydroxide and the mixture is filtered through Hyflo-Super Gel. The clear filtrate is adjusted to pH 6, concentrated under vacuum and subjected to fractional extraction: first with ether, then chloroform, and finally with chloroform-alcohol, 2:1 and 3:2. For isolation of glycosides of high solubility in water, the residual aqueous phase is half saturated with sodium sulfate and then extracted with chloroform-alcohol [20, 21]. The less polar fractions are separated by chromatography on neutral alumina [22]. The more polar fractions are usually chromatographed after acetylation or benzoylation and the free glycosides recovered by hydrolysis with bicarbonate.

Reversed phase column chromatography are widely accepted in many fields including HPLC of cardiac glycosides with RP-8 or RP-18 column and acetonitrile/water or methanol/water as an eluent, followed by UV detector at 220 nm [23]. The employment of HPLC techniques also led to the isolation of large number of cardiac glycosides [24–27]. The technique of DCCC has seen rapid expansion over the past few years. It was used to isolate three new glycosides from digitalis lanata using the solvent systems $CHCl_3$-MeOH-H_2O (5:6:4) and CH_2Cl_2-MeOH-H_2O (5:6:4) [28]. Four strophanthidin glycosides, out of a total of eight isolated compounds, were separated from one another by DCCC. The solvent systems $CHCl_3$-MeOH-PrnOH-H_2O (5:6:1:4) and $CHCl_3$-MeOH-PrnOH-H_2O (45:70:5:40) were used [29]. Further application of DCCC has been reported for the isolation of affinosides from *Anodendron affine* [30, 31]. Recently, Kopp et al. [32] used the technique of DCCC in successful application to isolate 41 bufadienolides after fractionation by column chromatography. Moreover, radial centrifugal chromatography gives a good resolution and ease of operation to isolate cardiac glycosides [33].

5. Chemical analysis

The analytical methods for cardiac glycosides can be divided into two groups, which are classical and sensitive methods. The classical methods (μg range) including photometry and chromatography have an importance in the pharmacopoeias and are widely employed in control laboratories for quantitative determination of the content and purity of glycoside preparations. Sensitive methods (ng range) include pharmacokinetic investigations, which require sophisticated apparatus. They comprise gas chromatography coupled to a mass spectrometer (GC-MS) and HPLC coupled to a sensitive detector (MS or fluorescence detector). Such method affords reliable measurements in the ng range [34], whereas the classical methods require preliminary purification, usually by chromatography [35].

In classical methods, direct measurement by UV led to the absorption maxima for cardenolides at 217 nm (εmol = 16,595) and for bufadienolides at 300 nm (εmol = 5250, εmol is the molar extinction coefficient). For qualitative and quantitative determination of the cardiac glycosides, it must therefore be converted into colored derivatives as shown in **Figure 4**. It can be converted into colored derivatives by reaction with polynitroaromatic derivatives in alkaline solution, with Keller-Kiliani or xanthydrolin acidic medium [34] or by treatment with strong acids and these can be measured by conventional photometers or fluorimeter [36, 37].

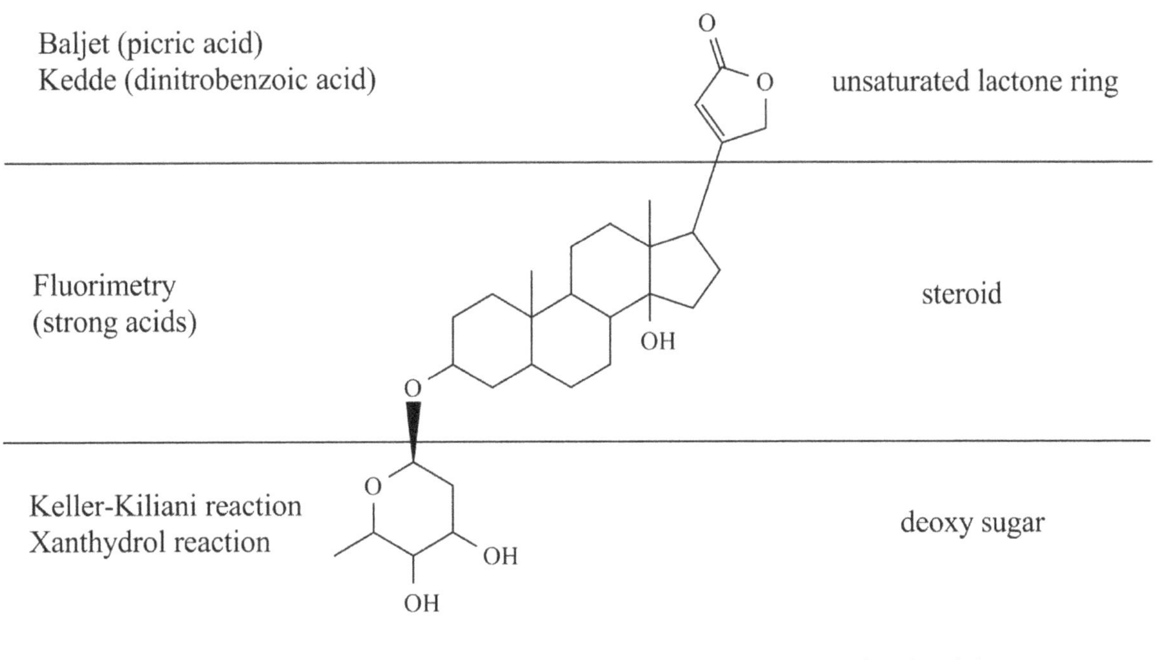

Figure 4. The chemical methods used for photometric and fluorimetric determination of cardenolides.

The reaction between cardenolides and polynitroaromatic derivatives in alkaline solution [38–41] are based on the C-C coupling of the unsaturated lactone ring with them to produce dye complexes which can be measured photometrically. The reagent may also be used as a spray reagent to visualize cardiac glycosides on TLC. The reagents that gained an established place are Baljet reagent (picric acid) [38], Kedde reagent (3,5-dinitrobenzoic acid) [40], and Rabitzsch reagent (tetranitrobiphenyl) [41]. However, the specificity of Baljet reagent is low because many other substances, e.g., ketones give intense color reaction with picric acid and alkali [34].

Various reaction mechanisms are suggested for the reaction of polynitroaromatic with cardiac glycosides [42]. According to the studies by Burns et al. [43] and Kovar et al. [42], splitting off of one proton at C21 produces a carbamine that consequently undergoes nucleophilic linkage to the polynitroaromatic molecule. The resulting complexes are cyclohexadienate type and known as Meisenheimer compounds [34], as shown in **Figure 5**.

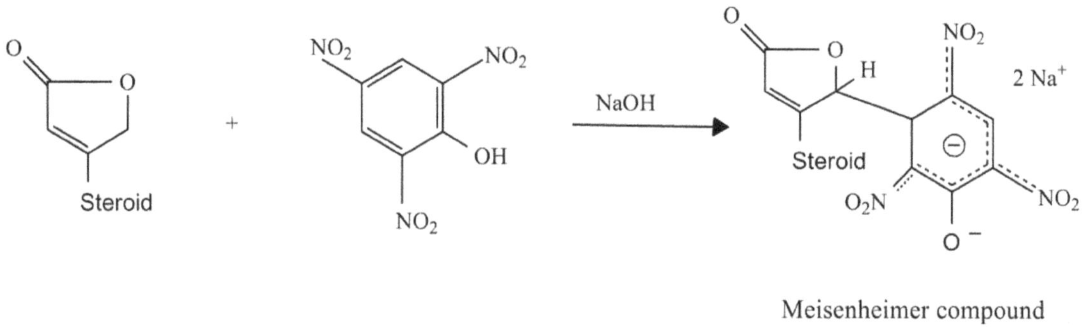

Figure 5. Meisenheimer complex formed of cardenolides with polynitroaromatic reagents.

Both the Keller-Kiliani and xanthydrol convert 2-deoxy-sugars into characteristic colored derivatives. In this way all digitoxose-containing glycosides can be qualitatively and quantitatively determined. All the acid reagents detect only those digitoxoses, which are easily hydrolyzed under the conditions of the test [34]. Keller-Kiliani reaction in acetic acid, ferric chloride, and sulfuric acid produces a blue coloration with absorption maxima at 470 and 590 nm. It is important to note that the color formation is dependent on time and it is affected by moisture content [37]. Xanthydrol reaction [44] in acetic acid/hydrochloric acid mixture produces red coloration with absorption maximum at 520 nm. However, the reagent is not very stable and decomposed products tend to interfere with the color reaction. Therefore, Pötter suggested the use or the more stable dixanthyl urea instead of xanthydrol [45].

Fluorescence spectroscopy is 10–100 times more sensitive than absorption photometry [46], so the reaction between cardiac glycosides and strong acids gives a restricted limit of detection in the ng range. For digoxin determinations, an activating wavelength of 340 nm is used and the emitted fluorescence is measured at 420 nm [47].

6. Structure elucidation

The earliest methods to determine the structure of cardiac glycosides depended on acid and/or enzymatic hydrolysis of the glycoside to the aglycone and sugar moieties followed by the identification of their nature. The method consumed a bigger quantity of the isolated glycoside, and consequently, it was only suitable for structure determination of the major constituents. The great development in the spectroscopic instruments and the analysis of the produced data in the last three decades was accompanied by a great jump in the study of structure and stereochemical behavior of the naturally occurring compounds. This development led to stabilize a clear relationship between the structure and the data obtained from the spectroscopic experiments.

Before developing the recent tools for chemical analysis of organic compounds, it was very difficult to elucidate the cardiac glycosides structures. In the past, it is important to perform acid hydrolysis [48–51] or enzymatic hydrolysis [52, 53] to obtain the sugar residues and the aglycone separately. Now, more sophisticated and accurate tools were used for identification the structure of cardiac glycosides with the stereochemistry determination, which give a powerful way to understand the mechanism of action and facilitate the structure activity relationship studies. Examples of these tools are mass spectroscopy, and FTIR and NMR.

6.1. Nuclear magnetic resonance (NMR)

No doubt that NMR is the most powerful tool for the structure determination of cardiotonic compounds. The advantage of pulsed Fourier transformation and two-dimensional NMR spectroscopy is that they provide information related to the carbon skeleton of the molecule and the structure environment of each hydrogen and carbon. Tori et al. [54] reported the first ^{13}C-NMR analysis of 10 cardenolides by employing single-frequency off-resonance, noise off-resonance decoupling, and the comparison with spectra of structurally related compounds. Later on, he used ^{13}C-NMR spectroscopy to determine the structure of thevetin A and B [55]. Robien et al. [56] reviewed ^{13}C NMR data of 36 bufadienolides. Later on, Kopp et al. [32] used ^{13}C NMR for elucidation of the structure of bufadienolides compounds isolated from *Urginea maritima*.

Cheung and Watson [57] briefly studied the ^{1}H and ^{13}C NMR of the compounds calactin, uscharidin, calotoxin, uscharin, and voruscharin and established their stereochemistry. The ^{13}C-chemical shift of C-19 also gives valuable information on the stereochemistry of both cardenolides and bufadienolides at C-5. In 5β-series, C-19 have its signal at 21.7 ± 2.5 ppm, whereas in 5α-series at 12.2 ± 0.4 ppm. Moreover, 5α-series show the deshielding of C-7 and C-9 by ~5.5 and 13 ppm, respectively. The number of sugar moieties could be determined from the number of anomeric carbons at the region of 95–103 ppm in its ^{13}C-NMR spectrum. Moreover, α- and β-sugars could be distinguished from each other by measuring the coupling constant of the anomeric hydrogen at the region of 4.4–5.3 ppm in its ^{1}H-NMR spectrum. The anomeric hydrogen of α-sugar is coupled with the adjacent hydrogen at 2–3 Hz, while of β-sugar is coupled at 7–8 Hz [58].

Elgamal et al. isolated and studied the structure of several cardiac glycosides [58–60]. Some of these compounds are shown in **Figure 6**. The structure elucidation of some example compounds, **A, B**, and **C**, was presented based on NMR spectral assignments [60], which were confirmed by DEPT, gs-COSY, TOCSY, *gs*-HMQC, ^{13}C-coupled *gs*-HMQC, ROESY, *gs*-HMBC, and 2D INAPT experiments. The ^{1}H and ^{13}C assignments are shown in **Table 2**. The stereochemistry of the steroid ring system and all substituents could be determined beyond doubt from the ^{1}H; ^{1}H coupling constants, as far as identifiable, and the ROESY cross-peaks. The ROE measurements are very informative to perform signal assignment and to determine the ring junction forms. In compound **B**, some ROESY cross-peaks gave evidence of the trans form of ring junctions A/B and B/C which revealed by H-2b/H-19, H-19/H-8b, and H-8b/H-18 cross-peaks, as shown in **Figure 7**. In addition, the ring junction C/D should be *cis*, as follows from the cross-peaks H-9/H-15a and H-12a/H-15a. The orientation of aglycone and glucose moiety in compound **C** was obtained from spatial proximities obtained from ROESY as shown in **Figure 8**.

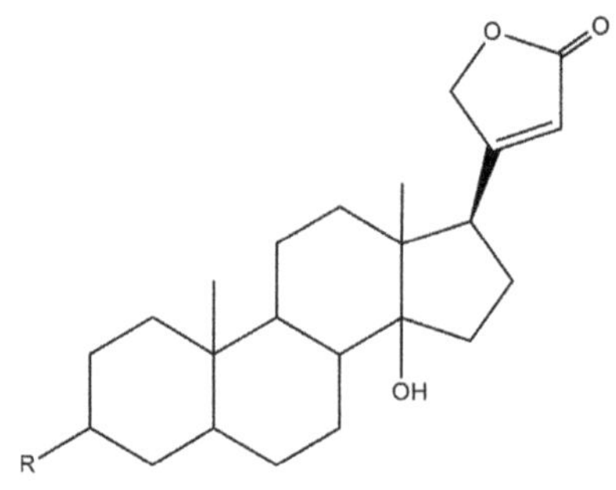

	R
A	=O
B	OH
C	O Glc

Figure 6. Structure of some cardenolides isolated from *Calotropis procera.*

		A		B		C	
		^1H	^{13}C	^1H	^{13}C	^1H	^{13}C
1	α	1.29	38.3	1.10	38.3	1.10	38.3
	β	1.96		1.84		1.85	
2	α	2.23	37.8	1.85	32.1	1.97	30.4
	β	2.32		1.47		1.62	
3	α	–	211.4	3.60	71.8	3.80	79.2
4	α	2.04	44.3	1.64	38.8	1.82	35.3
	β	2.21		1.36		1.41	
5	α	1.45	46.1	1.21	45.8	1.20	45.6
6	α	1.37	28.6	1.44	30.0	1.47	30.0
	β	1.23		1.35		1.38	
7	α	1.03	27.0	1.20	28.7	1.20	28.8
	β	1.96		2.13		2.13	
8	β	1.52	41.2	1.68	42.6	1.68	42.6
9	α	0.95	49.1	1.07	51.1	1.07	51.1
10		–	35.7	–	36.9	–	37.0
11	α	1.48	21.2	1.63	22.3	1.62	22.3
	β	1.30		1.38		1.38	
12	α	1.32	39.4	1.56	40.9	1.56	40.9
	β	1.45		1.56		1.56	
13		–	49.5	–	51.0	–	51.0

		A		B		C	
		^{1}H	^{13}C	^{1}H	^{13}C	^{1}H	^{13}C
14		–	84.7	–	86.3	–	86.3
15	α	1.98	32.7	2.20	33.4	2.20	33.4
	β	1.63		1.79		1.80	
16	α	2.07	26.7	2.23	28.0	2.23	28.0
	β	1.79		1.95		1.95	
17	α	2.72	50.7	2.91	52.1	2.90	52.1
18		0.84	15.7	0.97	16.4	0.97	16.4
19	a	0.94	11.2	0.91	12.6	0.92	12.6
	b	–		–		–	
20		–	174.8	–	178.4	–	178.4
21	a	4.76	73.3	5.01	75.3	5.00	75.4
	b	4.95		5.11		5.12	
22		5.81	117.4	5.98	117.8	5.98	117.8
23		–	174.4	–	177.2	–	177.3
1′						4.47 (7.8)	102.3
2′						3.22 (8.8)	75.2
3′						3.43 (8.8)	78.1
4′						3.35 (9.6)	71.7
5′						3.35 (5.1;1.5)	77.9
6′	a					3.73 (11.9;5.1)	62.8
	b					3.93 (11.9,1.5)	

Table 2. ^{1}H and ^{13}C NMR chemical shifts and characteristic *J* (H,H) couplings of three cardenolides **A–C**.

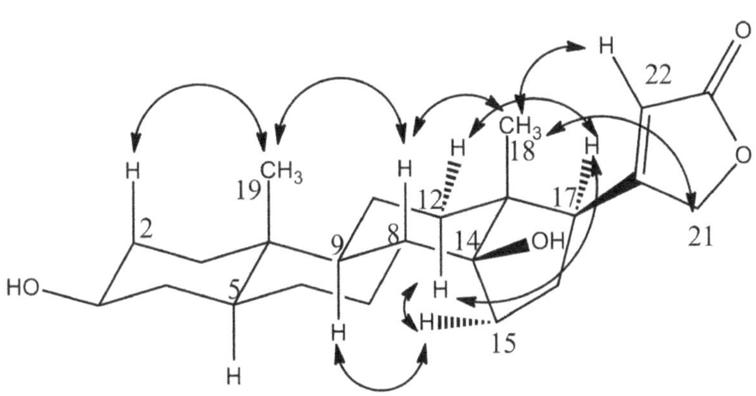

Figure 7. Stereostructure of **B**. The arrows indicate steric proximities (from ROESY experiment).

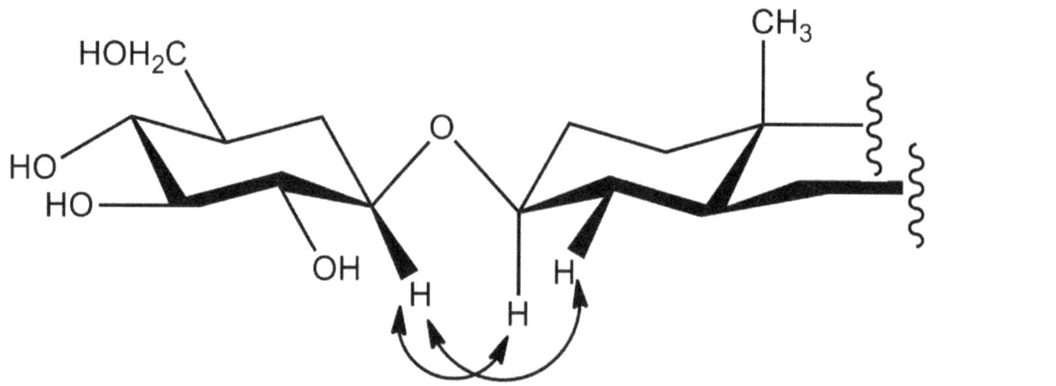

Figure 8. Relative orientation of the aglycone and the sugar moiety in **C**. The arrows refer to spatial proximities obtained from ROESY.

7. Pharmacological action of cardiac glycosides

The most important use of the cardiac glycosides is its effects in treatment of cardiac failure. In cardiac failure, or congestive heart failure, heart cannot pump sufficient blood to maintain body needs. During each heart contraction, there is an influx of Na^+ and an outflow of K^+. Before the next contraction, Na^+, K^+-ATPase must reestablish the concentration gradient pumping Na^+ into the cell against a concentration gradient. This process requires energy, which is obtained from hydrolysis of ATP to ADP by Na^+, K^+-ATPase. Cardiac glycosides inhibit Na^+, K^+-ATPase, and consequently increase the force of myocardial contraction [8]. On the other hand, some cardiac glycosides were investigated for their antitumor activity [61]. In addition, it has been reported that some cardiac glycosides display an inhibitory activity against rhinovirus [62].

8. Structure-activity relationship

In cardenolides, the steroidal part is considered the pharmacophoric moiety, responsible for the activity of these compounds [63]. Specifically, the 5β,14β-androstane-3β,14-diol skeleton has shown the same binding properties to the enzyme as digitalis compounds.

Furthermore, the bending in the structure as shown in *cis* junctions between A/B and C/D rings is very important to get the highest interaction energy. Any modification of A and/or B rings related to B-C plane, reduces the interaction energy [64]. In general, OH groups at any position of steroidal skeleton reduce the interaction energy, which depends on the position on the skeleton and the spatial location. This fact may be explained by the steric hindrance and the decreasing of steroidal positive potential field. Moreover, the OH group at position C14β is not an essential feature for inotropic activity, although when it is replaced by hydrogen atom, potency decreases considerably [65]. The change of the A/B junction does not mean a decrease of activity of aglycones but it decreases the activity of the corresponding glycosides. Thus, the main effect of A/B junction is revealed from its ability to put the sugar into its suitable position [66]. The lactone ring at C17β has been considered to be responsible for inotropic activity, bringing about conformational changes on the enzyme that would give rise to its inhibition [67]. Indeed, that is the most differentiating feature from steroid hormones, and its contribution to the interaction [68]. Sugar attachment to the steroid part modifies both pharmacokinetics as well as pharmacodynamics of digitalis glycosides. Free aglycones are absorbed faster than glycosides and they are easily metabolized to less active 3α-OH epimer. Thus, the action of free aglycone is fast and short lasting. The sugar moiety significance for digitalis activity is well established but sugar parts themselves do not show any activity [10].

Acknowledgements

I am thankful to my wife, Dr. Radwa Moustafa Elfaiomy, for her help and encouragement during this work.

Author details

Nagy Morsy

Address all correspondence to: namorsy@yahoo.com

1 Department of Chemistry, Faculty of Sciences and Arts, Khulais, University of Jeddah, Saudi Arabia

2 Department of Chemistry of Natural Compounds, National Research Centre, El-bohouth St., Dokki, Cairo, Egypt

References

[1] Akhtar N, Malik A, Ali SN, Kazmi SU. Proceragenin, an antibacterial cardenolide from *Calotropis procera*. Phytochemistry. 1992;31: 2821–2824.

[2] Brüschweiter F, Stöckel K, Reichstein T. supposed partial structure of Calotropis Glycosides. Glycosides and aglycones. Helvetica Chimica Acta. 1969;52: 2276–2303.

[3] Crout DHG, Curtis RF, Hassal CH, Jones TL. The cardiac glycosides of *Calotropis procera*. Tetrahedron Letters. 1963;4: 63–67.

[4] Prassas I, Diamandis EP. Novel therapeutic applications of cardiac glycosides. Reviews. 2008;7: 926–935.

[5] Shaker K, Morsy N, Zinecker H, Schneider B, Imhoff JF. Secondary metabolites from *Calotropis procera* R. BR. Phytochemistry Letters. 2010;3: 212–216.

[6] Haynes GS. The pharmacological action of Digitalis, Strophanthus, and Squill on the heart. Biochemical Journal. 1906;1: 62–87.

[7] Kelly RA. Cardiac glycosides and congestive heart failure. American Journal of Cardiology. 1990;65: 10–16.

[8] Farnsworth NF. Biological and phytochemical screening of plants. Journal of Pharmaceutical Sciences. 1966;55: 225–276.

[9] Pettit GR, Green B, Dasgupta AK, Whitehouse PA, Yardley JP. Bufadienolides. 3. A synthetic route to isocardenolides. Journal of organic Chemistry. 1970;35: 1381–1384.

[10] Melero CP, Medarde M, Feliciano AS. Short review on cardiotonic steroids and their aminoguanidine analogues. Molecule. 2000;5: 51–81.

[11] Reichstein T, Weiss E. The sugars of the cardiac glycosides. Advances in Carbohydrate Chemistry. 1962;17: 65–120.

[12] Hanessian S. Deoxy sugars. Advances in Carbohydrate Chemistry. 1966;21: 143–207.

[13] Zorbach WW, Bhat KV. Biosynthesis of ribose and deoxyribose. Advances in Carbohydrate Chemistry. 1966;21: 273–321.

[14] ReichsteinT. Cardenolide- and pregnanglycosides. Naturwissenschaften. 1967;54: 53–67.

[15] Singh B, Rastogi RP. Phytochemistry. Cardenolides—Glycosides and Genins. 1970;9: 315–331.

[16] Von Euw J, Hess H, Speiser P, Reichstein T. The glycosides of Strophanthus intermedius Pax. Glycosides and aglycones, 82. Mitteilung. Helvtica Chimica Acta. 1951;34: 1821–1833.

[17] Karawya MS, Abdel-Wahab SM, Niazi HM. Assay of cardinolides in Acokanthera spectabilis. Planta Medica. 1974;25: 17–21.

[18] Hollman A. Plants and cardiac glycosides. British Heart Journal. 1985;54: 258–261.

[19] Steyn PS, van Heerden RF. Bufadienolides of plant and animal origin. Natural Products Reports. 1998;15: 397–413.

[20] Bally PRO, Mohr K, Reichstein T. The glycosides of the root cortex of Acokanthera friesiorum Markgr. Helvetica Chimica Acta. 1952;35: 45–50.

[21] Muhr H, Hunger A, Reichstein T. The glycosides of the seeds of Acokanthera friesiorum Markgr. Helvetica Chimica Acta. 1954;37: 403–427.

[22] Von Euw J, Lardon A, Reichstein T. Partial synthesis of corticosterone. Helvetica Chimica Acta. 1944;27: 1287–1296.

[23] Castle MC. Isolation and quantitation of picomole quantities of digoxin, digitoxin and their metabolites by high-pressure liquid chromatography. Journal of Chromatography. 1975;115: 437–445.

[24] Linder W, Frei RW. Partition HPLC systems for the separation of digitalis glycosides of the cardenolide group. Journal of Chromatography. 1976;117: 81–86.

[25] El-Askary H, Holzl J, Hilal S, El-Kashoury E. Cardenolide glycosides from *Gomphocarpus sinaicus*. Phytochemistry. 1993;34: 1399–1402.

[26] Abdel-Azim NS, Hammouda FM, Hunkler D, Rimpler H. Re-investigation of the cardenolide glycosides from *Gomphocarpus sinaicus*. Phytochemistry. 1996;42 523-529.

[27] Abe F, Yamauchi T, Yahara S, Nohara T. Glycosides of 19-formylthevetiogenin and 5α-thevetiogenin from *Thevetia neriifolia*. Phytochemistry. 1994;37: 1429-1432.

[28] Krüger D, Junior P, Wichtl M. New cardiac glycosides from *Digitalis lanata*. Planta Medica. 1983;49: 74–78.

[29] Wagner H, Habermeier H, Schulten HR. The cardiac glycosides of the arrow poison of *Lophopetalum toxicum* Loher. Helvetica Chimica Acta. 1984;67: 54–64.

[30] Abe F, Yamauchi T. Affinoside A and companion glycosides from the stem and bark of *Anodendron affine*. Chemical and Pharmaceutical Bulletin. 1982;30: 1183–1193.

[31] Abe F, Yamauchi T. Affinosides S-I-S-VIII, cardenolide glycosides with a usual glycosidic linkage, from *Anodendron affine* (Anodendron. IV). Chemical and Pharmaceutical Bulletin. 1983;31 :1199–1206.

[32] Kopp B, Krenn L, Draxler M, Hoyer A, Terkola R, Vallaster P, Robin W. Bufadienolides from *Urginea maritima* from Egypt. Phytochemistry. 1966;42 :513–522.

[33] Martin RA, Lynch SP, Schmitz FJ, Pordesimo EO, Toth S Horten RY. Cardenolides from *Asclepias asperula* subsp. capricornu and *A. viridis*. Phytochemistry. 1991;30: 3935–3939.

[34] Clarke C.J, Cobb PH. Two-dimensional TLC of digitalis cardenolides using a continuous development technique. Journal of Chromatography. 1979;168: 541–549.

[35] Grade K, Förster W. An improved method for the isolation of heart glycosides from tissues by using Sephadex G 200. Biochemistry and Pharmacology. 1967;16: 1299–1303.

[36] Neuwald F. The photometric assay of digitoxin by the Baljet reaction. Journal of American Pharmacists Association. 1950;39: 172–174.

[37] Rowson JM, Dyer FJ. Studies in the genus Digitalis: Part II. A comparison of the colorimetric and biological methods for the evaluation of *Digitalis purpurea*. Journal of Pharmacy and Pharmacology. 1952;4: 831–843.

[38] Baljet H, Glycosides with digitalis effects. A new identity reaction. Pharmaceutisch weekblad. 1918;55: 457–463.

[39] Robert C. Anderson, K. K. Chen, The colorimetric assay of digitoxin by the modified raymond method. Journal of Pharmaceutical Sciences. 1946;13: 353–355.

[40] Kedde DL. Contribution to the chemical analysis of Digitalis preparations. Pharmaceutisch weekblad. 1947;82: 741–757.

[41] Rabitzsch G, Tambor U. Method for quantitative determination of cardiac glycosides and genins of cardenolide type with 2,4,2′,4′-tetranitrodiphenyl. Pharmazie. 1969;24: 262–269.

[42] Kovar KA, Frankas G, To the mechanism of the reactions according to Raymond, Kedde and Baljet. Archiv der Pharmazie 1977;310: 40–47.

[43] Burns LB, Stedmann RJ, Tuckerman MH. Polynitroaromatic compounds in analytical chemistry. I: Reaction with quabain and digitoxin. Journal of Pharmaceutical Sciences. 1977;66: 753–754.

[44] Pesez M. Xanthydrol reagent for desoxy sugars. Annales Pharmaceutiques Françaises. 1952;10: 104–108.

[45] Pötter H. Dixanthylurea, a new reagent for the quantitative determination of digitalis glycosides. Pharmazie. 1965;20: 737–737.

[46] Ringhardtz J. What does fluorescence spectroscopy do in biochemistry? Labor-Praxis. 1980;4: 32–39.

[47] Wells D, Katzung B, Megers FH. Spectrofluorometric analysis of cardiotonic steroids. Journal of Pharmacy and Pharmacology. 1961;13: 389–395.

[48] Voss W, Wachs W, On the alcoholysis of phenol glucoside. (1. Communication on Glycoside Cleavages in Non-Aqueous Media). Justus Liebig's Annalen der Chemie. 1936;522: 240–261.

[49] Mannich C, Siewert G. About g-Strophanthin (Ouabain) and g-Strophanthidin. Berichte der Deutschen Chemischen Gesellschaft. 1942;75: 737–750.

[50] Rosselet JP, Hunger A. Intermedioside (Substance No. 761). Helvetica Chimica Acta. 1951;34: 1036–1041.

[51] Kiliani H. About Digitalinum Verum. Berichte der Deutschen Chemischen Gesellschaft. 1930;63: 2866–2871.

[52] Stoll A, Pereira A, Renz J, About cardiac effective glycosides and aglycones of the seeds of Coronilla glauca. Helvetica Chimica Acta. 1949;32: 293–315.

[53] Stoll A, Renz J, Brack A. Cardiac glycosides. XXVIII. Preparation of scillarenin, the actual aglycon of scillaren A, with an adoptive enzyme. Helvetica Chimica Acta. 1951;34: 2301–2311.

[54] Tori K, Ishii H, Wolkowski ZW, Chachaty C, Sangaré M, Piriou F, Lukacs G. Carbon-13 nuclear magnetic resonance spectra of cardenolides. Tetrahedron Letters. 1973;14: 1077–1080.

[55] Tori K, Thang TT, Sangare M, Lukacs G. Application of carbon-13 NMR spectroscopy to structural determination of steroidal trisaccharides, thevetin A and B. Tetrahedron Letters. 1966;18: 717–720.

[56] Robien W, Kopp B, Schabl D, Schwartz H. Carbon-13 NMR spectroscopy of cardenolides and bufadienolides. Progress in Nuclear Magnetic Resonance Spectroscopy. 1987;19: 131–181.

[57] Cheung HTA, Watson TR. Stereochemistry of the hexosulose in cardenolide glycosides of the Asclepiadaceae. Journal of the Chemical Society, Perkin Transactions 1. 1980;10: 2162-2168.

[58] Hanna AG, Shalaby NMM, Morsy NAM, Simon A, Tóth G, Malik S, Duddeck H. Structure of calotropagenin-drived artifact from *Calotropis procera*. Magnetic Resonance in Chemistry. 2002;40: 599–602.

[59] Hanna AG, Elgamal MHA, Morsy NAM, Duddeck H, Kovàcs J, Tóth G. Two cardenolides from *Calotropis procera*. Magnetic Resonance in Chemistry. 1999;37: 754-757.

[60] Elgamal MHA, Hanna AG, Morsy NAM, Duddeck H, Simon A, Gàti T, Tóth G. Complete ^{1}H and ^{13}C signal assignment of 5 α-cardenolides isolated from *Calotropis procera* R. BR. Journal of Molecular Structure. 1999;477: 201–208.

[61] Doskotch RW, Malik MY, Hufford CD, Malik SN. Trent JE, Kubelka W. Antitumor agents. V: Cytotoxic cardenolides from *Cryptostegia grandiflora* (Roxb.) R. Br. Journal of Pharmaceutical Sciences. 1972;61: 570–573.

[62] Kamano Y, Satoth N, Nakayoshi H, Pettit GR, Smith CR. Rhinovirus inhibition by bufadienolides. Chemical & Pharmaceutical Bulletin. 1988;36: 326–332.

[63] Repke KRH. Novel developments in cardiac glycosides structure-activity relationship. Trends in Pharmacological Sciences. 1985;6: 275–278.

[64] Schönfeld W, Schönfeld R, Menke KH, Weiland J, Repke KRH. Origin of differences of inhibitory potency of cardiac glycosides in Na^{+}/K^{+}-transporting ATPase from human cardiac muscle, human brain cortex and guinea-pig cardiac muscle. Biochemical Pharmacology. 1986;35: 3221–3231.

[65] Shigei T, Tsuru H, Saito Y, Okada M. Structure-activity relationship of the cardenolide, with special reference to the substituents and configurations at C-14 and C-15. Experientia. 1973;29: 449–450.

[66] Melero PM, Medarde M, Feliciano AS. A short review on cardiotonic steroids and their aminoguanidine analogues. Molecules. 2000;5: 51–81.

[67] Smith P, Brown L, Boutagy J, Thomas R. Cardenolide analogues synthesis and biological activity of glucosides of C17b-modified derivatives of digitoxigenin. Journal of Medicinal Chemistry. 1982;25: 1222–1226.

[68] Schönfeld W, Repke KRH. A Free-Wilson analysis of 5β, 14β-androstane derivatives inhibiting the Na/K-ATPase from human heart. Quantitative Structure-Activity Relationships. 1988;7: 160–165.

13

Culture, History and Applications of Medicinal and Aromatic Plants in Japan

Maiko Inoue, Shinichiro Hayashi and Lyle E. Craker

Abstract

Historically, the Japanese began to use aromatic and medicinal plants for ritual activities, food flavor, and treatment of their bodies. The exotic plants, new ideas, and culture associated with medicinal and aromatic plants were introduced to Japan from other countries, primarily via Korea. In this way, experience and knowledge of uses were accumulated, and applications of aromatic and medicinal plants were expanded. The oldest Japanese medicine "Wa ho" leads the way to folk medicine today, and traditional Japanese medicine (Kampo) has spread into modern use. The elegance tradition of "Kodo," an incense ceremony of Japan, was developed because of the use of aromatic incensed wood in sixteenth century as recreation. Paired along with this ceremony is the Japanese sa-do tea ceremony that the spirituality and esthetic sense are inherited to Japanese today. Japanese green tea is becoming popular in many countries due to the constituent, catechins, that medically treats vascular disease, several cancers, and type II diabetes. Today, the Japanese medical system has new direction, integrating medicine with the adoption of modern western and alternative medicine. Scientific data must continue to be collected for interactions between the two medicinal systems for integrative medicine to be ideal for body, mind, and spirit of humans and nature.

Keywords: Kampo (traditional Japanese medicine), green tea, integrative medicine, body and spirit, phytotherapy

1. Introduction

Aromatic and medicinal plants fill a significant role in human societies that have helped improve the lives of people since ancient times. Ancient people became aware of the value and attractiveness of aromatic and medicinal plants, and the significance of historical books is a guide for the use of the plant material (**Table 1**) [1]. Initial books on use on medicinal and

Timeline	Book and author	Book about	Country
~500–300 BC	*Hippocratic corpus* written by Hippocrates; *De Causis Plantarum* and *Historia Plantarum* written by Theophrastis	Formalized medicine practices in diagnosis and treatments; list of medicinal plants and application	Greek
~150–100 BC	Huangdi Neijing (author unknown)	Theoretical foundation of Chinese medicine, diagnostic methods, and acupuncture	China
~100 BC-100 AC	Celsus wrote *De Medicina*; Dioscorides wrote *De Materia Medica*	Alexandrian medicine; pharmacopoeia of herbs and the medicines	Greek
~200–300 AC	*Shennong Bencaojing* (author unknown); *Shanghan Lun* written by Shang Zhongjing	Agriculture and medicinal plants; 113 herbal prescriptions and six stages of disease	China
~750–800 AC	Lu Yu wrote *The Classic of Tea*	Tea tree, making tea, and tea ceremony	China
~800–1000 AC	Avicenna writes *Book of Healing* and *Canon of Medicine*; Albucasis wrote *Kitab al-Tasrif*; Hildegard of Bingen wrote *Ohysica*; Averroes wrote *Kulliyat*	Clinical trials on medicines; Encyclopedia of medical practices; Scientific and medicinal properties of various plants; Medical encyclopedia	Arabic countries and Germany
~1000–1500 AC	Ibn al-Baitar wrote *Compendium on Simple Medicaments and Foods*	Pharmacopoeia listing 1400 plants	Arabic countries
~1500–1600 AC	John Gerard wrote *Herball, or Generall Historie of Plantes*	Heavily illustrated of 1000 plants	England
~1900–2000 AC	René-Maurice Gattefossé wrote *Aromathérapie*	Aroma and essential oil for Medicine	France

Table 1. Significant materials and books in history of medicinal plants and medicine [1].

aromatic plants were sourced in various parts of the world, such as the Middle East, Greece, China, and India, indicating that these ancient civilizations used indigenous aromatic and medicinal plants to improve lives in their own separate ways before ideas were shared. Japan is no exception; names of some local aromatic and medicinal plants were recorded in the oldest Japanese history book "Kojiki" written in 712 A.D. Aromatic and medicinal plants, however, continue to influence human life, culture, and history. Currently, an estimated 70,000 plant species are used in traditional medicine [2].

In Japan, most aromatic and medicinal plants have been used in the crude drug system, Kampo, the traditional Japanese medicine system, and in herbal tea as alternative or complemental medicines. The production value of Kampo was $1.38 billion, accounting for only two percent of all Japanese pharmaceuticals in 2011 [3], and although a total of 83.5% of 684 medical doctors were using Kampo for their prescriptions, according to web survey by the Japan Kampo Medicines Manufacturers Association (JKMA) in 2008 [4], the market for Kampo medicines increased by 23% over 5 years (2007–2011). In 2008, the usage of crude medicine for Kampo was 20,000 metric tons, of which a total of 83 percent was imported from China [5]. Almost 250 kinds of crude (not processed) medicines are used as Kampo materials in 2008, and the top 20 are listed as example (**Table 2**) [5].

Ranking	Common name	Spices	Family	Parts used	usage (kg)
1	Licorice	Glycyrrhiza uralinsis	Leguminosae	Root	1,267,395
2	Chinese Peony	Paeonia lactiflora	Paeoniaceae	Root	1,164,126
3	Cinnamon	Cinnamomum cassia	Lauraceae	Bark	1,033,793
4	Indian bread, tuckahoe	Poria cocos	Polyporaceae	Fungus	996,311
5	Jujube	Ziziphus jujuba	Rhamnaceae	Fruit	675,997
6	Pinellia	Pinellia ternata	Araceae	Tuber	629,063
7	Oriental Ginseng	Panax ginseng	Araliaceae	Root	610,092
8	Angelica acutiloba	Angelica acutiloba	Apiaceae	Root	580,607
9	Ephedra	Ephedra sinica	Ephedraceae	Stem	568,686
10	glutinous starch syrup	Oryza sativa	Gramineae	Seed	555,718
11	Kudzu vine, Japanese arrowroot	Pueraria lobata	Papilionaceae	Root	553,999
12	Atractylodes lancea	Atractylodes lancea	Asteraceae	Rhizome	501,647
13	Job's Tears	Coix lacryma-jobi	Gramineae	Seed	449,253
14	Sickle Hare's Ear	Bupleurum falcatum	Umbelliferae	Root	443,811
15	Rhubarb	Rheum palmatum	Polygonaceae	Rhizome	439,590
16	Atractylodes	Atractylodes japonica	Asteraceae	Rhizome	427,357
17	Alexandrian Senna	Senna alexandrina	Caesalpiniaceae	Leaves, pods	426,230
18	Chinese foxglove	Rehmannia glutinosa	Scrophulariaceae	Root	397,512
19	Baikal skullcap	Scutellaria baicalensis	Labiatae	Root	383,969
20	Gypsum				380,348

Table 2. Usage of top 20 crude medicines for Kampo in 2008 [5].

2. Introduction and opening: medical systems and recreations

Several of the plants were discovered to have medicinal effects and were spread throughout the world along with traditional medicines, and some of were being as indigenous. At first, traditional medicines were introduced to Japan from China via Korea from the seventh to ninth centuries which is called traditional Chinese medicine (TCM). Before TCM was introduced to Japan, an older medicine called "Wa ho" existed. As TCM started flourishing, Wa ho declined and will likely remain as a folk medicine. TCM influenced traditional Japanese medicine (TJM) known as Kampo, in terms of fundamental principle and diagnosis, such as Yin-Yang (two opposites form the whole), Qi (life energy), and the Five Elements (interactions and relationships). Many ancient thin wooden strips which were excavated from a 7th century ruin recorded Chinese medicinal plant names that indicated their use as medicines In 756, a total of 60 crude medicines, for example, pepper, cinnamon, licorice, rhubarb, betel nut palm, and croton, were contributed to Shosoin, where the treasure house that belongs to

Todai-ji, Nara, and 38 of them remained (**Figure 1**). At Shosoin, seven scent bags, included Borneo camphor, musk, and other fragrances from China also remained.

In 894, Japanese missions to Tang China were abolished by the imperial court of Japan, and the exchange of crude medicines, TCM, and culture was stopped. Thereby, medicine in Japan was developed uniquely until Sanki Tashiro (1465–1537) introduced Chinese medicine in 1498. Dosan Manase (1507–1594), Tashiro's apprentice, encouraged the more formal Chinese medicine, known as "gosei-ho," while Geni Nagoya (1625–1694), Gonzan Goto (1659–1733), Toyo Yamawaki (1705–1762), and Todo Yoshimasu (1702–1773) regarded "ko-ho" in which medicine should be clinical and adopted "*Shanghan Lun*" (*Treatise on Cold Damage Disorders*) for acute fever symptoms and "*Jin Gui Yao Lue*" (*Essential Prescriptions from the Golden Cabinet*) for pathology and treatments of various diseases which are the oldest complete clinical textbooks written by Zhang Zhongjing (150–219) [4, 6, 7]. Ko-ho put emphasis on abdominal palpation and is main stream of Kampo [8]. The word "Kampo" is used for comparison with "Rampo," a conventional western medicine introduced from the Netherlands in the 17th to 19th centuries. Kampo, however, was the main medicine in Japan until the end of the Edo era. In 1869, the Meiji administration decided that the national medicine system would be the German system, and then, in 1876, the government declared a regulation that passing a western medicine examination was necessary to become a medical doctor. This issue made Kampo usage decline rapidly, only a part of doctors, pharmacists, and medicine traders carried Kampo. After World War II, however, the side effects from using synthetic medicines happened frequently, thereby people returned to the idea of Kampo. At the same time, the Japan Society for Oriental Medicine (JSOM) was established to promote oriental medicine and contribute to the progress and dissemination of oriental medicine in 1950. The national health insurance started to cover Kampo in 1967, and therefore, the demands for Kampo increased. Finally, the medical specialist system of Kampo and pharmacist system were started in 1990 and 2000, respectively. Kampo was added to the core curriculum in medical education system in 2001. Thus, history indicates a U-turn movement for Kampo (**Figure 2**) [6, 8, 9].

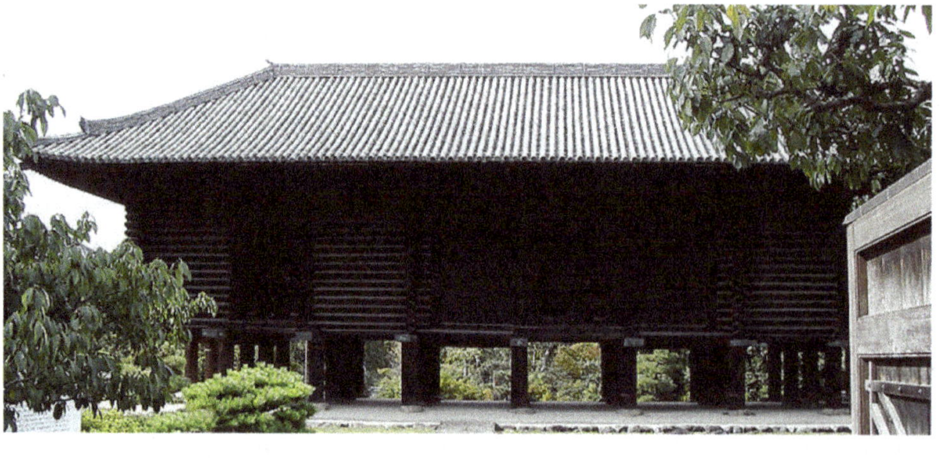

Figure 1. Shosoin treasure house that belongs to Todai-ji, Nara (Wikipedia).

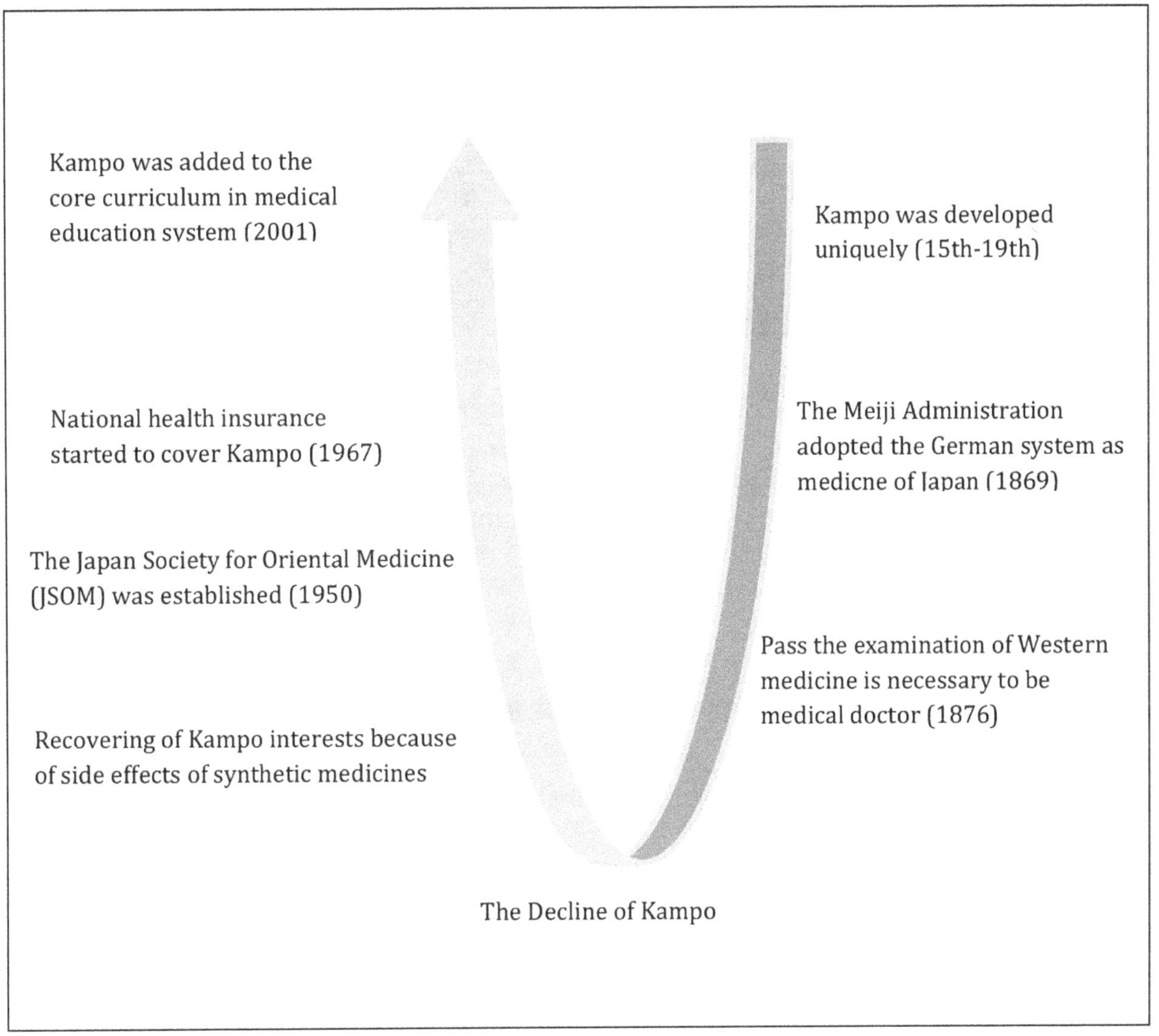

Figure 2. U-turn movement of Kampo in Japan.

According to "*Nihon Shoki*," the second oldest historical book in Japan, aloeswood (incense wood) drifted ashore on Awaji island of Japan in 595 A.D. Thus, incense in Japan started in the sixth century, with more brought from China, along with Buddhism. At first, the Japanese used incense wood in religious practices. *Ganjin*, the Chinese monk that arrived in Japan to propagate Buddhism, taught the people to make and use incense. Later, the Japanese started for transferring the elegant aroma to the robes and sutra books on Nara period. In the Heian period, aristocrats enjoyed mixing incense into their daily life with poems written about the incense, such as *The Tale of Genji* in the eleventh century [10].

In the late Muromachi period during the sixteenth century, samurai started to pursue a holistic approach, including the senses, human spirit, and nature. This new approach was the start of "*Ko-do*" (a way of incense or an elegant incense ceremony). In addition, *Ka-do* (*Ikebana*, Japanese flower arrangement) and *Sa-do* (Japanese tea ceremony). The incense, aloeswood, was made over time by the formation and ripeness of an aromatic resin. Usually, the incense

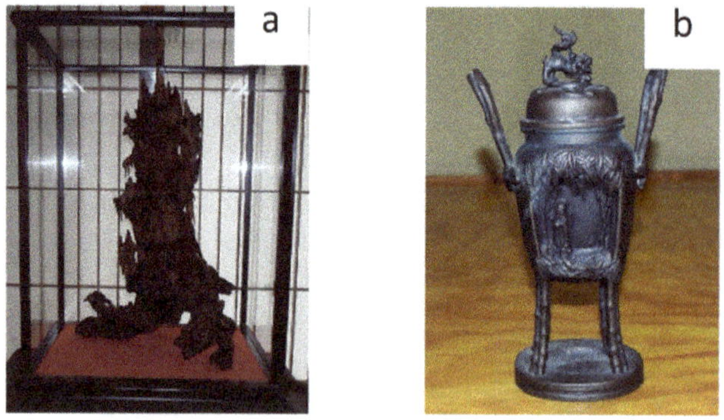

Figure 3. (a) Incense wood of Jinko; (b) Incense burner (Koro).

wood consists of three kinds, *Kyara, Jinko,* and *Byakudan* (**Figure 3a**). Raw materials such as aloes wood are costly because of the limited amount available and expensive equipment (**Figure 3b**). *Ko-do* has not spread widely due to the difficulty in obtaining raw materials as compared with the materials for *Ka-do* and *Sa-do*.

3. Conventional and modern uses: spirit and daily life

In the Edo era, Kampo was a medicine for wealthy people only as Kampo doctors visited a home by basket palanquin (a litter for one passenger) and treated patients using expensive Kampo materials. Therefore, the common people had to use Japanese folk medicines developed in earlier times. Such folk medicines exist today, but are not as popular as compared with modern western medicines and Kampo. Folk medicine, however, is an important cultural heritage that the Japanese ancestors left to future generations, including recipes of folk medicines, remedies for home use (**Table 3**). Some manufactured folk medicines are sold at pharmacy as quasi-drugs such as medicinal teas, cosmetics, medicinal bath, and supplements (**Figure 4a**).

The latest Japanese Pharmacopoeia (No. 17 issued 2016) included 324 crude medicines for Kampo [11]. Usually, Kampo medicines are a mix of several kinds of crude medicine, and each prescription has a name. Recently, many medical doctors prescribe Kampo medicines because of an increase in patients who prefer crude medicine rather than synthetic medicine. Patients can get Kampo medicines easily even without prescription (**Figure 4b**).

Aromatic and medicinal plants have spread broadly into Japanese spirit and daily life. The tea and aroma activities were simply an amusement for people until the Muromachi period that was started before the Japanese "sa-do" (tea ceremony) and "ko-do." At the end of the Muromachi period, Buddhist monks reformed the philosophy of tea to express conjointly with ethics and religion, changing the societal view about man and nature [12]. This innovative philosophy reflects the esthetics and world view of Japanese, for example, "wabi" and "sabi." Wabi expresses an esthetic of beauty of deficiency, in other words, senses which try to find sufficiency of mind from humble and deficiency. Sabi is beauty which could feel profoundness and richness inside of tranquility naturally. Subsequently, *Sen no rikyu* who is a

Japanese and common name	Scientific name	Medicinal effects	Uses	Part used
Hechima, Luffa	*Luffa cylindrica*	Heat rash, chapped skin, sunburn	Cosmetic	Water from fruit
Yomogi, Japanese mugwort	*Artemisia indica*	Dry skin, acne	Cosmetic	Leaf
Biwa, Loquat leaf	*Eriobotrya japonica*	Heat rash, eczema, insect bite, rash	Cosmetic	Leaf
Shiso, Perilla herb	*Perilla frutescens*	Eczema, acne, oily skin	Cosmetic	Leaf
Obako, Plantago seed	*Plantago asiatica*	Water metabolism, poor visibility, phlegm	Tea	Seed
Gobo, Burdock fruit	*Arctium lappa*	Heat diffusion, inflammation, promote eruption	Tea	Fruit
Dokudami, Houttuynia herb	*Houttuynia cordata*	Laxative, diuretic	Tea	Upper ground (flowering time)
Senna, Senna leaf	*Senna alexandrina*	Laxative	Tea	Leaf
Kuko, Lycium fruit	*Lycium chinense*	Weak constitution, fatigue, cold hands and feet, insomnia	Liquor	Fruit
Ninjin, Ginseng	*Panax ginseng*	Tonic	Liquor	Root
Toki, Japanese angelica root	*Angelica acutiloba*	Tonic, circulatory disorder, analgesic, sedative, compensate blood	Bath	Root
Senkyu, Cnidium Rhizome	*Cnidium officinale*	Anemia, cold hands and feet, menstrual irregularity	Bath	Rhizome
Kamitsure, German Chamomile	*Matricaria recutita*	Inflammation, sedative, calm spasm, excrete gas	Bath	Flower
Syobu, Calamus	*Acorus calamus*	Backache, neuralgia	Bath	Root, leaf
Yuzu, Yuzu	*Citrus junos*	Circulation improvement, cold prevention, backache, neuralgia	Bath	Fruit

Table 3. Plant materials, medicinal effects, and uses for folk medicines.

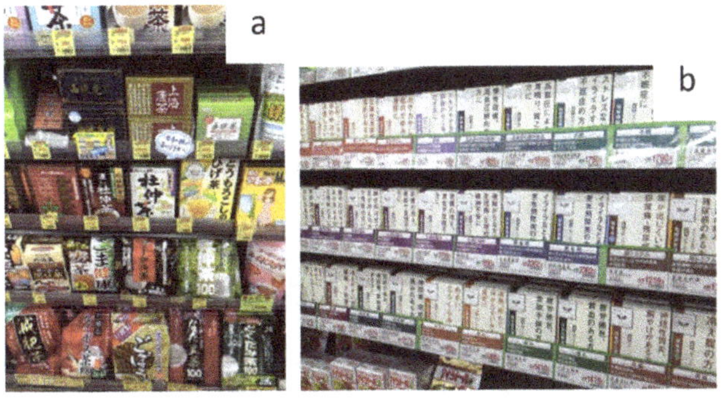

Figure 4. (a) Medicinal teas of folk medicine are sold at pharmacy; (b) Kampo medicines are sold at pharmacy.

famous tea master completed the foundation of present sa-do. The sense of wabi and sabi connects with Japanese spirit today, and sa-do is traditional practice for wholehearted hospitality for our daily life (**Figure 5**). A book "ALL ABOUT TEA" known as the encyclopedia of tea

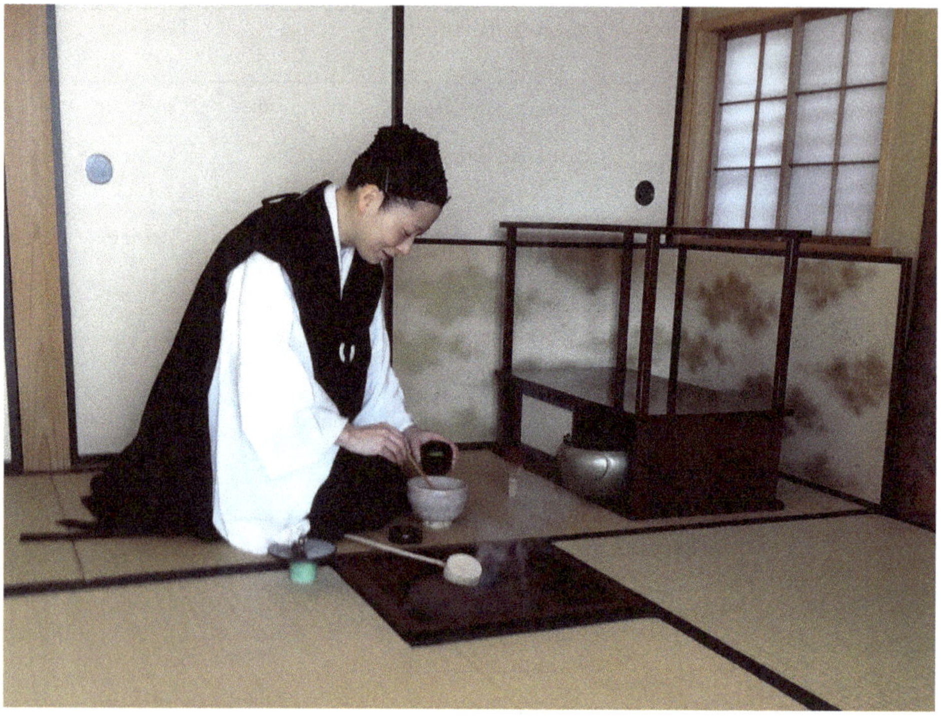

Figure 5. One of the sa-do practice called "otemae.".

describes the commercial side of tea including the production, cultivation technique, chemical constituent, distribution, trade, consumption, and cultural side related to the as history of drinking tea and the relationships among drinking tea, the literature, and art [13]. The book helps readers to comprehend sa-do as well.

In Japan, Buddhists worship ancestors with incense sticks as one of the traditional manners in appreciating all generations of family in daily life. The incense sticks are made from mixed lots of materials, including charcoals, incensed woods, crude medicines, and fragrances. Such incense sticks are used mostly in homes and temples (**Figure 6**).

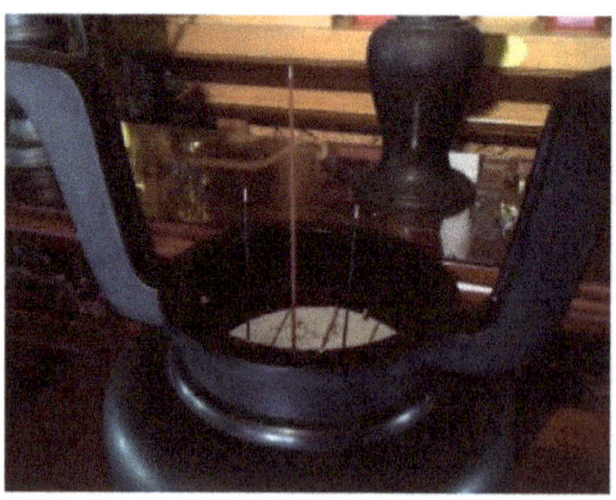

Figure 6. Incense sticks are offered to any Buddhist ceremony at temple.

4. Representative plant: Japanese green tea

Tea is the second consumed drink in the world after water. Tea is called by different names in different countries or areas. The origins, however, were split into two generally, "cha or chai" and "te or tea" depending the proximity to either China or Europe, respectively [14]. Almost all teas such as green, white, oolong, black, and pu'erh except maté and rooibos are made from *Camellia sinensis*, and the significant differences come from the processing of the leaves. Oxidation in leaves starts immediately after leaves are picked. Black tea is fully oxidized; oolong tea is half of oxidized; and green and white teas are barely oxidized at all.

As well-known, drinking tea was introduced from China by a Japanese Buddhist monk in seventh to eighth century. The manner became common among aristocrats and monks in ninth century at the time, and tea was hardened tea leaves like ball named "*dan cha*." In Song dynasty of China, the way of drinking tea was changed to use matcha and introduced to Japan. Buddhist monks drank matcha to avoid sleepiness and to concentrate their mentality for Zen practices. Chinese monk *Eisai* wrote "Kissa yojoki" was written about the medical effects of tea in 1211 [15]. In early fourteenth century, a game called "*To-cha*" was in fashion, people would first drink tea and then guess the area in which the tea was grown. In the late fifteenth century, *Jyuko Murata* (1423–1502) created "wabi-cha," based on the simplicity of Zen spirit and spirituality of "wabi." Subsequently, *Sen no rikyu* established sa-do. In 1830s, the finest quality green tea was "gyokuro," which tasted mellow, sweet, and full bodied, came into being in *Uji* area.

The most famous tea production area is Sizuoka prefecture, where tea is exposed to a strong wind and rain and cultivated on the hillside or riverside where other crops could not survive (**Figure 7**). The different quality of soil produces a different color and quality of tea leaf (**Figure 7**). In 2015, the total area of picked green tea was 35,600 ha, a one percent decline The yield of fresh leaf, 357,800 metric tons in 2015, declined by four percent from the previous year in Japan [16]. According to survey, more than 82% Japanese drink green tea every day [17]. In Japan, green tea is drunk in the morning after waking, after or during every meal, for break in the afternoon, to show hospitality whenever guests visit. Usually, Japanese enjoy many kinds of flavors and tastes, for example, "*sencha*," "*gyokuro*," "*matcha*," "*hojicha*," "*genmaicha*," and "bancha" have differences that come from the processing

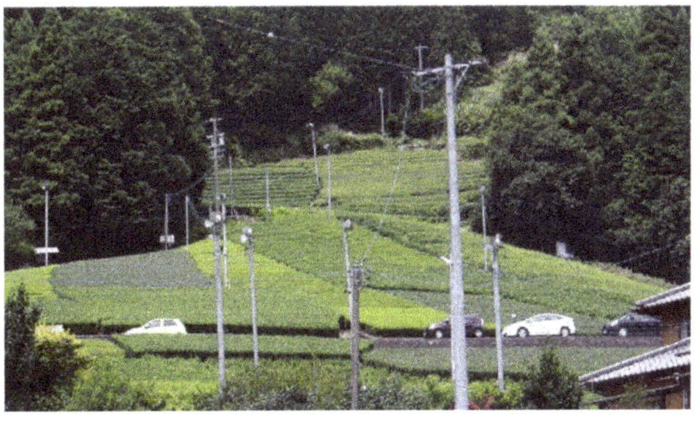

Figure 7. Green tea farms at Kawane honcho, Shizuoka.

methods of green tea (**Table 4**). The taste is a little bitterness and astringency, and it is perfectly refreshing your mouth after meals. Most distributed Japanese green tea is Sen-cha which accounts for 60% of all kinds of green tea [16].

green tea: Leaf / color	Name	Characteristic
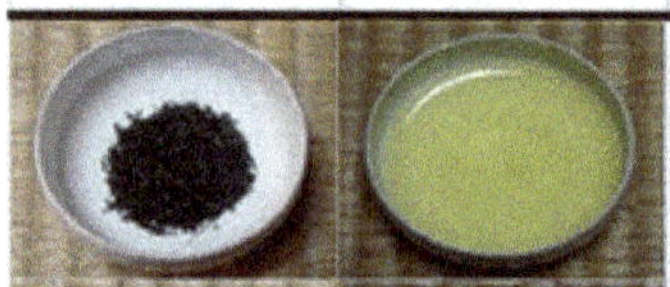	sen cha	young and soft leaves are hand-rolled, commonly drunk in Japan
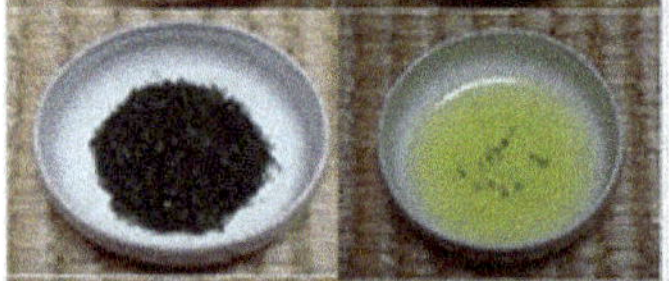	gyokuro	top quality of green tea, grown under tha shade for 20-30 days before harvested
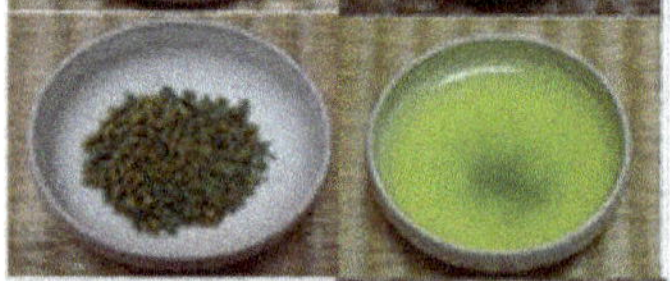	genmai cha	green tea with roasted brown rice, popularly as an alternative standard green tea
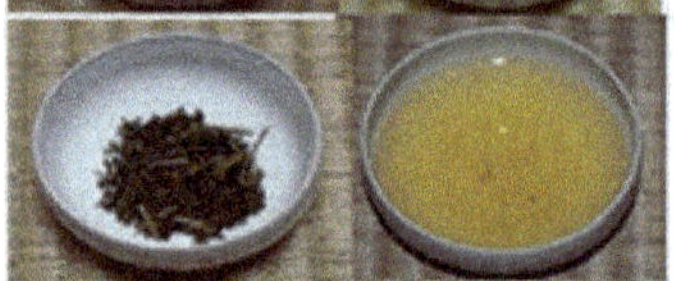	hoji cha	roasted green tea, good flavor of roased
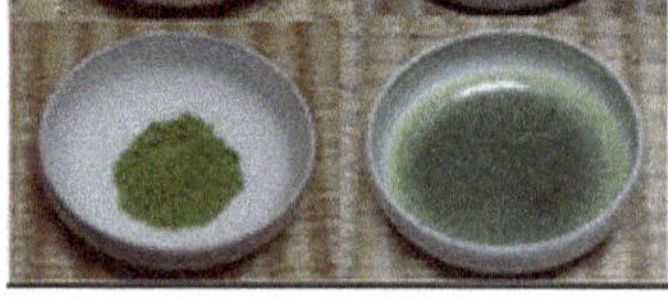	matcha	the finest tea buds of shade-grown grinded by mill stones, used in sa-do

Table 4. Different kinds of green tea.

Name of task	Action	Time (min)	Water contents (%)
Sassei (steam)	Fresh leaves are steamed at 100°C, and oxidation is stopped	0.5–1	100
Reikyaku (cool down)	Wait until room temperature and some water is removed from leaf surface	5	–
Sojyu (first hand-rolling)	Wield leaves and some mass of leaves come up by light hand-rolling at 35°C	60	40
Jyunen (second hand-rolling)	Push and make a mass bigger by knead hand-rolling and remove some water from inside of leaf at 100°C	20	–
Chujyu (third hand-rolling)	Loosen a mass up and twist leaf by hand-rolling at 95°C	30	30
Seijyu (forth hand-rolling)	Shape like needle and polish by hand-rolling at 85°C	60	10
Kansou (dry)	Dry at 65°C	120	5
Shiage (finishing)	Removed leaf powder and piece of stem with some heat for dry	–	4

Table 5. Processing sequences, action, and water contents for green tea manufacture.

Processing green tea is delicate and has several significant steps that require specialized skills. After the leaves are picked from the tree, a total of eight work sequences are necessary for ready to drink tea (**Table 5**).

Manufacturing Japanese green tea takes more than 5 h with much labor if all sequences are done by hand. Recently, most of the processing steps have become automated. Hand making tea, however, is still practiced by some processors as the hand-rolling technique is a cultural heritage (**Figure 8a–e**).

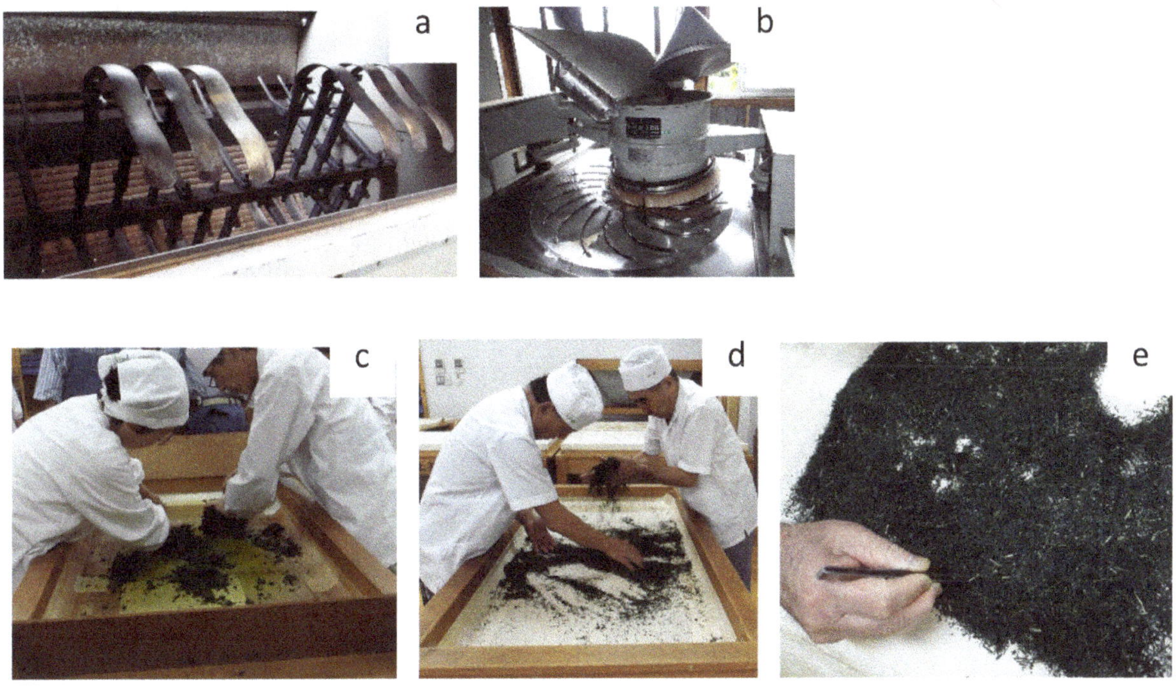

Figure 8. Processing machines, at Kawanehoncho, Shizuoka, (a) sojyu-ki, (b) jyunen-ki. Processing by hands, at Kawanehoncho, Shizuoka, (c) sojyu, (d) seijyu, and (e) shiage.

Recently, a number of scientific studies have suggested that green tea has medicinal effects, reducing high cholesterol and treating cancer, diabetes, and liver disease [18]. In the natural elements and nutrients in Japanese green teas, the most consumed *sencha* has the highest tannin (catechin), carbohydrate, and vitamin C, E, and B1 levels among *gyokuro, sencha, hojicha*, and *matcha* (**Table 6**) [19]. Catechins are one of the major polyphenolic compounds in green tea, which works on preventing various vascular diseases (**Figure 9**). Usually, catechin is very widespread, especially in woody plants and some medicinal plants, such as Agrimonia *eupatoria* (agrimony), *Crataegus laevigata* (hawthorn), *Salix alba* (white willow), and *Vaccinium myrtillus* (bilberry) contain catechin [20]. Significant effects of the catechins are antioxidative, antihypertensive, anti-inflammatory, antiproliferative, antithrombogenic, and lipid lowering actions that are important for maintaining vascular health [21]. The major catechin, epigallocatechin-3-gallate (EGCG), has been suggested to have great potential as a cancer preventative agent for liver, stomach, skin, lung, mammary gland, and colon cancer [22]. EGCG functions not only as a powerful antioxidant and preventing oxidative damage in healthy cells, but also an antiangiogenic and antitumor agent. EGCG stimulates telomere fragmentation by inhibiting telomerase activity. Some scientific articles suggest that green

	Gyokuro	Sencha	Houjicha	Matcha
Tannin (Catechin)	10.0	13.0	9.5	10.0
Caffeine	3.5	2.3	1.5	3.2
Theanine/Amino Acid	29.1	24.5	18.2	30.6
Fat	4.1	4.7	4.8	5.3
Carbohydrate	43.9	47.7	39.2	38.5
Fiber	11.1	10.6	18.7	10.0
Ash content	6.3	5.0	5.5	7.4
Vitamin A (μg)	21,000	13,000	6,700	29,000
C (mg)	110	260	44	60
E (mg)	16.6	68.1	-	28.1
B1 (mg)	0.30	0.36	0.10	0.60
B2 (mg)	1.16	1.43	0.82	1.35
Niacin (mg)	6.0	4.1	5.6	4.0

Table 6. Natural elements and nutrients in Japanese green tea [19].

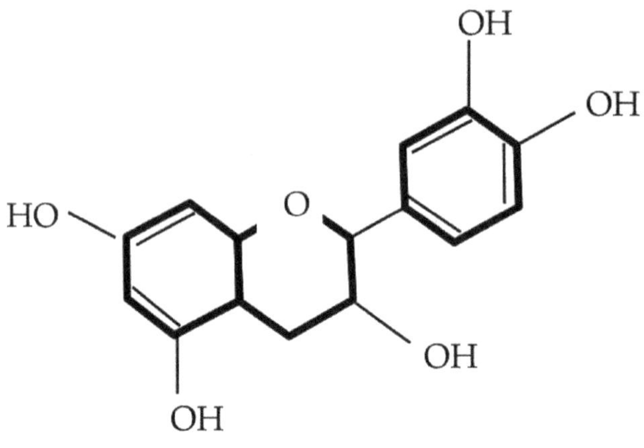

Figure 9. Catechin.

tea catechin may help in controlling type II diabetes by daily consumption [23–25]. EGCG blocks sodium-dependent glucose transporter 1 (SGLY1) and lipid micelle formation in the intestine.

Most convenience stores and supermarkets in Japan sell many kinds of bottled green tea. Some brands put a mark "food for specified health uses" indicating healthy effects, such as cholesterol reduction or gentle rising of blood sugar after meals, and have received approval for special marking from the Consumer Affairs Agency (**Figure 10**) [26]. These types of foods are used for sustaining health and preventing pre-symptomatic disease.

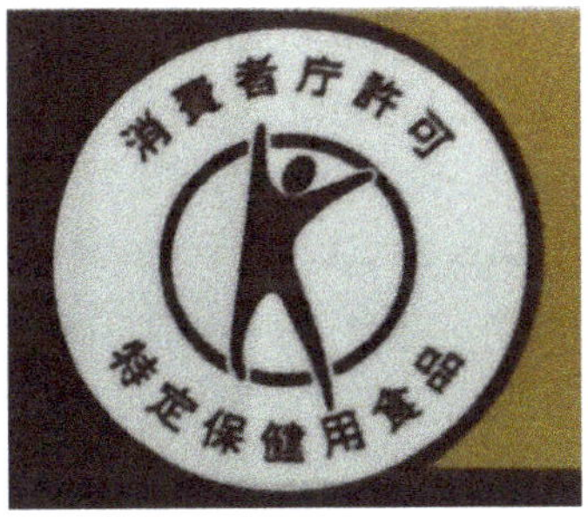

Figure 10. Food mark specifies green tea health uses.

5. Application

5.1. Integrative medicine

Integrative medicine is a person-centered care system that uses both modern western medicine, to take advantage of pharmaceuticals, operations, radiology, and other complementary and alternative medicines have become popular among advanced countries to change the structure of disease control. Many complementary and alternative medicine systems exist. Phytotherapy has been actively adapted into integrative medicine in United States because herbs and the origin of several pharmaceuticals and the accumulated scientific evidence are comprehended easily. For example, Dr. Andrew Weil of University of Arizona, a leading figure of integrative medicine, is an herbalist and prescribes medicinal plants for treatment [27].

Aromatherapy was introduced to Japan from the UK in 1985, and became popular as a relaxation technique. Subsequently, aromatherapy has become better known by medical professionals and researchers. This activity advanced clinical application in psychosomatic medicine, obstetrics and gynecology, and palliative care coupled with the spread of integrative medicine. In 2008, the Japanese Society of Integrative Medicine was established, a project team of integrative medicine in Ministry of Health, Labor, and Welfare was launched in 2010, and the Japanese Society of Phytotherapy was established in 2012 for study of medicinal herbs.

Although still controversial, functional mechanisms of complementary and alternative medicines are thought to have the improved the spontaneous healing power of humans. Currently, this understanding is compatible with oriental thought in a regimen and a balanced diet lead to a healthy body. Accumulation of scientific evidence, culture, and history exists behind the rapid spread of aromatherapy and medicinal herbs in Japan. The next generation of integrative medicine that creates inclusive correlation between body, mind, spirituality, natural environment, and local community can be expected to help those suffering from aging and improve the health of a maturing society.

5.2. Dietary supplements

In recent years, diffusion of dietary supplements is remarkably increasing worldwide, and the trend to use natural substances in healthcare and wellness will continue to rapidly expand dietary supplement markets. In one of the highest dietary supplement consuming countries, 53% of the adults in the United States used at least one dietary supplement each day in 2003–2006 [28]. This number was more than two times that of Japan [29], and comes from different systems of health insurance. To enter health insurance is not necessary for USA citizens have a relatively expensive medical care system, making individuals concerned about their health and wellness. In contrast, Japan citizens are basically mandated to enter a health insurance. According to various reports, some consumers in Japan have the wrong knowledge about dietary supplements. For example, an inappropriate meal is no problem if you take dietary supplements [30]. Nevertheless, the Japanese market of dietary supplement keeps growing rapidly, and the prospect of dietary supplement in Japan will continue to shift more to prevent disease and maintain health and wellness.

6. Conclusions

Medicinal and aromatic plants help people remain healthy and have influenced culture, nature, and history of humans from ancient times. Further study of medicinal and aromatic plants may discover new constituents that become future medicines. In future research, more clinical trial and interaction between medicinal plants and pharmaceuticals need to be examined and useful information shared throughout the world. The important thing is to appreciate the blessings of nature and sustain all of genetic resources. Today, the society of severe aging and maturity needs to shift from animalistic world view, such as the stronger prey upon the weaker in a high-growth period, to a cooperative vegetative world view with the key factor being medicinal and aromatic plants.

Author details

Maiko Inoue[1,*], Shinichiro Hayashi[2] and Lyle E. Craker[3]

*Address all correspondence to: den8mai@yhoo.co.jp

1 Specified Nonprofit Corporation of Horticulture Therapy and Zen, Hamamatsu, Japan

2 GREEN FLASK Inc., Tokyo, Japan

3 University of Massachusetts, Amherst, MA, USA

References

[1] Mamedov NA, Craker LE. Man and medicinal plants: a short review. Acta Hortic (ISHS). 2012;964:181–190.

[2] Farnsworth NR, Soejarto DD. Global importance of medicinal plants. In: Akereb O, Heywood V, Synge H editors. Conservation of Medicinal Plants. Cambridge University Press: Cambridge; 1991. p. 362. ISBN 0521392063, 9780521392068

[3] Ministry of Agriculture, Forestry, Fisheries. Medicinal crops program of Ministry of Agriculture, Forestry, Fisheries (in Japanese). [Internet]. 2013. Available from: http://www.maff.go.jp/j/keikaku/pdf/yakuyou_sesaku1.pdf [Accessed: 2016-08-10].

[4] Motoo Y, Seki T, Tsutani K. Traditional Japanese Medicine, Kampo: Its history and current status. The Chinese Journal of Integrated Traditional and Western Medicine. 2011;17(2):85–87.

[5] Japan Kampo Medicines Manufacturers Association. Report of usage of crude materials (in Japanese). [internet]. 2011. Available from http://www.nikkankyo.org/topix/news/111001/shiyouryou-chousa.pdf [Accessed: 2016-08-11].

[6] Sashida Y. Pharmacognocy. (in Japanese) Nankodo: Tokyo; 2002. p 394. ISBN978-4-524-40224-3

[7] Hatano T. Herbal drugs in traditional Japanese medicine. In: Sakagami H, editors. Alternative Medicine. InTech: Rijeka; 2012. p 306. doi:10.5772/53126

[8] Watanabe K, Matsuura K, Gao P, Hottenbacher L, Tokunaga H, Nishimura K, Imazu Y, Reissenweber H, Witt CM. Traditional Japanese Kampo medicine: Clinical research between modernity and traditional medicine – The state of research and methodological suggestions for the future. Evidence-Based Complementary and Alternative Medicine, Volume 2011. Hindawi Publishing Corporation: Cairo; 2011. ID 513842 doi:10.1093/ecam/neq067

[9] Irie Y. Kampo Medicine for Beginners (in Japanese). Sogensha: Osaka; 2008. p. 269. ISBN978-4-422-41078-4

[10] Pybus D. Kodo: The Way of Incense. Tuttle Publishing: North Clarendon; 2001. 96 p. ISBN13: 9780804832861

[11] The Japanese Pharmacopeia, 17th edition. Ministry of Health, Labour and Welfare [Internet]. 2016. Available from: http://jpdb.nihs.go.jp/jp17e/ [Accessed: 2016-08-25].

[12] Okakura K. The Book of Tea. Duffield & Company: New York; 1906. p. 160.

[13] Ukers WH. All About Tea. The Tea and Coffee Trade Journal Company. New York; 1935. p. 559.

[14] Yamada S, Tsunoyama S. Cha 108 Chapters-Culture Health Amenity (in Japanese). Fukujyuen: Kizugawa; 1990. p. 223.

[15] History of green tea. HIBIKI-AN [Internet]. 2004–2016. Available from: http://www.hibiki-an.com/contents.php/cnID/17 [Accessed: 2016-09-15].

[16] The area of green tea picked and the yield of fresh and *aracha* in 2015 (in Japanese). Statistics of Agriculture, Forestry and Fisheries [Internet]. 2015. Available from: http://www.maff.go.jp/j/tokei/kouhyou/sakumotu/sakkyou_kome/pdf/syukaku_1tya_15.pdf [Accessed: 2016-08-27].

[17] The actual consumed condition of green tea. (in Japanese) Ministry of Agriculture, Forestry, Fisheries [Internet]. 2005. Available from: http://www.maff.go.jp/j/heya/h_moniter/pdf/h1702.pdf [Accessed: 2016-09-15].

[18] Ehrlich S. Green tea. University of Maryland Medical Center [Internet]. 2015. Available from: http://umm.edu/health/medical/altmed/herb/green-tea [Accessed: 2016-08-25].

[19] Green tea for health. HIBIKI-AN [Internet]. 2004-2016. Available from: http://www.hibiki-an.com/contents.php/cnID/10 [Accessed: 2016-09-15].

[20] Hoffmann D, Ahgv F. Medical Herbalism: The Science and Practice of Herbal Medicine. Healing Arts Press: Rochester; 2003. p. 666. ISBN-978-089281749-8

[21] Velayutham P, Babu A, Liu D. Green tea catechins and cardiovascular health: An update. Current Medicinal Chemistry. 2008;15(18):1840–1850.

[22] Singh BN, Shankar S, Srivastava RK. Green tea catechin, epigallocatechin-3-gallate (EGCG): mechanisms, perspectives and clinical applications. Biochemical Pharmacology. 2011;15;82(12):1807–1821.

[23] Park JH, Bae JH, Im SS, Song DK. Green tea and type 2 diabetes. Integrative Medicine Research. 2014;3:4–10

[24] Fukino Y, Shimbo M, Aoki N, Okubo T, Iso H. Randomized controlled trial for an effect of green tea consumption on insulin resistance and inflammation markers. Journal of Nutritional Science and Vitaminology (Tokyo). 2005;51:335–42.

[25] Iso H, Date C, Wakai K, Fukui M, Tamakoshi A, JACC Study Group. The relationship between green tea and total caffeine intake and risk for self-reported type 2 diabetes among Japanese adults. Annals of Internal Medicine. 2006;144:554–62.

[26] Tanaka H, Kaneda F, Suguro R, Baba H. Current system for regulation of health foods in Japan. LMAJ. 2004;47(9):436–450.

[27] Weil A. Dr. Andrew Weil's Integrative Medicine Clinic. Healing Cancer [Internet]. Available from: http://www.healingcancer.info/ebook/andrew-weil [Accessed: 2016–09-13].

[28] Gahche J, Bailey R, Burt V, Hughes J, Yetley E, Dwyer J, Picciano MF, McDowell M, Sempos C. Dietary supplements use among U.S. adults has increased since NHANES III (1988-1994). NCHS Data Brief. 2011;Apr(61):1–8

[29] Situation of dietary supplements in Japan. (in Japanese) Holistic Health Academy [Internet]. 2013. Available from: http://h-h-a.com/archives/417/ [Accessed: 2016-09-04].

[30] Kaimoto T, Shibuya M, Maeda H. Study on dietary supplement use of university students: Comparative study between educational students and nutritional sciences students. (in Japanese) Bull. Shikoku Univ. 2012;35(B):23–27

14

Chemical Composition and Biological Activities of *Mentha* Species

Fatiha Brahmi, Madani Khodir,
Chibane Mohamed and Duez Pierre

Abstract

The genus *Mentha* L. (Lamiaceae) is distributed all over the world and can be found in many environments. *Mentha* species, one of the world's oldest and most popular herbs, are widely used in cooking, in cosmetics, and as alternative or complementary therapy, mainly for the treatment of gastrointestinal disorders like flatulence, indigestion, nausea, vomiting, anorexia, and ulcerative colitis. Furthermore, it is well documented that the essential oil and extracts of *Mentha* species possess antimicrobial, fungicidal, antiviral, insecticidal, and antioxidant properties. The economic importance of mints is also evident; mint oil and its constituents and derivatives are used as flavoring agents throughout the world in food, pharmaceutical, herbal, perfumery, and flavoring industry. To provide a scientific basis for their traditional uses, several studies have been conducted to determine the chemical composition of mints and assess their biological activities. This chapter describes the therapeutic effects and uses of *Mentha* species and their constituents, particularly essential oils and phenolic compounds; some additional biological activities will also be considered.

Keywords: *Mentha* sp., therapeutic effects, uses, composition, biological activities

1. Introduction

Mentha is a member of the Lamiaceae which was originally described and named by Jussieu (1789) who gave the family name Lamiaceae, due to the distinctive flowers with a prominent liplike lower petal. This family has almost cosmopolitan distribution, from temperate to tropical regions, but is primarily found in the Mediterranean Basin. Members of this family may be annual or perennial herbs, shrubs, and small trees. The Lamiaceae are closely allied to the Verbenaceae, and, in a recent family revision, several genera have been transferred to Lamiaceae [1]. As a result, the circumscription of the Lamiaceae has been changed to include eight subfamilies: Ajugoideae, Chloranthaceae, Lamioideae, Nepetoideae, Pogostemonoideae, Scutellarioideae, Teucrioideae, and Viticoideae. Nevertheless, over 47% of the Lamiaceae fall within the subfamily Nepetoideae [2].

This family includes about 260 genera and more than 7000 species. Their characteristic features include the stems which are quadrangular (square) in cross-section and the bisexual, zygomorphic bilaterally symmetrical flowers, composed of five united and deeply lobed petals and five united sepals; typically, the lower petal is larger than the others. The fruit is dry and woody, a schizocarp or drup. The distinctive strongly aromatic leaves are opposite with successive pairs at right angles (i.e., decussate) with margins entire or lobed. Many species of this family, such as mints, have important commercial uses for the culinary, pharmaceutical, herbal, and ornamental industries [1].

Throughout history, a number of mint species have been used around the globe for various properties. Peppermint oil is one of the world's oldest herbal medicines. The gathering of dried peppermint dates back to at least 1000 BC, and its use is documented in the ancient Egypt, Greece, and Rome; in traditional Chinese medicine, the use of a local mint species, *Mentha haplocalyx* Briq. called "bo he," has long been documented [3]. Peppermint (*Mentha piperita* L.) was not officially described until 1696, when the English botanist John Ray (1628–1705) first discovered this pepper-flavored mint. Entering the London Pharmacopoeia in 1721, peppermint has since been cultivated for its essential oil throughout Asia, Europe, and North America [4]. Mint history is colored by stories from ancient mythology. Proserpine, Pluto's wife, was said to have transformed a hated rival into a mint plant. Both the Latin "mentha" and the Greek "minthe" have come to be associated with metamorphosed beauty [5].

The taxonomy of the genus *Mentha* has been in a state of flux, with more than 3000 names published since 1753, most of them being synonyms or unresolved names [2], often referring to cultivars. The genus *Mentha* L. is widely distributed on all continents (except in South America and Antarctica). The centers of variety of this genus that groups spontaneous and cultivated forms are Europe, Australia, Central Asia, and North Africa [6].

Most *Mentha* grows best in wet environments and moist soils. Mints will grow 10–120 cm tall and can spread over an indeterminate-sized area. Due to the tendency to spread unchecked, mints are considered invasive. All mints prefer, and thrive in, cool, moist spots in partial shade. But, in general, mints tolerate a wide range of conditions and can also be grown in full sun. They are fast growing, extending their reach along surfaces through a network of runners [7]. According to the latest taxonomic treatment, the genus *Mentha* comprises 61 species [8] and about 100 varieties and cultivars, divided into five sections: *Audibertia, Eriodontes, Mentha, Preslia,* and *Pulegium*. The systematic of the genus is not fully elucidated because of the strong morphologic variations, levels of ploidy ($2n = 2x = 24$ to $2n = 6x = 96$) and hybridizations that can be intra- and interspecific and between spontaneous and cultivated forms [6].

Within the section *Mentha*, it has been suggested that the five basic species, *Mentha arvensis* L., *Mentha aquatica* L., *Mentha spicata* L., *Mentha longifolia* (L.) Huds, and *Mentha suaveolens* Ehrh. (**Figure 1**), have given rise to 11 naturally occurring and named hybrids. However, *M. spicata* and possibly *M. longifolia* are also of hybrid origin and incongruence of nuclear and plastid DNA-based phylogenies indicates that all species of this section may have experienced some extension of reticulate gene flow during their evolution [9].

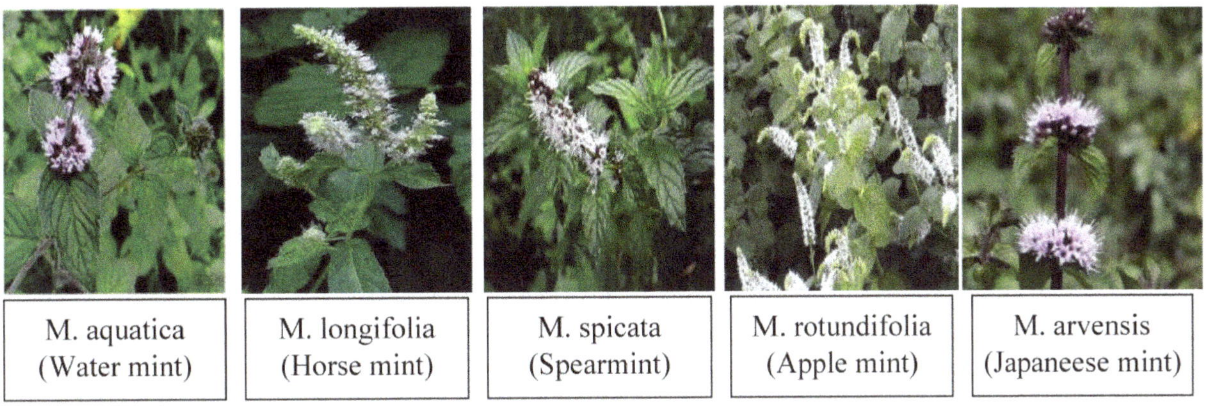
M. aquatica
(Water mint)
M. longifolia
(Horse mint)
M. spicata
(Spearmint)
M. rotundifolia
(Apple mint)
M. arvensis
(Japaneese mint)

Figure 1. The five basic species comprising the genus *Mentha* [10].

Šarić-Kundalić et al. [9] suggest a differentiation of the section *Mentha* into three basic lines, capitatae, spicatae, and verticillatae, based on inflorescence characters. The line "capitatae" includes all species with compact, headlike inflorescence; the type of species is *M. aquatica*. The "spicatae" species have a spike as shown by *M. spicata*, *M. longifolia*, and *M. suaveolens*. The third line is represented by *M. arvensis* having an inflorescence vertically partitioned into whorls.

2. Therapeutic effects and uses

Besides its culinary uses, mint is also used in traditional systems of medicine. Mints are mainly used to cure gastrointestinal disorders, but the spectrum of medical activities is broader [9]. Mint was originally used as a medicinal herb to treat stomachache and chest pains, and it is commonly used in the form of tea as a home remedy to stimulate digestion; alleviate stomach pain; and treat biliary disorders, dyspepsia, enteritis, flatulence, gastritis, gastric acidities, aerophagia, intestinal colic, and spasms of the bile duct, gallbladder, and gastrointestinal tract [7, 10, 11]. Mint also aids digestion, notably of fats; in recent years, it has been often recommended for treating obesity. Mint tea is also a strong diuretic [7].

The essential oil from *Mentha* spp. is used topically to treat oral mucosal inflammation and also an antimicrobial and an ingredient in many analgesic creams. Approved for internal use, the oil from *Mentha* spp. is also used to treat bile duct discomfort, irritable bowel syndrome, myalgia and neuralgia, inflammation of the oral mucosa, discomfort from menstrual cramps, secondary amenorrhea and oligomenorrhea, and diverticulitis and is used as an anti-inflammatory and expectorant [4, 12].

Other therapeutic effects attributed to a series of *Mentha* species are summarized in **Table 1**.

Species	Region	Indications	Reference
M. spicata	Brazil	For the expulsion of parasitic worms, mainly *Ascaris lumbricoides*	[13]
	Morocco	Leaf and stem infusion for headache and tiredness	[14]
	India	Stimulant, carminative, antispasmodic, fever, remedy in infantile troubles; the boiled leaves extract is used to relieve hiccup, flatulence, giddiness and as remedy for inflammation, bronchitis, to control vomiting during pregnancy	[15]
	Turkey	Three or four cups daily between meals can relieve gastrointestinal complaints. This herb is considered stimulant, carminative, antispasmodic, and antidote for poisons. It has been reported as a remedy for inflammation, fevers, bronchitis, infantile troubles, vomiting in pregnancy, and hysteria	[16]
	India	The boiled leave extract was counseled in the viral hepatitis, as analgesic known for its ability to enhance memory. Leaves are given for fever and bronchitis and are used as lotion in aphthae, as stomachic and diuretic, for gas pain, rheumatism, toothache, muscle pain, and mouthwash	[11]
	France	Acquires a very powerful action on the nervous system	[17]
	India	The plant is typically used in the treatment of loss of appetite, common cold, bronchitis, sinusitis, fever, nausea, and vomiting	[10]
M. pulegium	Brazil	For expulsion of parasitic worms; mainly *Ascaris lumbricoides*, *Entamoeba histolytica*, and *Giardia lamblia*; renal calculus; fever; bad cold; cough; bronchitis; bellyache; and bad cold	[13]
	Algeria	Stomachic, carminative, antiemetic, antispasmodic, tonic, antitussive, and insecticidal	[18]
	Iran	Antiseptic for treatment of cold, sinusitis, cholera, food poisoning, bronchitis, and tuberculosis	[19]

Species	Region	Indications	Reference
M. rotundifolia	Iran	In the treatment of flatulent dyspepsia and intestinal colic	[7]
	Spain	Hypotensive	[20]
	Morocco	Leaf and stem decoction was used in cold and for system digestive	[14]
	France	Tonic, stimulative, stomachic, carminative, analgesic, choleretic, antispasmodic, anti-inflammatory, sedative, hypotensive, and insecticidal	[21]
M. longifolia	Iran	Different parts of the plant (leaves, flower, stem, bark, and seeds) have been used as antimicrobial, carminative, stimulant, antispasmodic, antirheumatic, anticatarrhal, wound healing, deworming, insect repellent, antiemetic, sedative, diuretic, aphrodisiac, blood purifier and for the treatment of headaches, digestive disorders, tonsillitis, diarrhea, dysentery, abdominal disorders, constipation, gall stone, jaundice, toothache, flatulence, asthma, cough, dyspnea, common cold, fever, headache, general weakness, and bladder and kidney stones	[22]
M. piperita	India	Peppermint oil (as well as peppermint leaf) has been used internally as an antispasmodic (upper gastrointestinal tract and bile ducts) and to treat irritable bowel syndrome, catarrh of the respiratory tract, and inflammation of the oral mucosa. Externally, peppermint oil has been used for myalgia and neuralgia To relieve menstrual cramps and used externally for neuralgia, myalgia, headaches, migraines, and chicken pox	[23]
	India	Peppermint plants have been used for many conditions, including loss of appetite, common cold, bronchitis, sinusitis, fever, nausea, vomiting, and indigestion	[10]
	Finland	Peppermint uses include irritable bowel syndrome, flatulence, indigestion, nausea, vomiting, cough, and bronchitis	[24]
	USA	The odors of peppermint serve as central nervous system stimulant and are used to decrease fatigue	[25]

Species	Region	Indications	Reference
M. arvensis	India	Possess abortifacient property	[10]
M. australis	Australia	Decoctions were used to treat colds and coughs while inhaling the crushed mint to relieve headaches; the plant is also used as an abortifacient	[26]
M. haplocalyx	China	Various parts of the plant are used to treat sores and rashes on the skin, headache, red eyes, common cold, superficial visual obstructions, sore throat, mouth ulcers, and distension and oppression in the chest and the hypochondrium	[27, 28]

Table 1. Traditional indications of some *Mentha* species.

Mint is also used for buccodental prevention. During the middle ages, powdered mint leaves were used to whiten teeth [7]. Fresh mint leaves are used in chewing, for mouth burns; in decoction, it is used as mouthwashes to reduce gingival pain [29]. Mint is used in making oral dentifrices as it can provide overall freshness in breath. More studies are being done as to whether or not it directly contributes to preventing caries and plaque; however, it is confirmed that it does create an unfavorable environment for bacteria [23]. Moreover, peppermint applied to the gums of teething babies can help relieve distress and clean teeth [4].

Mint oil and its constituents and derivatives are also used as flavoring agents throughout the world in food, pharmaceutical, perfumery, and flavoring industry [23]. Essential oils isolated from *Mentha* plants have a long history of use as improving the flavor of foods like confectionaries (such as candies and chewing gums) and beverages. Mint flavor, which includes spearmint, peppermint, and corn mint, is probably the third most important flavor used after vanilla and citrus. As a result, *Mentha* plants are among the most important commercial herbs cultivated for dry leaf production in Germany, Spain, Poland, Bulgaria, Egypt, Morocco, Greece, Israel, United Kingdom, Turkey, Nigeria, and China [12, 30].

3. Adverse and toxic effects

Although some healthcare professionals believe that herbal medicines, such as the essential oil from *Mentha* spp., are relatively safe as they are "natural," recent publications have highlighted potentially severe side effects [4]. Contact allergy to the leaves of *Mentha spicata* has been reported, and cases of contact cheilitis from its essential oil, as toothpaste flavoring, have been described. The main allergens appear to be carvone and limonene. Spearmint and peppermint tea can cause iron deficiency anemia [16]. Besides, the essential oil from peppermint is associated with adverse effects such as heartburn, nausea, vomiting, allergic reactions, flushing, and headaches [4]. Potentially toxic compounds in peppermint are pulegone and menthol. Pulegone and its metabolite menthofuran, the probable hepatotoxic compounds in pennyroyal mint (*Mentha pulegium* L.), are also found in peppermint in much smaller proportions [23].

On the basis of recent rodent chronic studies [31], target organs for pulegone and menthofuran are the liver and kidney, and a plausible mechanism for toxicity is the formation of reactive metabolites, which is also supported by in vitro experimental data. According to the Committee of Experts on Flavoring Substances (CEFS), provisional consumption limits were established for pulegone at 20 mg/kg in food and beverages [32].

Menthol causes hepatocellular changes in rats. Inhalation of menthol can cause apnea and laryngeal constriction, a risk for infants. Contact sensitivity to menthol and peppermint with oral symptoms including burning mouth syndrome, recurrent oral ulceration, or a lichenoid reaction has been reported. The excessive inhalation of mentholated preparation has caused reversible nausea, anorexia, cardiac problems, ataxia, and other central nervous system (CNS) problems. Peppermint oil is contraindicated in obstruction of the bile ducts, gallbladder inflammation, and severe liver failure [23].

Dose-dependent hepatotoxicity and nephrotoxicity were reported for *M. piperita* and *M. spicata* in rats as well as decreased plasma testosterone and increased plasma LH and FSH levels affecting spermatogenetic activity; extensive degenerative changes in germinal epithelium and spermatogenesis arrest were observed in testicular biopsies. The exact *Mentha* compounds that cause these effects are not known [33].

In Wistar rats, depending on dosage, the *M. longifolia* leaves' essential oil increased the population of neutrophils, monocytes, and large unstained cells; the liver-body weight ratio; and the serum cholesterol, HDL cholesterol, triglyceride, inorganic phosphate, total and conjugated bilirubin, alkaline phosphatase activity, total proteins, and albumin; it reduced the serum urea and atherogenic index. The oil, at 500 μL/kg of body weight, also increased the kidney-body weight ratio [22].

Due to the major decrease of the potentially harmful pulegone and menthone by oven-drying, it is recommended that this herb should be oven-dried or cooked before consumption in order to reduce toxicity. Eating of the raw plant should be discouraged, particularly in patients with a history of liver disease or those taking cytochrome P450-inducing drugs [22].

4. Composition of *Mentha* species

The majority of studies on mint constituents focus on essential oils. Indeed, these compounds are widely used in different industries. Moreover, major polyphenols have also been investigated for interesting biological properties.

4.1. Essential oils

Essential oils are natural and volatile secondary metabolites characterized by a strong odor and a complex composition. They are usually obtained by steam or hydro-distillation from various aromatic plants, generally localized in temperate to warm countries like Mediterranean and tropical countries where they represent an important part of the traditional pharmacopoeia [34].

Several species of *Mentha* are cultivated for the production of essential oil. Indeed, mint oils are among the most important essential oils produced in the world, and their values are exceeding 400 million of US dollar/year. For instance, *M. canadensis* L. produces corn mint oil which represents the most important source of (–) menthol; *M. piperita* L. produces peppermint oil, constituted of menthol, menthone, and menthyl acetate as main components; *M. spicata* ssp., *M. viridis* (native spearmint), and *M. gracilis* (scotch spearmint) produce mostly carvone-rich oils, although different compositions have been reported; *M. citrata* is a source of linalool and linalyl acetate; *M. pulegium* produces the so-called pennyroyal oil, which is a pulegone-rich oil; the composition of *M. aquatica* oils is dominated by menthofuran [21]; *M. haplocalyx* could be classified into six chemotypes, including linalool, pulegone, menthone, carvone, menthol, and piperitenone oxide [35].

Peppermint leaves typically contain 1.2–3.9% (v/w) of essential oil, with more than 300 identified compounds. The terpenic class is the most represented, comprising about 52% of monoterpenes and 9% of sesquiterpenes, whereas other groups, such as aldehydes (9%), aromatic hydrocarbons (9%), miscellaneous (8%), lactones (7%), and alcohols (6%), have been shown to be present in a smaller proportion. Among monoterpenes, menthol is the major constituent (35–60%), followed by menthone (2–44%), menthyl acetate (0.7–23%), 1,8-cineole (eucalyptol) (1–13%), menthofuran (0.3–14%), isomenthone (2–5%), neomenthol (3–4%), and limonene (0.1–6%), whereas β-caryophyllene is the main sesquiterpene (1.6–1.8%) [36]. Most of peppermint oil medicinal properties are ascribed to menthol, their major active component, while esters, such as menthyl acetate, provide the familiar minty taste and associated aroma [4].

Table 2 presents published compositions of some widespread mint essential oils with a more limited commercial interest, including *M. pulegium*, the source of the essential oil "pennyroyal" rich in pulegone; *M. spicata*, dominated by carvone; and *M. rotundifolia* and *longifolia* of varied composition.

Species	Component	Origin (% in the oil)	Reference
M. spicata	Carvone	Tunisia (50), China (47–65), Greece (59), Japan(62), Israel(58), India (73), Portugal (76),South Africa (55), India (50–77), Serbia (50), Pakistan (60–63), Turkey (50), Algeria (59), Morocco (29), India (49), Algeria (49)	[6, 35, 37–51]
	Pulegone	Brazil (55)	[52]
	Piperitenone oxide	Greece (36)	[53]
	Piperitone	Turkey (22–28)	[54]
M. pulegium	Pulegone	Portugal (35), Algeria (39), Japan (51), Switzerland (20–35),Greece (45–50), Portugal (78–81), Uruguay (73), Morocco (80),Iran (38), Greece (33–76), India (66–83), Bulgaria (27–50), Egypt (44), Algeria (4–87), Spain (41–42), Tunisia (61),Iran (41), Morocco (70), Algeria, Bejaia (70); Algeria, Bouira (71)	[41, 47, 55–72]

Species	Component	Origin (% in the oil)	Reference
	Menthone	Portugal (36)	[73]
	Piperitone	Austria (70), Iran (38)	[19, 74]
	Piperitenone	Greece (84–97)	[75]
	Menthol	Tunisia (41–52), Greece (61–78)	[76, 77]
M. rotundifolia	Carvone	Argentina (43), Finland (62),	[78, 79]
	Trans-piperitone oxide	Italy (41), Japan (18–26)	[80, 81]
	Cis-piperitone oxide	Algeria (28–31)	[82]
	Piperitol	Spain (58)	[83]
	Piperitenone oxide	Japan (46), Japan (8–84), Morocco (0.9–56), Algeria (24–39)	[38, 84–86]
	Lippione	Senegal (80)	[87]
	Pulegone	Morocco (85), Tunisia (32)	[88, 89]
	2,4(8),6-p-Menthatrien-2,3-diol	Cuba (15)	[90]
	Menthol	Morocco (41)	[91]
	Piperitenone	Algeria (55)	[86]
	Trans-piperitone epoxide	Algeria, Bejaia (30)	[71]
M. longifolia	Piperitone	Yugoslavia (39)	[92]
	Pulegone	Tunisia (47), Senegal (52 and 42)	[12, 68]
	Cis-piperitone epoxide	Turkey (18)	[93]

Table 2. Major constituents of the essential oils of some *Mentha* species described in the literature.

4.2. Phenolic compounds

Phenolic compounds, secondary metabolites ubiquitously distributed in plants, include a large group of biologically active compounds, with over 8000 molecules, either small or large and complex molecules, presenting at least one aromatic ring with one or more hydroxyl groups attached. These compounds often appear in their natural sources as esters and glycosides [94].

Species of the genus *Mentha* have been reported to contain a range of components, including cinnamic acids and aglycon, glycoside, and/or acylated flavonoids [95]. Triantaphyllou et al. [96] reported that water extracts from *Mentha* contain esters of phenolic acids and flavonoid derivatives and glycosidic flavonoids hydroxylated in position 3 or 5.

Regarding phenolic acids, the genus *Mentha* is particularly rich in caffeic acid and its derivatives, chlorogenic and rosmarinic acid [24, 25, 36, 94, 95, 97–99], the latter accounting for 60–80% of total phenolic compounds. In addition, seven salvianolic acids have been described in *Mentha* plants, such as salvianolic acid H/I, salvianolic acid E, salvianolic acid B, and isosalvianolic acid A (caffeate trimers) [30].

Mentha plants are rich in flavonoids, particularly in flavones and flavanones. Luteolin and its derivatives are the main flavones described in *Mentha* species [30]. The components eriocitrin, luteolin-7-*O*-glucoside, naringenin-7-*O*-glucoside, isorhoifolin, eriodictyol, luteolin, and apigenin were identified in aqueous extracts from *Mentha* species, hybrids, varieties, and cultivars [95]. Besides, Areias et al. [97] have reported the main component in aqueous *Mentha* extracts to be the glycoside eriocitrin.

In an older study, external lipophilic methylated flavonoids have been extracted from dried leaves of *Mentha aquatica, M. spicata, M. x piperita,* and *M. citrata*. Twenty flavonoids have been identified. 5,6-Dihydroxy-7,8,3′,4′-tetramethoxyflavone was identified as major flavonoid of *M. spicata* and *M. x piperita* and 5-hydroxy-6,7,8,4′-tetramethoxyflavone (gardenin B) as a major compound of *M. citrata* and *M. aquatica* [100].

The phenolic composition of other species of different origins is summarized in **Table 3**.

Class of compounds	Identified compounds	Origin	Reference
M. spicata			
Phenolic acids	Rosmarinic acid	Japan	[101]
	Veratric acid	China	[102]
	Vanillic, homovanillic, hydroxybenzoic, syringic, 4-hydroxy cinnamic, trans-hydroxy cinnamic, 2-hydroxy cinnamic, and ferulic acids	Greece	[103]
	Gallic acid	Greece	[104]
	Protocatechuic acid	China	[105]
	Gallic, chlorogenic, caffeic, vanillic, syringic, *p*-coumaric, ferulic, and rosmarinic acids	Finland	[106]
	Protocatechuic and vanillic acids	China	[107]
	4-Hydroxy benzoic, caffeic, *p*-coumaric, chlorogenic, and rosmarinic acids	Algeria	[99]
Flavonoids	Diosmetin, diosmin, diosmin-7-glucoside	India	[108]
	6,4′-trihydroxy-7,3′-dimethoxyflavone	Spain	[109]
	5-Desmethoxynobiletin, 5,6-dihydroxy-7,8,3′,4′-tetramethoxyflavone, thymonin, sideritiflavone	Japan	[101]
	5-Hydroxy-3′,4′,6,7-tetramethoxyflavone and thymonin	China	[102]
	Naringenin, luteolin	Greece	[103]
	Apigenin, rutin, catechin	Greece	[104]
	Chrysoeriol, 5, 6-dihydroxy-7, 8, 3′, 4′-tetramethoxyflavone and nodifloretin	China	[105]
	Rutin, quercetin, luteolin	Greece	[110]

Class of compounds	Identified compounds	Origin	Reference
	Rutin, scopoletin	Czech Republic	[111]
	Catechin, epicatechin, rutin, myricetin, luteolin, apigenin, naringenin	Malaysia	[112]
	Rutin, naringin, luteolin, diosmin, naringenin, kaempferol, and diosmetin	Algeria	[99]
Lignans	Spicatolignan A and spicatolignan B	China	[113]
M. piperita			
Phenolic acids	Rosmarinic acid	France	[114]
	Rosmarinic, caffeic, and lithospermic acids	Poland	[115]
	Rosmarinic and lithospermic acids	Poland	[116]
	Rosmarinic, salvianolic, and dehydro-salvianolic acids		[117]
	Caffeic, syringic, gallic, vanillic, *p*-coumaric, and ferulic acids	USA	[25]
	Caffeic acid, salvianolic acid B, protocatechuic acid glucoside, isosalvianolic acid A, prolithospermic acid, salvianolic acids (E and H/I), danshensu	Iran	[118]
	Protocatechuic acid glucoside, caffeic, chlorogenic, rosmarinic, prolithospermic acids, salvianolic acid H/I, isosalvianolic acid A, salvianolic acid B, salvianolic acid E, and danshensu	Different origins	[24, 30]
	Caffeic, vanillic, ferulic, and chlorogenic acids	Iran	[119]
	Caffeic, *p*-coumaric, sinapic, shikimic, rosmarinic acids	Mexico	[98]
	Rosmarinic, caffeic, gallic, syringic, *p*-hydroxybenzoic, o-coumaric, and cinnamic acids	Croatia	[120]
	Caffeic, chlorogenic, 3-O-caffeoylquinic acids, salvianolic acid B, and salvianolic acid L	Portugal	[94]
Flavonoids	Luteolin 7-O-rutinoside, isorhoifolin, eriodictyol 7-O-glucoside, hesperidin, eriocitrin, narirutin, diosmin	France	[114]
	5,6-Dihydroxy-7,8,3′,4′-tetramethoxyflavone, sorbifolin, thymosin, thymonin, sideritoflavone, ladanein, xanthomicrol, acacetin, salvigenin, 5-O-demethylnobiletin	France	[121]
	Luteolin 7-O-β-glucuronide, luteolin 7-O-rutinoside, isorhoifolin, eriodictyol, eriodictyol 7-O-β-glucoside, hesperidin, eriocitrin, narirutin, naringenin-7-O-β-glucoside	Poland	[115]
	Luteolin 7-O-glucuronide	Poland	[116]
	Luteolin 7-glucoside, luteolin 7-O-rutinoside, isorhoifolin, pebrellin, eriodictyol 7-O-glucoside, eriodictyol-7-rutinoside, 5,6-dihydroxy-7,8,3′,4′-tetramethoxyflavone	Portugal	[97]

Class of compounds	Identified compounds	Origin	Reference
	Luteolin O-diglucuronide, luteolin O-glucuronide, methylated luteolin-glucuronide, luteolin-glucopyranosyl-rhamnopyranoside, eriodictyol-glucopyranosyl-rhamnopyranoside	Poland	[117]
	Luteolin, luteolin 7-O-neohesperidoside, tricetin 3′-O-glucoside, 5′-O-rhamnoside, pebrellin, hesperidin, eriocitrin, narirutin, eriodictyol-7-rutinoside, gardenin D, isosafrole, kaempferol 7-O-rutinoside, 4′-methoxykaempferol-7-O-rutinoside	USA	[122]
	Catechin, (−)-epigallocatechin gallate	USA	[25]
	Luteolin O-diglucuronide, luteolin O-glucuronide, luteolin O-rutinoside, eriocitrin, narirutin, diosmin, myricetin O-glucoside	Iran	[118]
	Luteolin-di-O-glucuronide, eriocitrin, luteolin-O-glucuronide, luteolin-O-rutinoside, narirutin, apigenin-O-rutinoside, diosmin, luteolin-O-glucuronide, myricetin-O-glucoside	Different origins	[24]
	Rutin	Iran	[119]
	Catechin, quercetin-4′-glucoside, (−)-epicatechin	Croatia	[120]
	Gallocatechin-gallate, rutin, quercetin, naringin, hesperidin	Mexico	[98]
	Luteolin-7-O-rutinoside, luteolin-7-O-glucuronide, luteolin-O-diglucuronide, eriodictyol-O-rutinoside and eriodictyol-O-hexoside, naringenin-7-O-rutinoside, eriodictyol-7-O-rutinoside	Portugal	[94]
Lignans	Medioresinol, medioresinol sulfate	Iran	[118]
Stilbenes	Trans-resveratrol	Croatia	[120]
M. pulegium			
Phenolic acids	Caffeic acid	Egypt	[123]
	Caffeic, vanillic, and ferulic acids	Greece	[104]
	4-Hydroxy benzoic, caffeic, *p*-coumaric, chlorogenic, and rosmarinic acids	Algeria	[99]
Flavonoids	Diosmin	France	[124]
	Thymonin, jaceosidin, pectolinaringenin, ladanein, sorbifolin, pedalitin, 5,6,4′-trihydroxy-7,3′-dimethoxyflavone; 5,6-dihydroxy-7,3′,4′-trimethoxyflavone; 5-hydroxy-6,7,3′,4′-tetramethoxyflavone, apigenin, luteolin, chrysoeriol	Algeria	[125]
	Acacetin 5-O-α-L-rhamnopyranosyl(1-2)-O-α-L-rhamnopyranoside, 7-O-α-rutinosides of apigenin and luteolin, vicenin, 5-hydroxy-6,7,3′,4′-tetramethoxyflavone	Egypt	[123]
	Luteolin, diosmin, and kaempferol	Algeria	[99]
	Apigenin, luteolin, naringenin, catechin	Greece	[104]

Class of compounds	Identified compounds	Origin	Reference
M. rotundifolia			
Phenolic acids	Caffeic, *p*-hydroxybenzoic, ferulic, and *p*-coumaric acids	Spain	[126]
	Caffeic, *p*-coumaric, chlorogenic, and rosmarinic acids	Algeria	[99]
Flavonoids	Apigenin, luteolinidin, elargonidin, cyanidin, delphinidin, petunidin, luteolin	Spain	[126]
	Thymonin, thymosin, 5,6-dihydroxy-7,8,3′,4′-tetramethoxyflavone, jaceosidin, hispidulin, ladanein, sorbifolin, nodifloretin, apigenin, luteolin, genkwanin	Algeria	[125]
	Esculetin	Czech Republic	[127]
	Luteolin, diosmin, naringenin, kaempferol, and diosmetin	Algeria	[99]
M. longifolia			
Phenolic acids	Rosmarinic, salvianolic acid L, dedihydro-salvianolic acid	Poland	[117]
Flavonoids	Luteolin-glucuronide, luteolin-diglucuronide, luteolin-glucopyranosyl-rhamnopyranoside, eriodictyol-glucopyranosyl-rhamnopyranoside, methylated luteolin-glucuronide	Poland	[117]
	5-Hydroxy-6,7,3′,4′-tetramethoxyflavone	Turkey	[128]
M. australis			
Phenolic acids	Rosmarinic, chlorogenic, and caffeic acids	Australia	[26]
Flavonoids	Neoponcirin, narirutin, biochanin A, apigenin, hesperetin, and naringenin	Australia	[26]
M. haplocalyx			
Phenolic acids	Rosmarinic, caffeic acid	China, Finland	[27, 129]
	Cis-salvianolic acid J, salvianolic acid J, lithospermic acid, rosmarinic acid, lithospermic acid B, magnesium lithospermate B, sodium lithospermate B, and danshensu	China	[130]
Flavonoids	Isoraifolin, luteolin-7-glucoside, menthoside	China	[27]
	Eriocitrin, luteolin-7-*O*-glucoside	Finland	[129]

Table 3. Phenolic composition of *Mentha* species reported in the literature.

4.3. Other compounds

Various other classes of compounds have been characterized and quantified in the mints. *M. spicata* and *M. piperita* contain different trace elements [46, 131]. Maffei and Scannerini [132] studied the variability of the triacylglycerol, diacylglycerol, and free fatty acids in some *Mentha* species. They found a high level of C_{18}:3 only in the leaves of certain species (*M. longifolia, M. crispa,* and *M. sachalinensis*). Among the major components found in peppermint leaves are fatty acids such as linoleic, linolenic, and palmitic acid [98]. In addition, recent studies identified two new ceramides from the methanolic extract of *M. longifolia*, longifoamides A and B [10].

Triterpenoids and steroids were also isolated from mints. So, two triterpenoids ursolic acid and uvaol and three steroids stigmast-5-en-3-β-yl formate, stigmast-5-en-3-one, and β-sitosterol were isolated from the aerial parts of *M. longifolia* subsp. *noeana* [128].

On the other hand, different pigments were identified and quantified in *Mentha* species. The analysis of *M. spicata* revealed the presence of xanthophylls (neoxanthin, violaxanthin, and lutein, zeaxanthin), carotenes (α-carotene) [133], and chlorophylls (chlorophylls a and b) [134, 135]. Carotenoids (lutein and β-carotene isomers) were determined in dry peppermint tea, but only lutein was found in infusion [36]. Among vitamins, α-tocopherols and ascorbic acid were present in mints [36, 98, 135].

Mint was also reported to contain sugars, saponins, alkaloids, anthraquinones, and quinines [136], but these absolutely surprising HPTLC-based phytochemical data as well as the identity/purity of investigated samples should be thoroughly verified.

5. Biological activities

The research over the past several years has shown that mint and its constituents possess different biological activities including antioxidant, antimicrobial, insecticidal, anticancer, and anti-inflammatory properties [10].

5.1. Antioxidant activity

Various types of compounds from aromatic and medicinal plants are receiving particular attention due to their radical scavenging properties. Reactive oxygen species (ROS) are chemical species formed in the body during metabolism that are highly reactive and may have one or more unpaired electrons. Oxidative stress, i.e., an imbalance between ROS and antioxidant defenses, has deleterious effects, such as the peroxidation of membrane lipids and the attack on biomolecules (proteins, membrane enzymes, carbohydrates, and DNA) [137].

Various *Mentha* species and their extracts or essential oils have been shown to possess antioxidant activity [30]. Phenolic acids (e.g., rosmarinic and caffeic acids), flavones (e.g., luteolin derivatives), and flavanones (e.g., eriocitrin derivatives) are possibly the major antioxidants. Vitamin antioxidants (e.g., ascorbic acid and carotenoids) are minor contributors to the overall antioxidant potential. In essential oils, unsaturated terpenes having a cyclohexadiene structure (e.g., terpinene) and minor cyclic oxygenated terpenes (e.g., thymol) may contribute to antioxidant potential, while acyclic unsaturated oxygenated monoterpenes (e.g., linalool) may act as pro-oxidants [36].

Mentha extracts are widely known to act as free radical scavengers in vitro. The acetonic extract and essential oil of peppermint act as scavengers of hydroxyl radical (•OH) [25, 138], the hydroalcoholic extract of *M. piperita* [139] and peppermint essential oil [140] as scavengers of nitric oxide (•NO), and the ethanolic and water extracts of *M. pulegium* [141] as scavengers of hydrogen peroxide (H_2O_2). Besides, different fractions of the ethanol extract of *M. spicata* [142]; the ethanolic extracts from *M. spicata, M. pulegium,* and *M. rotundifolia* [99]; the methanolic extract of *M. pulegium* [68, 143] and *M. longifolia* [68] were shown to quench superoxide ($O_2•^-$) radicals.

Mentha plants have also been reported for antioxidant activities in several functional tests. The DPPH test, a test widely used to measure the ability to donate hydrogen atoms [41], was applied to measure the antioxidant capacities of *Mentha* species extracted by different solvent systems; these include the ethanol extracts of *M. longifolia, M. piperita* [144], *M. pulegium* [73, 99, 141, 144], *M. spicata,* and *M. rotundifolia* [96, 144]; the methanol extracts from *M. pulegium* [68, 69, 143, 145], *M. longifolia* [68, 93], *M. aquatica, M. arvensis, M. piperita, M. rotundifolia,* and *M. villosa* [145]; the water extracts from *M. pulegium* [69, 73, 141]; and the acetonic extracts from peppermint [25] and *M. spicata* [146]. DPPH was also used to evaluate the antioxidant activity of the essential oils from *M. aquatica* [92], *M. longifolia* [6, 68, 92, 93], *M. spicata* [6, 46, 51], *M. pulegium* [68, 69, 72, 73], *M. rotundifolia* [89, 147], and *M. piperita* [46, 92, 138, 140].

Other tests are less used in literature to evaluate the antioxidant potential/radical scavenger capacity of *Mentha* species polar extracts and essential oils (**Table 4**).

Species	Type of extract	Reference
Test measuring the quenching of ABTS⁺		
M. spicata, M. piperita, M. longifolia, M. pulegium, M. rotundifolia	Ethanolic	[99, 144, 148]
M. longifolia, M. viridis	Essential oil	[6]
M. spicata, M. pulegium, M. rotundifolia	Essential oil	[51, 71, 147]
Measurement of lipid peroxidation inhibition		
M. pulegium	Water Essential oil	[69]
M. aquatica, M. pulegium, M. suaveolens, M. piperita	Methanolic	[145, 149]
M. longifolia	Methanolic	[149]
M. arvensis, M. villosa	Methanolic	[145]
M. piperita	Essential oil	[140]
M. spicata, M. pulegium, M. rotundifolia	Ethanolic	[150]
Measurement of iron chelating activity		
M. spicata	Ethanolic	[142]
M. piperita	Ethanol/water	[139]
M. aquatica, M. arvensis, M. piperita, M. pulegium, M. rotundifolia, and M. villosa	Methanolic	[145]

Species	Type of extract	Reference
Measurement of iron(III) to iron(II) reducing activity		
M. spicata	Ethanolic	[142]
M. longifolia	Methanolic	[151]
M. piperita	Essential oil	[138]
M. pulegium	Ethanolic, water	[141]
Measurement of total antioxidant activity (TAA) by the phosphomolybdenum method		
M. spicata	Acetone, acetone/water methanol, methanol/water, ethanol, ethanol/water	[146]
M. piperita	Essential oil	[138]
M. pulegium	Ethanol, water	[141]
Measurement of oxygen radical absorbance capacity (ORAC)		
M. piperita	Acetonic	[25]
Kit Radicaux Libres (KRL) assay		
M. spicata, M. pulegium, M. rotundifolia	Essential oils	[51, 71]
Clinical tests measuring the ferric reducing ability of plasma (FRAP test)		
M. longifolia		[151]
M. pulegium	Water, ethanolic	[73, 141]
M. pulegium	Essential oil	[73]
M. rotundifolia	Essential oil	[89]

Table 4. Different methods applied to evaluate the antioxidant properties of *Mentha* species.

The most studied species are *M. spicata, M. piperita, M. longifolia, M. pulegium, M. rotundifolia, M. arvensis,* and *M. aquatica*. *M. piperita* and *M. spicata* extracts showed good antioxidant activities in several in vitro assay systems compared to other species [95, 99, 144, 149]. The antioxidant compounds present in these extracts act as hydrogen- or electron-donating agents and/or metal chelators. Moreover, as expected from their composition, the polar extracts of *Mentha* species showed much better activity than the essential oils [6, 41, 69, 93].

5.2. Antimicrobial activity

The antibacterial and antifungal activities of *Mentha* species have been studied on various bacteria and fungi [30]. These studies indicate that essential oils are more efficient antifungals and antibacterials compared to the polar extracts [6, 68, 73]. *Mentha* essential oils showed remarkable antimicrobial activity against bacteria and other microorganisms, such as yeasts and periodontopathogens [4], mainly due to the presence of oxygenated monoterpenes in their chemical compositions [22]. Bactericidal and bacteriostatic activities are observed in the 1/1 to 1/1000 (V/V) and 1–5 mg/mL concentration ranges, respectively.

Thus, *M. rotundifolia* oils showed effect against *Bacillus subtilis, B. cereus, Escherichia coli, Proteus mirabilis, Salmonella typhimurium,* and *Staphylococcus aureus* [21, 88, 89, 152]. The pulegone-rich essential oil of *M. suaveolens* efficiently inhibited all the microorganisms (20 stains) tested by Oumzil et al. [85]. Furthermore, according to Brahmi et al. [71], *M. rotundifolia* essential oils exhibited stronger antimicrobial effect than *M. pulegium* oils against all the microorganisms studied (three Gram$^+$, three Gram$^-$, two fungal, and one yeast). Nevertheless, *M. pulegium* oil showed good antimicrobial activity against 11 bacteria (3 Gram$^+$ and 8 Gram$^-$) and 2 yeasts [72].

M. pulegium presents an appreciable activity toward all microorganisms (five Gram$^+$, five Gram$^-$, and six fungal strains) tested by Hadjlaoui et al. [68] and *Streptococcus pyogenes* [47]. Similarly, they showed the best bacteriostatic and bactericidal effect compared to tested medicinal and aromatic plants from other genera [70]. Besides, the essential oil of the flowering aerial parts of *M. pulegium* showed a significant activity against microorganisms especially Gram-positive bacteria [19].

The essential oil of *M. spicata* has an appreciable activity against *Streptococcus pyogenes* [47], *E. coli, S. aureus, S. pyogenes* [46], and *C. albicans* [46, 51]. Oils of *Mentha longifolia* showed strong antimicrobial activity against all 16 microorganisms tested by Hadjlaoui et al. [68] and against *Escherichia coli, Shigella sonnei,* and *Micrococcus flavus.* These bacteria were also inhibited by the essential oils from *M. aquatica* and *M. piperita* [92]. Of the *Mentha* essential oils tested by Hussain et al., the oil from *M. arvensis* showed relatively higher antimicrobial activity [45]; the essential oils of *Mentha officinalis* totally inhibited *E. coli, Bacillus aureus, Streptococcus lactis,* and *S. aureus* [153].

Besides, the essential oils from *Mentha* spp. have been considered a safe ingredient for the development of antibiofilm agents that could find a role in the pharmaceutical industry [4].

The antibacterial or antifungal activity of *Mentha* plant polar extracts have been studied to a much lesser extent; bactericidal and bacteriostatic activities are observed in the 2–4 mg/mL and 100–250 μg/mL concentration ranges, respectively, and at 6 μg/disk. The extracts were shown to possess antibacterial and antifungal activity [30]. Methanolic extracts of *M. viridis* and *M. pulegium* showed slight antimicrobial capacity against *S. enteritidis* and *E. coli,* respectively [104]; infusions of *M. piperita* and *M. spicata* were active on *Vibrio parahaemolyticus* [154]. Fractions from *M. spicata* ethanol extract showed effective antibacterial activity against *Escherichia coli, Salmonella paratyphi, Shigella boydii, Staphylococcus aureus,* and *Vibrio cholerae* [142]. Peppermint tea extracts were active against *Chlamydia pneumoniae* [24].

5.3. Insecticidal activity

Mint is also known to exhibit insecticidal activity against a wide variety of insects. *Mentha* has been used as insecticides mainly in the form of essential oils [155]. *M. spicata, M. pulegium,* and *M. rotundifolia* oils demonstrated insecticidal properties against adults of *Rhyzopertha dominica,* in contact and fumigation bioassays and repellency [51, 71]. *M. pulegium* and *M. rotundifolia* oils were also very toxic in the first 24 h in a contact toxicity bioassay against the same pest [156].

M. arvensis oil was toxic against *Sitophilus oryzae* (LC_{50}, 45.5 μL/L) [157, 158]. Similarly, the essential oil of *M. microphylla* gave remarkable activity against this insect (LC_{50}, 0.2 μL/L) in fumigation bioassays and in contact bioassays (24 h; LC_{50}, 0.01 mg/cm^2) [159], and the ethanolic extract of *M. longifolia* was also efficient against it (24.2% repellency) [160]. Additionally, *M. pulegium* oil was toxic against *Sitophilus granarius* (contact LD_{50}, 9.1 μL/mL) [72], and *M. longifolia* essential oil has 100% repellence against *Sitophilus zeamais* [22].

Varma and Dubey [158] reported complete inhibition of *Tribolium castaneum*, through the treatment of wheat samples with *M. arvensis* essential oil. The essential oil of *M. microphylla* gave remarkable activity against adults of this insect (LC_{50}, 4.5 μL/L) in fumigation bioassays [159]. Furthermore, the insecticidal properties of *M. longifolia* essential oil against this pest have been attributed to piperitenone oxide (LC_{50}, 9.95 mg/L) [22]. In another study, Lee et al. [157] observed that *M. piperita* (LD_{50}, 25.8 μL/L) was a slightly better fumigant than *M. spicata* (LD_{50}, 33.1 μL/L) against *T. castaneum*. Besides, in both contact and fumigation assays, the *M. rotundifolia* oil samples rich in pulegone and menthone, compared to other chemotypes, exhibited superior insecticidal activity against the adults of the same insect [161].

Mentha essential oils and polar extracts showed also insecticidal properties toward other insect species. The ethanolic extract of *M. longifolia* was efficient against third- and fourth-instar larvae of *Culex pipiens* (LC_{50}-26.8 ppm). *M. arvensis* oil efficiently repelled (85%) *Callosobruchus chinensis* [160]. Feeding on *M. longifolia* caused death in *Chrysolina herbacea* [22]. *M. pulegium* L. oil also caused 100% mortality of *Mayetiola destructor* [162]. Studies have shown that essential oils of spearmint were effective against *Lycoriella ingenua* at 20 × 10^{-3} mg/mL [10]; fumigation allowed controlling all stages of *Callosobruchus maculatus*; and the egg stage was the most susceptible stage [163]. Also, compared to *M. pulegium*, a *M. suaveolens* hydrosol showed higher insecticidal activity toward an insect pest of citrus, *Toxoptera aurantii* [164].

5.4. Cytotoxicity

Several studies have indicated that *Mentha* plants contain constituents with cytotoxic properties that may find use in developing anticancer agents. For example, *M. arvensis, M. longifolia, M. spicata,* and *M. viridis* methanolic and aqueous extracts showed antiproliferative effect against various cancer cell lines in vitro at a concentration of 100 μg/mL [165]. Similarly, in Yi and Wetzstein [166] study, spearmint and peppermint methanolic extracts significantly inhibited SW-480 colon cancer cell growth (IC_{50s}: 143.6 ± 25.6 μg/mL for spearmint and 92.3 ± 17.8 μg/mL for peppermint). The cytotoxic effect of the essential oil of *M. pulegium* on ovarian adenocarcinoma (SK-OV-3), human malignant cervix carcinoma (HeLa), and human lung carcinoma (A549) cell lines has been shown by other investigators (IC_{50}s ranging from 14.10 to 59.10 μg/mL) [167]. In an in vitro screening for the tumoricidal properties of international medicinal herbs, *M. spicata* and *M. piperita* exhibited extremely weak tumoricidal effects (LC_{50} > 5.0 mg/mL), while *M. pulegium* showed a weak activity (LC_{50}, 1.2–2.5 mg/mL) [168].

The cytotoxicity of essential oils from four *Mentha* species (*M. arvensis, M. piperita, M. longifolia,* and *M. spicata*) was tested on breast cancer (MCF-7) and prostate cancer (LNCaP) cell lines using the MTT assay. The tested *Mentha* essential oils showed prominent cytotoxic activity against both cancer cell lines (IC_{50}s ranging from 43.5 ± 2.1–95.7 ± 4.5 μg/mL) [45].

In another study, aqueous extract of *M. spicata* significantly reduced the proliferation of Wehi-164 and U937 cells dose and time dependently (LD_{50}s ranging from 4.63 to 5.97 mg/mL) [169]. Jain et al. [170] examined the possible molecular mechanisms underlying the cytotoxicity and anticarcinogenic potential of *Mentha piperita* leaf extracts on six human cancer (HeLa, MCF-7, Jurkat, T24, HT-29, MIA PaCa-2). The chloroform and ethyl acetate extracts showed significant dose- and time-dependent anticarcinogenic activity, leading to G1 cell cycle arrest and mitochondrial-mediated apoptosis, perturbation of oxidative balance, upregulation of Bax gene, elevated expression of p53 and p21 in the treated cells, and acquisition of senescence phenotype (effective doses ranging from 10 × (10 μg/μL) to 100 × (100 μg/μL)).

Lv et al. [25] also evaluated the antiproliferative activity of a peppermint extract against the human tumor cell line HT-29 (effective doses 250 and 500 μg/mL). Similarly, the cytotoxic effect of *Mentha piperita* essential oil was assessed against four human cancer cells. It was found to be significantly active against human lung carcinoma SPC-A1, human leukemia K562, and human gastric cancer SGC-7901 cells, with IC_{50} values of 10.9, 16.2, and 38.8 μg/mL, respectively [138].

M. longifolia methanolic extract and *M. piperita* ethanolic extract presented a cytotoxic activity, respectively, against human breast cancer (IC_{50} = 191.2 μg/mL) [171] and human laryngeal epidermoid carcinoma (IC_{50} = 94 μg/mL) [172]. Besides, peppermint extract showed cytotoxicity against four human tumor cell lines (MCF-7, NCI-H460, HeLa, and HepG2; IC_{50}s ranging from 98 ± 9 to 226 ± 11 μg/mL) [94].

5.5. Anti-inflammatory properties

Mentha extracts contain numerous constituents which could have anti-inflammatory effects. In vitro, the anti-inflammatory activity of the *M. piperita* essential oil has been determined by 5-lipoxygenase (5-LOX) inhibition assay (IC_{50}s ranging from 0.03 ± 0.01–0.08 ± 0.01 μg/mL) [140]. It could also effectively inhibit nitric oxide (•NO) and prostaglandin E2 (PGE2) production in lipopolysaccharide (LPS)-activated RAW 264.7 macrophages [138]. Lv et al. [25] using J774A.1 mouse macrophage cells showed that peppermint extracts were efficient in inhibiting IL-1 and COX-2 expression and have inhibitory effect on IL-6 and MCP-1 (IC_{50}s ranging from 50 to 100 μg/mL).

In vivo, pretreatment of albino mice and female Wistar rats with *M. suaveolens* methanol extract induced an anti-inflammatory effect [173]. The anti-inflammatory effects of aqueous, chloroform, ethyl acetate, and hexane extracts of *M. spicata* ethyl acetate and aqueous fractions were both effective in reducing the chronic and acute inflammation of *Wistar albino* rats [11]. In addition, edema reduction was also observed by topic use of *M. aquatica* L. alcohol extract on Male CD-1 mice [174]. The *M. piperita* essential oil exhibited potent anti-inflammatory activities in a croton oil-induced mouse ear edema model. The oil reduced the edematous response by 5.77, 7.37, and 30.24% at the dose of 200, 400, and 800 μg, respectively [138].

Author details

Fatiha Brahmi[1*], Madani Khodir[1], Chibane Mohamed[2] and Duez Pierre[3]

*Address all correspondence to: fatiha.brahmi@univ-bejaia.dz

1 3BS Laboratory, Faculty of Natural Sciences and Life, University of Bejaia, Bejaia, Algeria

2 Faculty of Natural, Life and Earth Sciences, Akli Mohand Oulhadj University, Bouira, Algeria

3 Medicinal Chemistry and Pharmacognosy Department, Faculty of Medicine and Pharmacy, University of Mons (UMONS), Belgium

References

[1] De Judicibus M. Botanical notebook. UoM Custom Book Centre; Printed by Custom Book Centre, University of Melbourne, March 2010 Australia. 2011. 232 p.

[2] Lawrence B.M. Mint: the genus *Mentha*. Medicinal and aromatic plants -industrial profiles. CRC Press/Taylor & Francis, Boca Raton, FL; 2007.

[3] Qing W. *Mentha*'s historical textual research and clinical new application, Journal of Haidian University. 2002;02.

[4] Peixoto I.T.A., Furlanetti V.F., Anibal P.C., Duarte M.C.T., Höfling J.F. Potential pharmacological and toxicological basis of the essential oil from *Mentha* spp. Rev Ciênc Farm Básica Apl. 2009;**30**(3):235–239.

[5] Sutour S. Study of the chemical composition of essential oils and extracts of mints from Corsica and Kumquants. Doctorat thesis in organic and analytical chemistry. University of Corsica. 2010; 221 p.

[6] Mkaddem M., Bouajila J., Ennajar M., Lebrihi A., Mathieu F., Romdhane M. Chemical composition and antimicrobial and antioxidant activities of *Mentha* (*longifolia* L. and *viridis*) essential oils. Journal of Food Science. 2009;**74**: 358–363.

[7] Abbaszadeh B., Valadabadi S.A., Farahani H.A., Darvishi H.H. Studying of essential oil variations in leaves of *Mentha* species. African Journal of Plant Science. 2009;**3**(10): 217–221.

[8] Kew. 2010. The Plant list: http://www.theplantlist.org/tpl/search=Mentha+species

[9] Saric-Kundalic B., Fialova S., Dobes C., Olzant S., Tekelova D., Grancai D., Reznicek G., Saukel J.. Multivariate numerical taxonomy of *Mentha* species hybrids varieties and cultivars. Sci Pharm. 2009;**77**: 851–876.

[10] Kunnumakkara A.B., Chung J.G., Koca C., Dey S. Mint and its constituants. In Aggarwal B.B., Kunnumakkara A.B.: Molecular targets and therapeutic uses of spices. World Scientific, Singapore; Hackensack, NJ; 2009; pp.373–401.

[11] Arumugam P., Gayatri Priya N., Subathra M., Ramesh A. Anti-inflammatory activity of four solvent fractions of ethanol extract of *Mentha spicata* L. investigated on acute and chronic inflammation induced rats. Environmental Toxicology and Pharmacology. 2008;**26**: 92–95.

[12] Diop S.M., Guèye M.T., Ndiaye I., Ndiaye E.B., Diop M.B., Heuskin S., Fauconnier M.L., Lognay G. Chemical composition of essential oils and floral waters of *Mentha longifolia* (L.) Huds. from Senegal. American Journal of Essential Oils and Natural Products. 2016;**4**(1): 46–49.

[13] Di Stasi L.C., Oliveira G.P., Carvalhaes M.A., Queiroz-Junior M., Tien O.S., Kakinami S.H., Reis M.S. Medicinal plants popularly used in the Brazilian tropical atlantic forest. Fitoterapia. 2002;**73**: 69–91.

[14] El-Hilaly J., Hmammouchi M., Lyoussi B. Ethnobotanical studies and economic evaluation of medicinal plants in Taounate province (Northern Morocco). Journal of Ethnopharmacology. 2003;**86**: 149–158.

[15] Kumar A., Chattopadhyay S. DNA damage protecting activity and antioxidant potential of pudina extract. Food Chemistry. 2007;**100**: 1377–1384.

[16] Akdogan M., Tamer M.N., Cure E., Cure M.C., Korolu B.K., Delibat N. Effect of spearmint (*Mentha spicata* Labiatae) teas on androgen levels in women with Hirsutism. Phytotherapy Research. 2007;**21**: 444–447.

[17] Bruneton J. Pharmacognosy phytochemistry. Medicinal plants, fourth ed. Tec and Doc, Paris; 2009;1269 p.

[18] Delille L. The medicinal plants of Algeria. Berti Editions, Alger; 2007;240 p.

[19] Mahboubi M., Haghi G. Antimicrobial activity and chemical composition of *Mentha pulegium* L. essential oil. Journal of Ethnopharmacology. 2008;**119**: 325–327.

[20] Bello R., Calatayud S., Beltran B., Primo-Yufera E., Esplugues J. Cardiovascular effects of the methanol and dichloromethanol extracts from *Mentha suaveolens* Ehrh. Phytotherapy Research. 2001;**15**: 447–448.

[21] Sutour S., Bradesi P., de Rocca-Serra D., Casanova J, Tomi F. Chemical composition and antibacterial activity of the essential oil from *Mentha suaveolens* ssp. Insularis (Req.) Greuter. Flavour and Fragrance Journal. 2008;**23**: 107–114.

[22] Mikaili P., Mojaverrostami S., Moloudizargari M., Aghajanshakeri S. Pharmacological and therapeutic effects of *Mentha Longifolia* L. and its main constituent, menthol. Ancient Science of Life. 2013;**33**: 129–136.

[23] Balakrishnan A. Therapeutic uses of peppermint—a review. Journal of Pharmaceutical Sciences and Research. 2015;**7**(7): 474–476.

[24] Kapp K., Hakala E., Orav A., Pohjala L., Vuorela P., Püssa T., Vuorela H., Raal A. Commercial peppermint (*Mentha* × *piperita* L.) teas: antichlamydial effect and polyphenolic composition. Food Research International. 2013;**53**:758–766.

[25] Lv J., Huang H., Yua L., Whent M., Niu Y., Shi H., Wang T.T.Y., Luthria D., Charles D., Yu L.C. Phenolic composition and nutraceutical properties of organic and conventional cinnamon and peppermint. Food Chemistry. 2012;**132**: 1442–1450.

[26] Tang K.S.C., Konczak I., Zhao J. Identification and quantification of phenolics in Australian native mint (Mentha australis R. Br.). Food Chemistry. 2016;**192**: 698–705.

[27] Bensky D., Clavey S., Stoger E. Chinese herbal medicine: materia medica, 3rd ed. Eastland Press, Inc., Seatle, WA, USA; 2004;47–49pp.

[28] Chinese Pharmacopoeia Commission. Pharmacopoeia of the People's Republic of China. 1. China Medical Science Press. 2010;pp 278–279.

[29] Lamendin H., Toscano G., Requirand P. Buccodental phytotherapy and aromatherapy. EMC-Dentisterie 2004;**1**: 179–192.

[30] Kapp K. Polyphenolic and essential oil composition of *Mentha* and their antimicrobial effect. Academic Dissertation. Faculty of Pharmacy of the University of Helsinki. 2015;90 p.

[31] NTP 2011. Toxicology and carcinogenesis studies of pulegone (CAS No. 89-82-7) in F344/N rats and B6C3F1 mice (gavage studies). Natl Toxicol Program Tech Rep Ser. 2011;563: 1–201.

[32] European Commission. Regulation (EC) No 1334/2008 of the European Parliament and of the 550 Council of 16 December 2008 on flavourings and certain food ingredients with flavouring properties for 551 use in and on foods and amending Council Regulation (EEC) No 1601/91, Regulations (EC) No 2232/96 552 and (EC) No 110/2008 and Directive 2000/13/EC. Official Journal of the European Union Lex. 2008;354:34.

[33] Akdogan M., Ozguner M., Kocak A., Oncu M., Cicek E. Effects of peppermint teas on plasma testosterone, follicle-stimulating hormone, and luteinizing hormone levels and testicular tissue in rats. Urology. 2004;**64**: 394–398.

[34] Bakkali F., Averbeck S., Averbeck D., Idaomar M. Biological effects of essential oils—a review. Food and Chemical Toxicology. 2008;**46**: 446–475.

[35] Zhao D., Xu Y.W., Yang G.L., Husaini A.M., Wu W. Variation of essential oil of *Mentha haplocalyx* Briq. and *Mentha spicata* L. from China. Industrial Crops and Products. 2013;**42**: 251–260.

[36] Riachi L.G., De Maria C.A.B. Peppermint antioxidants revisited. Food Chemistry. 2015;**176**: 72–81.

[37] Adam K., Sivropoulou A., Kokkini S., Lanaras T., Arsenakis M. Antifungal activities of *Origanum vulgare* subsp. hirtum, *Mentha spicata, Lavandula angustifolia,* and *Salvia fruticosa* essential oils against human pathogenic fungi. Journal of Agricultural and Food Chemistry. 1998;**46**: 1739–1745.

[38] Miyazawa M., Watanabe H., Umemoto K., Kameoka H. Inhibition of acetylcholinesterase activity by essential oils of *Mentha* species. Journal of Agricultural and Food Chemistry. 1998;**46**: 3431–3434.

[39] Oka Y., Nacar S., Putievsky E., Ravid U., Yaniv Z., Spiegel Y. Nematicidal activity of essential oils and their components against the root-knot nematode. Phytopathology. 2000;**90**: 710–715.

[40] Chowdhury J.U., Nandi N.C., Uddin M., Rahman M. Chemical constituents of essential oils from two types of spearmint (*Mentha spicata* L. and *M. cardiaca* L.) introduced in Bangladesh. Bangladesh. Journal of Scientific and Industrial Research. 2007;**42**: 79–82.

[41] Mata A.T., Proenc C., Ferreira A.R., Serralheiro M.L.M., Nogueira J.M.F., Araújo M.E.M. Antioxidant and anti-acetylcholinesterase activities of five plants used as Portuguese food spices. Food Chemistry. 2007;**103**: 778–786.

[42] Mkolo N.M., Olowoyo J.O., Sako K.B., Mdakane S.T.R., Mitonga M.M.A., Magano S.R. Repellency and toxicity of essential oils of *Mentha piperita* and *Mentha spicata* on larvae and adult of *Amblyomma Hebraeum* (Acari: Ixodidae). Science Journal of Microbiology. 2011;7 p.

[43] Chauhan R.S., Kaul M.K., Shahi A.K., Kumar A., Ram G., Tawa A. Chemical composition of essential oils in *Mentha spicata* L. accession [IIIM(J)26] from North-West Himalayan region, India. Industrial Crops and Products. 2009;**29**: 654–656.

[44] Sokovic M.D., Vukojevic J., Marin P.D., Brkić D.D., Vajs V., Van Griensven L.J. Chemical composition of essential oils of *Thymus* and *Mentha* species and their antifungal activities. Molecules. 2009;**14**(1): 238–249.

[45] Hussain A.I., Anwar F., Nigam P.S., Ashraf M., Gilani A.H. Seasonal variation in content, chemical composition and antimicrobial and cytotoxic activities of essential oils from four *Mentha* species. Journal of the Science of Food and Agriculture. 2010;**90**(11): 1827–1836.

[46] Kizil S., Hasimi N., Tolan V., Kilinç E., Yuksel U. Mineral content, essential oil components and biological activity of two *Mentha* species (*M. piperita* L., *M. spicata* L.). Turkish Journal of Field Crops. 2010; **15**(6): 148–153.

[47] Boukhebti H., Chaker A.N., Belhadj H., Sahli F., Ramdhani M., Laouer H., Harzallah D. Chemical composition and antibacterial activity of *Mentha pulegium* L. and *Mentha spicata* L. essential oils. Der Pharmacia Lettre. 2011;**3**: 267–275.

[48] Znini M., Bouklah M., Majidi L., Kharchouf S., Aouniti A., Bouyanzer A., Hammouti B., Costa J., Al-Deyab S.S. Chemical composition and inhibitory effect of *Mentha spicata* essential oil on the corrosion of steel in molar hydrochloric acid. International Journal of Electrochemical Science. 2011;6: 691–704.

[49] Govindarajan M., Sivakumar R., Rajeswari M., Yogalakshmi K. Chemical composition and larvicidal activity of essential oil from *Mentha spicata* (Linn.) against three mosquito species. Parasitology Research. 2012;**110**: 2023–2032.

[50] Allali H., Chikhi I., Dib M.E., Muselli A., Fekih N., Meliani N., Kamal M.A., Tabti B., Costa J. Antioxidant activity and chemical analysis of *Mentha spicata* cultivated from

west northern region of Algeria by headspace solid phase micro-extraction and hydro-distillation. Natural Products: An Indian Journal. 2013;**9**(6): 258–263.

[51] Brahmi F., Adjaoud A., Marongiu B., Falconieri D., Yalaoui-Guellal D., Madani K., Chibane M. Chemical and biological profiles of essential oils from *Mentha spicata* L. leaf from Bejaia in Algeria. Journal of Essential Oil Research. 2016;http://dx.doi.org/10.1080/10412905.2015.1118411.

[52] Gonçalves R.S., Battistin A., Pauletti G, Rota L., Serafini L.A. Antioxidant properties of essential oils from *Mentha* species evidenced by electrochemical methods. Revista Brasileria de Plantas Medicinais. 2009;**11**(4): 372–382.

[53] Koliopoulos G., Pitarokili D., Kioulos E., Michaelakis A., Tzakou O. Chemical composition and larvicidal evaluation of *Mentha, Salvia,* and *Melissa* essential oils against the West Nile virus mosquito *Culex pipiens*. Parasitology Research 2010;**107**: 327–335.

[54] Telci I., Demirtas I., Bayram E., Arabaci O., Kacar O. Environmental variation on aroma components of pulegone/piperitone rich spearmint (*Mentha spicata* L.). Industrial Crops and Products. 2010;**32**: 588–592.

[55] Fujita Y., Fujita S.I. Essential oil of *Mentha pulegium* and *M. grattefossei* view from the standpoint of comparative biocheistry. Nippon Kagaku Zasshi. 1967;**88**: 767–768.

[56] Sticher O., Fluck H. The composition of genuine, extracted and distilled essential oils of some *Mentha* species. Pharmaceutica Acta Helvetiae. 1968;**43**: 411–446.

[57] Sivropoulou A., Kokkini S., Lanaras T., Arsenakis M.. Antimicrobial activity of mint essential oils. Journal of Agricultural and Food Chemistry. 1995;**43**: 2384–2388.

[58] Reis-Vasco E.M.C., Coelho J.A.P., Palavra A.M.F. Comparison of pennyroyal oils obtained by supercritical CO_2 extraction and hydrodistillation. Flavour and Fragrance Journal. 1999;**14**: 156–160.

[59] Lorenzo D., Paz D., Dellacassa E., Davies P., Vila R., Canigueral S. Essential oils of *Mentha pulegium* and *Mentha rotundifolia* from Uruguay. Brazilian Archives Boilogy and Technology. 2002;**45**(4): 519–524.

[60] Aghel N., Yamini Y., Hadjiakhoondi A., Pourmortazavi S.M. Supercritical carbon dioxide extraction of *Mentha pulegium* L. essential oil. Talanta. 2004;**62**: 407–411.

[61] Bouchra C., Achouri M., Idrissi Hassani LM., Hmamouchi M. Chemical composition and antifungal activity of essential oils of seven Moroccan Labiatae against *Botrytis cinerea Pers*: Fr. Phytochemistry. 2003; 89: 165–69.

[62] Kokkini S., Handilou E., Karouscou R. Clinal variation of *Mentha pulegium* essential oils along the climatic gradient of Greece. Journal of Essential Oil Research. 2004;**16**: 588–593.

[63] Agnihotri V.K., Agarwal S.G., Dhar P.L., Thappa Baleshwar R.K., Kapahi B.K., Saxena R.K., Qazi G.N. Essential oil composition of *Mentha pulegium* L. growing wild in the north-western Himalayas India. Flavour and Fragrance Journal. 2005;**20**: 607–610.

[64] Stoyanova A., Georgie V., Kula J., Majda T. Chemical composition of the essential oil of *Mentha pulegium* L. from Bulgaria. Journal of Essential Oil Research. 2005;**17**: 475–477.

[65] El-Ghorab A.H. The chemical composition of *Mentha pulegium* L. essential oil from Egypt and its antioxidant activity. Journal of Essential Oil Bearing Plants. 2006;**9**: 183–195.

[66] Beghidja N., Bouslimani N., Benayache F., Benayache S., Chalchat J. Composition of the oils from *Mentha pulegium* grown in different areas of the east of Algeria. Chemistry of Natural Compounds. 2007;**43**: 481–483.

[67] Diaz-Maroto M.C., Castillo N., Castro-Vazquez L., Gonzalez-Vinas M.Á., Perez-Coello M.S. Volatile composition and olfactory profile of pennyroyal (*Mentha pulegium*) plants. Flavour and Fragrance Journal. 2007;**22**: 114–118.

[68] Hajlaoui H., Trabelsi N., Noumi E., Snoussi M., Fallah H., Ksouri R., Bakhrouf A. Biological activities of the essential oils and methanol extract of tow cultivated mint species (*Mentha longifolia* and *Mentha pulegium*) used in the Tunisian folkloric medicine. World Journal of Microbiology and Biotechnology. 2009;**25**: 2227–2238.

[69] Kamkar A., Jebelli Javan A., Asadi F., Kamalinejad M. The antioxidative effect of Iranian *Mentha pulegium* extracts and essential oil in sunflower oil. Food and Chemical Toxicology. 2010;**48**: 1796–1800.

[70] Ait-Ouazzou A., Lorán S., Arakrak A., Laglaoui A., Rota C., Herrera A., Pagán R., Conchello P. Evaluation of the chemical composition and antimicrobial activity of *Mentha pulegium, Juniperus phoenicea,* and *Cyperus longus* essential oils from Morocco. Food Research International. 2012;**45**: 313–319.

[71] Brahmi F., Abdenour A., Bruno M., Silvia P., Alessandra P., Danilo F., Yalaoui-Guellal D., Elsebai M.F., Madani K., Chibane M. Chemical composition and *in vitro* antimicrobial, insecticidal and antioxidant activities of the essential oils of *Mentha pulegium* L. and *Mentha rotundifolia* (L.) Huds growing in Algeria. Industrial Crops and Products. 2016;**88**: 96–105.

[72] Abdelli M., Moghrani H., Aboun A., Maachi R. Algerian *Mentha pulegium* L. leaves essential oil: chemical composition, antimicrobial, insecticidal and antioxidant activities. Industrial Crops and Products. 2016;**94**: 197–205.

[73] Teixeira B., Marques A., Ramos C., Batista I., Serrano C., Matos O., Neng N.R., Nogueira, J.M.F., Saraiva J.A., Nunes M.L. European pennyroyal (*Mentha pulegium*) from Portugal: chemical composition of essential oil and antioxidant and antimicrobial properties of extracts and essential oil. Industrial Crops and Products. 2012;**36**: 81–87.

[74] Zwaving J.H., Smith D. Composition of the essential oil of Austrian *Mentha pulegium*. Phytochemistry. 1971;**10**: 1951–1953.

[75] Kokkini S., Handilou E., Karousou R., Lanaras T. Variations of pulegone content in pennyroyal (*Mentha pulegium* L.) plants growing wild in Greece. Journal of Essential Oil Research. 2002;**14**: 224–227.

[76] Marzouk B., Fredj M.B.H., Chraief I., Mastouri M., Boukef K., Marzouk Z. Chemical composition and antimicrobial activity of essential oils from Tunisian *Mentha pulegium* L. Journal of Food, Agriculture and Environment. 2008;**6**: 78–82.

[77] Petrakis E.A., Kimbaris A.C., Pappas C.S., Tarantilis P.A., Polissiou M.G. Quantitative determination of pulegone in pennyroyal oil by FT-IR spectroscopy. Journal of Agricultural and Food Chemistry. 2009;**57**: 10044–10048.

[78] De la Torre C.P., Torres O.A. Essential oil of *Mentha rotundifolia*. Arch Bioquim Quim Farm. 1977;**20**: 85–88.

[79] Galambosi B., Aflatuni A., Sorvari K. Effect of cultivation techniques on mint oils in northern Finland. Perfumer and Flavorist. 1998;**23**: 27–31.

[80] Avato P., Sgarra G., Casadoro G. Chemical composition of the essential oils of *Mentha* species cultivated in Italy. Scientia Pharmaceutica. 1995;**63**: 223–230.

[81] Umemoto K., Arai T., Nii H., Furukawa K. Chemical constituents of wild mints. Part XX. Essential oil of self-pollinated plants of *Mentha aquatica* with sesquiterpene alcohols as major components. Nippon Nogei Kagaku Kaishi. 1994;**68**: 1567.

[82] Brada M., Bezzina M., Marlier M., Lognay G.C. Chemical composition of the leaf oil of *Mentha rotundifolia* (L.) from Algeria. Journal of Essential Oil Research. 2006;**18**: 663–665.

[83] Perez Raya M.D., Utrilla M.P., Navarro M.C., Jiménez J. CNS activity of *Mentha rotundifolia* and *Mentha longifolia* essential oil in mice and rats. Phytotherapy Research. 1990;**4**: 232–234.

[84] Fujita S., Nakano T., Fujita Y. Studies on the essential oils of the genus *Mentha*. Part X. On the components of the essential oils of *Mentha rotundifolia* (Linn.) Huds. Nippon Nogei Kagaku Kaishi. 1977;**51**: 699–702.

[85] Oumzil H., Ghoulami S., Rhajaoui M., Ilidrissi A., Fkih-Tetouani S., Faid M., Ben-jouad A. Antibacterial and antifungal activity of essential oils of *Mentha suaveolens*. EHRH Phytotherapy Research. 2002;**16**: 723–731.

[86] Brada M., Bezzina M., Marlier M., Carlier A., Lognay G. Variabilité de la composition chimique des huiles essentielles de *Mentha rotundifolia* du Nord de l'Algérie. Journal of Biotechnology, Agronomy, Societyand Environment. 2007;**11**: 3–7.

[87] Koyalta D., Sanokho A., Miralles J., Bassene E. Essential oil composition of three Senegalese mint species, 4. Rivista Italiana EPPOS. 1993;4: 544–547.

[88] El Arch M., Satrani B., Farah A., Bennani L., Boriky D., Fechtal M., Blaghen M., Talbi M. Chemical composition, antimicrobial and insecticide activities of Mentha rotundifolia essential oil from Morocco. Acta Botanica Gallica. 2003;**150**: 267–274.

[89] Riahi L., Elferchichi M., Ghazghazi H., Jebali J., Ziadi S., Aouadhi C., Chograni H., Zaouali, Y., Zoghlami N., Mliki A. Phytochemistry: antioxidant and antimicrobial activities of the essential oils of *Mentha rotundifolia* L. in Tunisia. Industrial Crops and Products. 2013;**49**: 883–889.

[90] Pino J.A., Rosado A., Fuentes V. Chemical composition of the leaf oil of *Mentha rotundifolia* (L.) Hudson from Cuba. Journal of Essential Oil Research. 1999;**11**: 241–242.

[91] Derwich E., Benziane Z., Boukir A. Antibacterial activity and chemical composition of the leaf essential oil of *Mentha rotundifolia* from Morocco. Electronic Journal of Environmental Agricultural and Food Chemistry. 2010;**9**: 19–28.

[92] Mimica-Dukic N., Bozin B., Sokovic M., Mihajlovic B., Matavulj M. Antimicrobial and antioxidant activities of three *Mentha* species essential oils. Planta Medica. 2003;**69**:413–419.

[93] Gulluce M., Sahin F., Sokmen M., Ozer H., Daferera D., Sokmen A., Polissiou M., Adiguzel A., Ozkan H. Antimicrobial and antioxidant properties of the essential oils and methanol extract from *Mentha longifolia* L. ssp. *longifolia*. Food Chemistry. 2007;**103**: 1449–1456.

[94] Pereira E., Pimenta A.I., Calhelha R.C., Antonio A.L., Verde S.C., Barros L., Santos-Buelga C., Ferreira I.C.F.R. Effects of gamma irradiation on cytotoxicity and phenolic compounds of *Thymus vulgaris* L. and *Mentha x piperita* L. LWT—Food Science and Technology. 2016;**71**: 370–377.

[95] Dorman H.J.D., Kosar M., Kahlos K., Holm Y., Hiltunen R. Antioxidant properties and composition of aqueous extracts from *Mentha* species, hybrids, varieties, and cultivars. Journal of Agricultural and Food Chemistry. 2003;**51**: 4563–4569.

[96] Triantaphyllou K., Blekas G., Boskou D. Antioxidative properties of water extracts obtained from herbs of the species Lamiaceae. International Journal of Food Sciences and Nutrition. 2001;**52**: 313–317.

[97] Areias F.M., Valentao P., Andrade P.B., Ferreres F., Seabra R.M. Phenolic fingerprint of peppermint leaves. Food Chemistry. 2001;**73**: 307–311.

[98] Pérez M.G.F., Rocha-Guzmán N.E., Mercado-Silva E., Loarca-Piña G., Rosalía Reynoso-Camacho R. Effect of chemical elicitors on peppermint (*Mentha piperita*) plants and their impact on the metabolite profile and antioxidant capacity of resulting infusions. Food Chemistry. 2014;**156**: 273–278.

[99] Brahmi F., Hauchard D., Guendouze N., Madani K., Kiendrebeogo M., Kamagaju L., Stévigny C., Chibane M., Duez P. Phenolic composition, *in vitro* antioxidant effects and tyrosinase inhibitory activity of three Algerian *Mentha* species: *M. spicata* (L.) *M. pulegium* (L.) and *M. rotundifolia* (L.) Huds (Lamiaceae). Industrial Crops and Products. 2015;**74**: 722–730.

[100] Voirin B., Bayet C., Faure O., Jullien F. Free flavonoid aglycones as markers of parentage in *Mentha aquatica, M. citrata, M. spicata* and *M. x piperita*. Phytochemistry. 1999;**50**: 1189–1193.

[101] Yamamura S., Ozawa K., Ohtani K., Kasai R., Yamasaki K. Antihistaminic flavones and aliphatic glycosides from *Mentha spicata*. Phytochemistry. 1998;**48**(1): 131–136.

[102] Zheng J., Zhao D.S., Wu B., Wu L.J. Study on chemical constituents in the herb of *Mentha spicata*. Zhongguo Zhong Yao Za Zhi= Zhongguo Zhongyao Zazhi= China Journal of Chinese Materia Medica. 2002;**27**(10): 749–751.

[103] Fiamegos Y.C., Nanos C.G., Vervoort J., Stalikas C.D. Analytical procedure for the in-vial derivatization-extraction of phenolic acids and flavonoids in methanolic and aqueous plant extracts followed by gas chromatography with mass-selective detection. Journal of Chromatography. 2004;**1041**: 11–18.

[104] Proestos C., Chorianopoulos N., Nychas G.J.E., Komaitis M. RP-HPLC analysis of the phenolic compounds of plant extracts: investigation of their antioxidant capacity and antimicrobial activity. Journal of Agricultural and Food Chemistry. 2005;**53**: 1190–1195.

[105] Chen G., Gao H., Zheng J., Wu B., Yang X., Wu L. Study of chemical constituents in active parts of *Mentha spicata* III. Zhongguo Zhong Yao Za Zhi= Zhongguo Zhongyao Zazhi= China Journal of Chinese Materia Medica. 2006; **31**(7): 560–562.

[106] Kivilompolo M., Hyotylainen T. Comprehensive two-dimensional liquid chromatography in analysis of Lamiaceae herbs: characterisation and quantification of antioxidant phenolic acids. Journal of Chromatography. 2007;**1145**: 155–164.

[107] Song Y., Chen G.T., Sun B.H., Huang J., Li X., Wu L.J. Study of chemical constituents in active parts of *Mentha spicata* Shenyang Yaoke Daxue Xuebao. 2008; **25**(9): 705–707.

[108] Sankara Subramanian S., Nair A.G.R. Flavonoids of the leaves of *Mentha spicata* and *Anzsochzlus carnosus*. Phytochemistry. 1972;**11**: 452–453.

[109] Tomas-Barberan F.A., Husain S.Z., Gil M.I. Distribution of methylated flavones in the Lamiaceae. Biochemical Systematics Ecology. 1988;**16**(1): 43–46.

[110] Papageorgiou V., Mallouchos A., Komaitis M. Investigation of the antioxidant behavior of air- and freeze-dried aromatic plant materials in relation to their phenolic content and vegetative cycle. Journal of Agricultural and Food Chemistry. 2008;**56**: 5743–5752.

[111] Adam M., Dobias P., Eisner A., Ventura K. Extraction of antioxidants from plants using ultrasonic methods and their antioxidant capacity. Journal of Separation Science. 2009;**32**: 288–294.

[112] Bimakr M., Abdul Rahman R., Saleena Taip F., Ganjloo A., Md Salleh L., Selamat J., Hamid A., Zaidul I.S.M. Comparison of different extraction methods for the extraction of major bioactive flavonoid compounds from spearmint (*Mentha spicata* L) leaves. Food and Bioproducts Processing. 2011;**89**: 67–72.

[113] Zheng J., Chen G.T., Gao H.Y., Wu B., Wu L.J. Two new lignans from *Mentha spicata* L. Journal of Asian Natural Products Research. 2007;**9**(3–5): 431–435.

[114] Guedon D.J., Pasquier B.P. Analysis and distribution of flavonoid glycosides and rosmarinic acid in 40 *Mentha piperita* clones. Journal of Agricultural and Food Chemistry. 1994;**42**: 679–684.

[115] Fecka I., Turek S. Determination of water soluble polyphenolic compounds in commercial herbal teas from Lamiaceae: peppermint, melissa, and sage. Journal of Agricultural and Food Chemistry. 2007;**55**: 10908–10917.

[116] Fecka I., Raj D., Krauze-Baranowska M. Quantitative determination of four water-soluble compounds in herbal drugs from Lamiaceae using different chromatographic techniques. Chromatographia. 2007;**66**: 87–93.

[117] Krzyzanowska J., Janda B., Pecio L., Stochmal A., Oleszek W., Czubacka A., et al. Determination of polyphenols in *Mentha longifolia* and *M. piperita* field-grown and *in vitro* plant samples using UPLC-TQ-MS. Journal of AOAC International. 2011;**94**(1): 43–50.

[118] Hadjmohammadi M., Karimiyan H., Sharifi V. Hollow fibre-based liquid phase microextraction combined with high-performance liquid chromatography for the analysis of flavonoids in *Echinophora platyloba* DC and *Mentha piperita*. Food Chemistry. 2013;**141**: 731–735.

[119] Farnad N., Heidari R., Aslanipour B. Phenolic composition and comparison of antioxidant activity of alcoholic extracts of peppermint (*Mentha piperita*). Journal of Food Measurement and Characterization. 2014;**8**: 113–121.

[120] Mekinic I.G., Skroza D., Ljubenkov I., Simat V., Mozina S.S., Katalinic V. *In vitro* antioxidant and antibacterial activity of Lamiaceae phenolic extracts: a correlation study. Food Technology and Biotechnology. 2014;**52**(1): 119–127.

[121] Voirin B., Saunois A., Bayet C. Free flavonoid aglycones from *Mentha piperita*: developmental, chemotaxonomical and physiological aspects. Biochemical Systematics and Ecology. 1994;**22**(1): 95–99.

[122] Gao B., Lu Y., Qin F., Chen P., Shi H., Charles D., et al. Differentiating organic from conventional peppermints using chromatographic and flow injection mass spectrometric (FIMS) fingerprints. Journal of Agricultural and Food Chemistry. 2012;**60**: 11987–11994.

[123] Shalaby N.M.M., Moharram F.A., El-Toumy S.A.A., Marzoyk M.S.A., Ahmed A.A.E. Phytochemical and pharmacological studies of *Mentha pulegium* L. Bulletin of Faculty of Pharmacy, Cairo University, Department of Natural Products, National Research Centre, Cairo, Egypt. 2000;**38**(2): 143–151.

[124] Ramos T., Groubert A., Pellecuer J. Diosmine analysis from several plant origins. Institut National de la Recherche Agronomique, Faculté de Pharmacie, Université Montpellier I, Montpellier, Fr. Colloques, 69 (Polyphenols 94); 1995. pp. 311–12. CODEN: COLIEZ ISSN: 0293-1915.

[125] Zaidi F., Voirin B., Jay M., Viricel M.R. Free flavonoid aglycones from leaves of *Mentha pulegium* and *Mentha suaveolens* (Labiatae). Phytochemistry. 1998;**48**(6): 991.

[126] Marin Pares E. A pharmacognostic study on *Mentha rotundifolia* (L.) Hudson Circle Farm. 1983;**41**(279): 133–152.

[127] Dobias P., Pavlikova P., Adam M., Eisner A., Benova B., Ventura K. Comparison of pressurised fluid and ultrasonic extraction methods for analysis of plant antioxidants and their antioxidant capacity. Central European Journal of Chemistry. 2010;**8**(1):87–895.

[128] Ertaş A., Gören A.C., Haşimi N., Tolan V., Kolak U. Evaluation of antioxidant, cholinesterase inhibitory and antimicrobial properties of *Mentha longifolia* subsp. *noeana* and its secondary metabolites. Records of Natural Products. 2015;**9**(1): 105–115.

[129] Kosar M., Dorman H.J.D., Baser K.H.C., Hiltunen R. Screening of free radical scavenging compounds in water extracts of *Mentha* samples using a postcolumn derivatization method. Journal of Agricultural and Food Chemistry. 2004;**52**(16): 5004–5010.

[130] She G.M., Xu C., Liu B., Shi, R.B. Polyphenolic acids from mint (the aerial of *Mentha haplocalyx* Briq.) with DPPH radical scavenging activity. Journal of Food Science. 2010;**75**(4): C359–C362.

[131] Choudhury R.P., Kumar A., Garg A.N. Analysis of Indian mint (*Mentha spicata*) for essential, trace and toxic elements and its antioxidant behavior. Journal of Pharmaceutical and Biomedical Analysis. 2006;**41**: 825–832.

[132] Maffei M., Scannerini S. Fatty acid variability in some *Mentha* species. Biochemical Systematics and Ecology. 1992;**20**(6): 573–582.

[133] Raju M., Varakumar S., Lakshminarayana R., Krishnakantha T.P., Baskaran V. Carotenoid composition and vitamin A activity of medicinally important green leafy vegetables. Food Chemistry. 2007;**101**: 1598–1605.

[134] Curutchet A., Dellacassa E., Ringuelet J.A., Chaves A.R., Vina S.Z. Nutritional and sensory quality during refrigerated storage of fresh-cut mints (*Mentha × piperita* and *M. spicata*). Food Chemistry. 2014;**143**: 231–238.

[135] Dambrauskienė E., Viškelis P., Karklelienė R. Productivity and biochemical composition of Mentha piperita L. of different origin. Biologija. 2008;**54**(2): 105–107.

[136] Padmini E., Prema K., Geetha B.V., Rani M.U. Comparative study on composition and antioxidant properties of mint and black tea extract. International Journal of Food Science and Technology. 2008;**43**: 1887–1895.

[137] de Sousa Barros A., de Morais S.M., Travassos Ferreira P.A., Pinto Vieira I.G., Craveiro A.A., dos Santos Fontenelle R.O., de Menezes J.E.S.A., Ferreira da Silva F.W., de Sousa H.A. Chemical composition and functional properties of essential oils from *Mentha* species. Industrial Crops and Products. 2015;**76**: 557–564.

[138] Sun Z., Wang H., Wang J., Zhou L., Yang, P. Chemical composition and anti- inflammatory, cytotoxic and Antioxidant activities of essential oil from leaves of *Mentha piperita* grown in China. PLoS One. 2014;9(12).

[139] Ebrahimzadeh M.A., Nabavi S.M., Nabavi S.F. Antioxidant and antihemolytic activities of *Mentha longifolia*. Pharmacologyonline. 2010;**2**:464–471

[140] Tsai M.L., Wu C.T., Lin T.F., Lin W.C., Huang Y.C., Yang C.H. Chemical composition and biological properties of essential oils of two mint species. Tropical Journal of Pharmaceutical Research. 2013;**12**(4): 577–582.

[141] Brahmi F., Boulekbache-Makhlouf L., Yalaoui-Guellal D., Chibane M., Madani K. Comparative study on the antioxidant effect of aqueous and ethanolic extracts of *Mentha pulegium* L. grown at two different locations. PhytoChem BioSub Journal. 2014;**8** (3): 138–149.

[142] Arumugam P., Murugan R., Subathra M., Ramesh A. Superoxide radical scavenging and antibacterial activities of different fractions of ethanol extract of *Mentha spicata* (L.). Medicinal Chemistry Research. 2010;**19**: 664–673.

[143] Karray-Bouraoui N., Ksouri R., Falleh H., Rabhi M., Abdul Jaleel C., Grignon C., Lachaâl M. Effects of environment and development stage on phenolic content and antioxidant activities of *Mentha pulegium* L. Journal of Food Biochemistry 2010;**34**: 79–89.

[144] Nickavar B., Alinaghi A., Kamalinejad M. Evaluation of the antioxidant properties of five *Mentha* species. Iranian Journal of Pharmaceutical Research. 2008;**7**(3): 203–209.

[145] Benabdallah A., Rahmoune C., Boumendjel M., Aissi O., Messaoud C. Total phenolic content and antioxidant activity of six wild *Mentha* species (Lamiaceae) from northeast of Algeria. Asian Pacific Journal of Tropical Biomedicine. 2016;**6**(9): 760–766.

[146] Brahmi F., Madani K., Dahmoune F., Rahmani T., Bousbaa K., Oukmanou S., Chibane, M. Optimization of solvent extraction of antioxidants (phenolic compounds) from Algerian mint (*Mentha spicata* L.). Pharmacognosy Communications. 2012;**2** (4):72–86.

[147] Brahmi F., Madani K., Djerrada N., Idir S., Harfi F., Chibane M., Brada M. Assessment of the chemical composition and *in vitro* antioxidant activity of *Mentha rotundifolia* (L.) Huds essential oil from Algeria. Journal of Essential Oil Bearing. Plants. 2016;**19**(5): 1251–1260, DOI: 10.1080/0972060X.2015.1108878.

[148] Arumugam P., Ramamurthy P., Santhiya S.T., Ramesh A. Antioxidant activity measured in different solvent fractions obtained from *Mentha spicata* Linn.: an analysis by $ABTS^{+}$ decolorization assay. Asia Pacific Journal of Clinical Nutrition. 2006;119–124.

[149] Lopez V., Martín S., Gómez-Serranillos M.P., Carretero M.E., Jäger A.K., Calvo M.I. Neuroprotective and neurochemical properties of mint extracts. Phytotherapy Research. 2010;**24**: 869–874.

[150] Brahmi F., Madani K., Stévigny C., Chibane M., Duez P. Algerian mint species: HPTLC quantitative determination of rosmarinic acid and *in vitro* inhibitory effects on linoleic acid peroxidation. Journal of Coastal Life Medicine. 2014;**2**(12):986–992.

[151] Raj J.X., Bajpjpai P.K., Kumar P.G., Murugan P.M., Kumar J., Chaurasia O.P., et al. Determination of total phenols, free radical scavenging and antibacterial activities of *Mentha longifolia* Linn. Hudson from the cold desert, Ladakh, India. Pharmacognosy Journal. 2010;**2**: 470–475.

[152] Ladjel S., Gherraf N., Hamada D. Antimicrobial effect of essential oils from the Algerian medicinal plant *Mentha rotundifolia* L. Journal of Applied Sciences Research. 2011;7(11): 1665–1667.

[153] Justin K., Protais M., Rose N., Viateur U. Chemical composition and in vitro antibacterial activity of the leaf essential oil of *Mentha officinalis* from Rwanda. Journal of Chemistry Chemical Engineering. 2012;**6**: 401–409.

[154] Yano Y., Satomi M., Oikawa H. Antimicrobial effect of spices and herbs on *Vibrio parahaemolyticus*. International Journal of Food Microbiology. 2006;**111**: 6–11.

[155] Kumar P., Mishra S., Malik A., Satya S. Insecticidal properties of *Mentha* species: a review. Industrial Crops and Products. 2011; **34**(1): 802–817.

[156] Benayad N., Ebrahim W., Hakiki A., Mahjouba Mosaddak M. Chemical characterization and insecticidal evaluation of the essential oil of *Mentha suaveolens* L. and *Mentha pulegium* L. growing in Morocco. Scientific Study and Research. 2012;**13**(1): 027–032.

[157] Lee S.E., Lee B.H., Choi W.S., Park B.S., Kim J.G., Campbell B.C. Fumigant toxicity of volatile natural products from Korean spices and medicinal plants towards the rice weevil *Sitophilus oryzae* (L.). Pest Management Science. 2001;**57**: 548–553.

[158] Varma J., Dubey N.K. Efficacy of essential oils of *Caesulia axillaris* and *Mentha arvensis* against some storage pests causing biodeterioration of food commodities. International Journal of Food Microbiology. 2001;**68**: 207–210.

[159] Mohamed M.I.E., Abdelgaleil A.M.S. Chemical composition and insecticidal potential of essential oils from Egyptian plants against *Sitophilus oryzae* (L.) (Coleoptera: curculionidae) and *Tribolium castaneum* (Herbst) (Coleoptera:Tenebrionidae). Applied Entomology and Zoology. 2008;**43**: 599–607.

[160] Kumar A., Shukla R., Singh P., Singh A.K., Dubey N.K. Use of essential oil from *Mentha arvensis* L. to control storage moulds and insects in stored chickpea. Journal of the Science of Food and Agriculture. 2009;**89**: 2643–2649.

[161] Kasrati A., Alaoui Jamali C., Bekkouche K., Spooner-Hart R., Leach D., Abbad A. Chemical characterization and insecticidal properties of essential oils from different wild populations of *Mentha suaveolens* subsp. timija (Briq.) Harley from Morocco. Chemistry & Biodiversity. 2015;**12**: 823–831.

[162] Lamiri A., Lhaloui S., Benjilali B., Berrada M. Insecticidal effects of Hessian fly against Mayetiola destructor (Say). Field Crops Research. 2001;**71**: 9–15.

[163] El Nagar T.F.K., Abdel Fattah H.M., Khaled A.S., Aly S.A. Efficiency of peppermint oil fumigant on controlling *Callosobruchus maculates* F. infesting cow pea seeds. Life Science Journal. 2012;**9**(2): 375–383.

[164] Zekri N., Handaq N., El Caidi A., Zair T., El Belghiti M.A. Insecticidal effect of *Mentha pulegium* L. and *Mentha suaveolens* Ehrh. hydrosols against a pest of citrus *Toxoptera aurantii* (Aphididae). Research on Chemical Intermediates. 2015;1–11, http://dx.doi.org/10.1007/s11164-015-2108-0.

[165] Sharma V., Shabir H., Moni G., Kumar S.A. *In vitro* cancer activity of extracts of *Mentha* spp. against human cancer cells. Indian Journal of Biochemistry and Biophysics. 2014;**51**(5): 416–419.

[166] Yi W., Ywetzstein H. Anti-tumorigenic activity of five culinary and medicinal herbs grown under greenhouse conditions and their combination effects. Journal of Science and Food Agriculture. 2011;**91**: 1849–1854.

[167] Shirazi F.H., Ahmadi N., Kamalinejad M. Evaluation of northern Iran *Mentha pulegium* L. cytotoxicity. Daru Journal of Pharmaceutical Sciences. 2004;**2**(3): 106–110.

[168] Mazzio E.A., Soliman K.F.A. *In vitro* screening for the tumoricidal properties of international medicinal herbs. Phytotherapy Research. 2009;**23**: 385–398.

[169] Hajighasemi F., Hashemi V., Khoshzaban F. Cytotoxic effect of *Mentha spicata* aqueous extract on cancerous cell lines *in vitro*. Journal of Medical Plants Research. 2011;**5**(20): 5142–5147.

[170] Jain D., Pathak N., Khan S., Venkata Raghuram G., Bhargava A., Samarth R., Kumar Mishra P. Evaluation of cytotoxicity and anticarcinogenic potential of *Mentha* leaf extracts. International Journal of Toxicology. 2011;**30**(2): 225–236.

[171] Al-Ali K.H., El-Beshbishy H.A., El-Badry A.A., Alkhalaf M. Cytotoxic activity of methanolic extract of *Mentha longifolia* and *Ocimum basilicum* against human breast cancer. Pakistan Journal of BiologicalScience. 2013;**16**(23): 1744–1750.

[172] Abirami S.K.G., Nirmala P. A comparative—*in vitro* study of anticancer effect of *Mentha piperita, Ocimum Basilicum* and *Coleus aromaticus* against human laryngeal epidermoid carcinoma (HEP-2) cell lines. Journal of Medical Plants and Studies 2014;**2**(1): 2320–3862.

[173] Moreno L., Bello R., Primo-Yufera E., Esplugues J. Pharmacological properties of the methanol extract from *Mentha suaveolens* Ehrh. Phytotherapy Research. 2002;**16**: S10–S13.

[174] Conforti F., Sosa S., Marrelli M., Menichini F., Statti G.A., Uzunov D., Tubaro A., Menichini F., Loggia R.D. *In vivo* anti-inflammatory and *in vivo* antioxidant activities of Mediterranean dietary plants. Journal of Ethnopharmacology. 2008;**116**(1): 144–151.

Permissions

All chapters in this book were first published in AMP, by InTech Open; hereby published with permission under the Creative Commons Attribution License or equivalent. Every chapter published in this book has been scrutinized by our experts. Their significance has been extensively debated. The topics covered herein carry significant findings which will fuel the growth of the discipline. They may even be implemented as practical applications or may be referred to as a beginning point for another development.

The contributors of this book come from diverse backgrounds, making this book a truly international effort. This book will bring forth new frontiers with its revolutionizing research information and detailed analysis of the nascent developments around the world.

We would like to thank all the contributing authors for lending their expertise to make the book truly unique. They have played a crucial role in the development of this book. Without their invaluable contributions this book wouldn't have been possible. They have made vital efforts to compile up to date information on the varied aspects of this subject to make this book a valuable addition to the collection of many professionals and students.

This book was conceptualized with the vision of imparting up-to-date information and advanced data in this field. To ensure the same, a matchless editorial board was set up. Every individual on the board went through rigorous rounds of assessment to prove their worth. After which they invested a large part of their time researching and compiling the most relevant data for our readers.

The editorial board has been involved in producing this book since its inception. They have spent rigorous hours researching and exploring the diverse topics which have resulted in the successful publishing of this book. They have passed on their knowledge of decades through this book. To expedite this challenging task, the publisher supported the team at every step. A small team of assistant editors was also appointed to further simplify the editing procedure and attain best results for the readers.

Apart from the editorial board, the designing team has also invested a significant amount of their time in understanding the subject and creating the most relevant covers. They scrutinized every image to scout for the most suitable representation of the subject and create an appropriate cover for the book.

The publishing team has been an ardent support to the editorial, designing and production team. Their endless efforts to recruit the best for this project, has resulted in the accomplishment of this book. They are a veteran in the field of academics and their pool of knowledge is as vast as their experience in printing. Their expertise and guidance has proved useful at every step. Their uncompromising quality standards have made this book an exceptional effort. Their encouragement from time to time has been an inspiration for everyone.

The publisher and the editorial board hope that this book will prove to be a valuable piece of knowledge for researchers, students, practitioners and scholars across the globe.

List of Contributors

Adebayo Taiwo Ezekiel Jolayemi
Department of Anaesthesia and ICU, Goulburn Base Hospital, Australia National University, Golburn City, Australia

Mayela Govea-Salas and Jésus Morlett-Chávez
Clinical Analysis and Molecular Biology Laboratory, School of Chemistry, Autonomous University of Coahuila, Saltillo, Coahuila, Mexico
Cellular Biology Laboratory, School of Chemistry, Autonomous University of Coahuila, Saltillo, Coahuila, Mexico

Raúl Rodriguez-Herrera and Juan Ascacio-Valdés
Food Science and Technology Department, School of Chemistry, Autonomous University of Coahuila, Saltillo, Coahuila, Mexico

Busisiwe Ndawonde
University of Johannesburg, Johannesburg, South Africa

Sitwala Namwinji Imenda
University of Zululand, KwaDlangezwa, South Africa

Humbulani Nancy Mutshaeni
University of Venda, Thohoyandou, South Africa

Renata Takeara, Regiane Gonçalves, Vanessa Farias dos Santos Ayres and Anderson Cavalcante Guimarães
Federal University of Amazonas, Institute of Science and Technology, Itacoatiara, AM, Brazil

Imad Hadi Hameed
Department of Nursing, Babylon University, Hilla City, Hillah, Iraq

Ghaidaa Jihadi Mohammed
College of Science, Al-Qadisiya University, Al Diwaniyah, Iraq

Ngozichukwuka P. Igoli
Centre for Food Technology and Research, Benue State University, Makurdi, Nigeria

John O. Igoli
University of Agriculture, Makurdi, Nigeria

Sofija M. Djordjevic
Institute for Medicinal Plant Research "Dr Josif Pancic", Belgrade, Republic of Serbia

Dennis R.A. Mans, Deeksha Ganga and Joëlle Kartopawiro
Department of Pharmacology, Anton de Kom University of Suriname, Paramaribo, Suriname

Radu Claudiu Fierascu and Irina Fierascu
The National Institute for Chemistry and Petrochemistry—ICECHIM, Bucharest, Romania

Alina Ortan
University of Agronomic Sciences and Veterinary Medicine, Bucharest, Romania

Sorin Marius Avramescu
University of Bucharest, Research Centre for Environmental Protection and Waste Management, Bucharest, Romania

Cristina Elena Dinu-Pirvu
"Carol Davila" University of Medicine and Pharmacy, Bucharest, Romania

Daniela Ionescu
S.C. HOFIGAL EXPORT IMPORT S.A., Bucharest, Romania

Tian Ling
Gansu University of Chinese Medicine, Lanzhou, PR China

Liu Dongling
Gansu University of Chinese Medicine, Lanzhou, PR China
Key Laboratory of Traditional Chinese Medicine Quality and Standard, Lanzhou, PR China

Shinichiro Hayashi
GREEN FLASK Inc., Tokyo, Japan

Wang Yinquan
Gansu University of Chinese Medicine, Lanzhou, PR China
Northwest Collaborative Innovation Center for Chinese Medicine, Lanzhou, PR China

Nagy Morsy
Department of Chemistry, Faculty of Sciences and Arts, Khulais, University of Jeddah, Saudi Arabia
Department of Chemistry of Natural Compounds, National Research Centre, El-bohouth St., Dokki, Cairo, Egypt

Maiko Inoue
Specified Nonprofit Corporation of Horticulture Therapy and Zen, Hamamatsu, Japan

Lyle E. Craker
University of Massachusetts, Amherst, MA, USA

Fatiha Brahmi and Madani Khodir
3BS Laboratory, Faculty of Natural Sciences and Life, University of Bejaia, Bejaia, Algeria

Chibane Mohamed
Faculty of Natural, Life and Earth Sciences, Akli Mohand Oulhadj University, Bouira, Algeria

Duez Pierre
Medicinal Chemistry and Pharmacognosy Department, Faculty of Medicine and Pharmacy, University of Mons (UMONS), Belgium

Index

www.ingramcontent.com/pod-product-compliance
Lightning Source LLC
LaVergne TN
LVHW080914210926
848485LV00004B/653